Get ahead!

Specialties

100 EMQs for finals

Get ahead!
Specialties
100 EMQs for finals

Peter Cartledge
Specialist Trainee in Paediatrics
Leeds General Infirmary, Leeds, UK

Mary Watson
Foundation Year House Officer
Academic Psychiatry
Leeds General Infirmary, Leeds, UK

Rebecca Cairns
GP Registrar
Bradford VTS, Bradford, UK

Fiona Bach
Specialist Trainee in Obstetrics and Gynaecology
Leeds General Infirmary, Leeds, UK

The ROYAL
SOCIETY *of*
MEDICINE
PRESS *Limited*

Published by the Royal Society of Medicine Press Ltd
1 Wimpole Street, London W1G 0AE, UK
Tel: +44 (0)20 7290 2921
Fax: +44 (0)20 7290 2929
Email: publishing@rsm.ac.uk
Website: www.rsmpress.co.uk

British Library Cataloguing in Publication Data
A catalogue record for this book is available from the British Library

ISBN 978-1-85315-722-6

Distribution in Europe and Rest of World:

Marston Book Services Ltd
PO Box 269
Abingdon
Oxon OX14 4YN, UK
Tel: +44 (0)1235 465500
Fax: +44 (0)1235 465555
Email: direct.order@marston.co.uk

Distribution in the USA and Canada:

Royal Society of Medicine Press Ltd
c/o BookMasters Inc
30 Amberwood Parkway
Ashland, OH 44805, USA
Tel: +1 800 247 6553/+1 800 266 5564
Fax: +1 419 281 6883
Email: orders@bookmasters.com

Distribution in Australia and New Zealand:

Elsevier Australia
30-52 Smidmore Street
Marrickville NSW 2204, Australia
Tel: +61 2 9517 8999
Fax: +61 2 9517 2249
Email: service@elsevier.com.au

Typeset by IMH(Cartrif), Loanhead, Scotland
Printed by Bell & Bain, Glasgow

Contents

Welcome to *Get ahead! Specialties*. This book contains 100 EMQ themes, each with five stems, covering obstetrics, gynaecology, paediatrics and psychiatry. The EMQs are arranged by specialty as ten practice papers, each of which should take no longer than 90 minutes to complete. You can either work through the practice papers systematically or dip in and out of the book using the EMQ index as a guide to where questions on a specific topic can be found. We have tried to include all the main conditions about which you can be expected to know, as well as some more detailed knowledge suitable for candidates aiming towards distinction. As in the real exam, these papers have no preset pass mark. Whether you pass or fail depends on the distribution of scores across the whole year group, but around 60% should be sufficient.

We hope this book fulfils its aim in being a useful, informative revision aid. If you have any feedback or suggestions please let us know (RevisionForMedicalFinals@gmail.com).

We would like to acknowledge the assistance of Elizabeth Mills, for helping to review the manuscript, and David Capewell, for his helpful additions to the explanations.

Finally, we would like to thank Sarah Vasey and Sarah Burrows, both of the Royal Society of Medicine Press, for their support and guidance throughout this project.

Peter Cartledge
Mary Watson
Rebecca Cairns
Fiona Bach
Saran Shantikumar (Series Editor)

Get ahead!

Extended matching questions (EMQs) are becoming more popular as a method of assessment in summative medical school examinations. EMQs have the advantage of testing candidates' knowledge of clinical scenarios rather than their ability at detailed factual recall. However, they do not always parallel real-life situations and are no comparison to clinical decision-making. Either way, the EMQ is here to stay.

The *Get ahead!* series is aimed primarily at undergraduate finalists. Much like the real exam, we have endeavoured to include commonly asked questions as well as a generous proportion of harder stems, appropriate for the more ambitious student aiming for honours. The Universities Medical Assessment Partnership (UMAP) is a collaboration of 14 medical schools in the UK that is compiling a bank of EMQs to be used in summative examinations. The questions in the *Get ahead!* series are written to closely follow the 'house-style' of the UMAP EMQs, and hence are of a similar format to what many of you can expect in your exams. All the questions in the *Get ahead!* series are accompanied by explanatory answers, including a succinct summary of the key features of each condition. Even when you get an answer right, I strongly suggest that you read these – I guarantee that you'll learn something. For added interest, we have included some details of eponymous conditions ('eponymous' from Greek *epi* = upon + *onyma* = name; 'giving name'), and, as you have just seen, some derivations of words from the original Latin or Greek.

How to pass your exams

Exam EMQs are intended to be based on 'house officer knowledge'. Sadly, this is not always the case, and you shouldn't be surprised when you get a question concerning the management of various stages of prostate cancer (as I was). So start revising early and don't restrict yourself to the given syllabus if you can avoid it. If your exam is only two weeks away then CRAM, CRAM, CRAM – you'll be surprised at how much you can learn in a fortnight.

During the exam ...

1. Try to answer the questions without looking at the responses first – the questions are written such that this should be possible.

2. Take your time to read the questions fully. There are no bonus marks for finishing the paper early.

3. If you get stuck on a question then make sure that you mark down your best guess before you move on. You may not have time to return to it at the end.

4. Answer all the questions – there is no negative marking. If you are unsure, go with your instinct – it's probably going to be your best guess.

5. Never think that the examiner is trying to catch you out. Red herrings are not allowed, so don't assume that there is one. If a question looks easy, it probably is!

But all this is obvious and there is no substitute for learning the material thoroughly and practising as many questions as you can. With this book, you're off to a good start!

A final word ...

The *Get ahead!* series is written by junior doctors who have recently finished finals and who have experience teaching students. As such, I hope that the books cover information that is valuable and relevant to you as undergraduates who are about to sit finals.

I wish you the best of luck in your exams!

Saran Shantikumar
Series Editor, *Get ahead!*

Theme 1: Antenatal screening

Options

- A. Amniocentesis
- B. Cardiotocography
- C. Chorionic villus sampling
- D. Fetal blood sampling
- E. Fetal echocardiography
- F. Fetal electrocardiography
- G. Fetal tissue sampling
- H. First-trimester ultrasound scan
- I. Nuchal translucency test
- J. Second-trimester ultrasound scan
- K. Serum 'triple test'
- L. Uterine artery Doppler ultrasound

For each of the following scenarios, select the most appropriate screening test. Each option may be used once, more than once or not at all.

1. A 42-year-old woman and a 51-year-old man have conceived their first child together with a gestation of 11 weeks. They are very concerned about the possibility of Down's syndrome. They would like a test that would give them the definitive diagnosis as to whether their baby has Down's syndrome, as they may consider terminating the pregnancy if an abnormality is found.

2. A 24-year-old woman is at 12 weeks' gestation. She would like to know whether there are any gross anatomical deformities of the fetus. Also, her sister has twins, and she would like to know if her current pregnancy involves more than one baby.

3. A 35-year-old woman and a 45-year-old man have been given a result of 1:200 for a triple test done at 17 weeks' gestation. They would like definite clarification as to whether or not the baby will be born with Down's syndrome.

4. A 25-year-old woman would like a non-invasive initial assessment for Down's syndrome and spina bifida. She is at 16 weeks' gestation.

5. A 34-year-old pregnant woman had congenital heart disease as a child. She would like to have her baby's heart investigated for a similar problem.

Theme 2: Chronic pelvic pain

Options

A. Adhesions from surgery
B. Chronic pelvic inflammatory disease
C. Constipation
D. Endometriosis
E. Fibroid degeneration
F. Functional pain
G. Irritable bowel syndrome
H. Ovarian cysts
I. Primary dysmenorrhoea
J. Primary menorrhagia
K. Renal calculus
L. Secondary dysmenorrhoea
M. Secondary menorrhagia

For each of the following scenarios, select the most likely underlying cause. Each option may be used once, more than once or not at all.

1. A 35-year-old accountant presents with heavy, painful periods and pain on intercourse. She reports intermenstrual bleeding and postcoital bleeding with occasional rectal bleeding. She had a caesarean section 3 years ago for fetal distress after having difficulty conceiving.

2. A 31-year-old actress complains of feeling generally unwell, with constant lower abdominal pain and pain on intercourse. She and her current partner have been trying to conceive for 2 years without success. She complains of irregular bleeding and postcoital bleeding. Her observations include heart rate 82 beats/min, blood pressure 124/88 mmHg and temperature 37.4°C.

3. A 33-year-old manager presents with colicky lower abdominal pain, loin pain and pain on passing water. She also admits to passing bloodstained urine. Her observations are pulse 68 beats/min, blood pressure 128/92 mmHg and temperature 36.8°C. She has never been in hospital before.

4. A 37-year-old shop assistant complains of very painful periods since a LLETZ (large loop excision of the transformation zone) procedure. The pain generally starts on the day of, or the day before, menstruation, and lasts for 2 days.

5. A 42-year-old teacher has been attending the gynaecology clinic for 7 years complaining of pelvic pain and dyspareunia, which has not improved despite various medications. She has had two laparoscopies, three hysteroscopies and multiple ultrasound scans, all of which revealed no pathology. She is convinced that her partner is unfaithful and she has contracted an infection because of this, but multiple swabs have revealed no evidence of infection.

Theme 3: Cardiotocography

Options

A. Accelerations
B. Baseline bradycardia
C. Early decelerations
D. Late decelerations
E. Normal baseline fetal heart rate
F. Normal variability
G. Pseudosinusoidal pattern
H. Reduced variability
I. Sinusoidal pattern
J. Sustained tachycardia
K. Variable decelerations

For each of the following scenarios, select the most appropriate description of a cardiotocogram. Each option may be used once, more than once or not at all.

1. A pattern that is associated with maternal pyrexia.

2. This feature is associated with fetal sleep.

3. On a cardiotocogram tracing, a dip in the fetal heart rate of 20 beats/min is seen. It starts at the same time as contractions and recovers to normal by the end of the contraction.

4. This reassuring sign, although not always present, occurs with contractions in a healthy fetus.

5. This pattern is often seen in cord compression, particularly in oligohydramnios.

Theme 4: Sexually transmitted infections 1

Options

A. Bacterial vaginosis
B. Cervical cancer
C. Chancroid
D. Chlamydia
E. Epstein–Barr virus
F. Genital candidiasis
G. Genital herpes
H. Genital warts
I. Gonorrhoea
J. Granuloma inguinale (donovanosis)
K. HIV
L. Lymphogranuloma venereum
M. Molluscum contagiosum
N. Phthiriasis
O. Reiter's syndrome
P. Scabies
Q. Syphilis
R. Trichomoniasis

For each of the following scenarios, select the most likely diagnosis. Each option may be used once, more than once or not at all.

1. A 35-year-old man presents with a 3-day history of left knee pain and dysuria. On examination, his temperature is 37.2°C and you notice that his eyes are red.

2. A 45-year-old woman who is HIV positive presents with multiple lesions on her face. The lesions are raised and shiny, non-tender, non-erythematous and around 3 mm in diameter. They have an umbilicated centre.

3. A 34-year-old woman presents to her GP with pain on passing urine and increased frequency. She is started on a course of trimethoprim and a urine sample is sent to the laboratory. She returns 4 days later complaining of an 'extreme itching down there' and pain when having sexual intercourse. On speculum examination, there is redness of the vulva and a thick white discharge is seen within the vagina.

4. A 30-year-old man presents with a single ulcer on his penis which he says developed from a spot. He denies any pain in the area. On examination, lymphadenopathy is palpable in the left groin, with evidence of a discharging sinus. A culture of the discharge reveals *Chlamydia trachomatis*.

5. A 45-year-old woman attends the GP with a persistent headache. She has recently finished a 10-year round-the-world expedition. On examination, you notice that her pupils are small, irregular and unequal in size. The light reflex is absent.

Theme 5: Hormones of menstruation

Options

    A. Activin
    B. Follicle-stimulating hormone
    C. Inhibin
    D. Luteinizing hormone
    E. Luteinizing hormone and follicle-stimulating hormone
    F. Estradiol
    G. Progesterone
    H. Progesterone and estradiol

For each of the following descriptions, select the most appropriate hormone(s). Each option may be used once, more than once or not at all.

1. It is the surge in this hormone that stimulates ovulation.

2. This hormone would continue to rise to maintain pregnancy if the ovum were fertilized.

3. This hormone stimulates the growth of 6–12 primary follicles each month.

4. This steroid hormone stimulates proliferation of glandular and stromal elements of the endometrium. It also encourages production of thin cervical mucus that is easily penetrable by sperm.

5. Hormone(s) released by the pituitary gland.

Theme 6: Pain in pregnancy

Options

    A. Acute fatty liver of pregnancy
    B. Acute pyelonephritis
    C. Braxton Hicks contractions
    D. Cholecystitis
    E. Chorioamnionitis
    F. HELLP syndrome
    G. Labour
    H. Obstetric cholestasis
    I. Placental abruption
    J. Round ligament stretching
    K. Symphysis pubis dysfunction
    L. Urinary tract infection
    M. Uterine rupture

For each of the following scenarios, select the most likely diagnosis. Each option may be used once, more than once or not at all.

1. A 32-year-old woman of 39+6 gestation attends the antenatal day unit feeling very unwell with sudden-onset epigastric pain associated with nausea and vomiting. Her temperature is 36.7°C. On examination, she is found to be tender over the right upper quadrant. Her blood results show mild anaemia, low platelets, elevated liver enzymes and haemolysis.

2. A 32-year-old woman of 38+2 gestation complains of feeling unwell with fever, rigors and abdominal pains. The pain was initially located in her lower abdomen and was associated with urinary frequency and dysuria. The pain has now become more generalized, specifically radiating to her right loin. She says that she has felt occasional 'uterine tightenings'. A CTG is reassuring.

3. A 32-year-old woman para 3 of 39+3 gestation reports having had spontaneous rupture of membranes 4 days ago. She did not attend the delivery suite, as she knew what would happen and had already decided on a home birth. Today, she feels very hot and sweaty. She thought that she was starting to have labour pains, but she describes the pain as more constant. On examination, her uterus is tender throughout. Blood tests show a raised CRP and white cell count.

4. A 32-year-old woman of 40+3 gestation attends the antenatal day unit with sudden-onset epigastric pain with nausea and vomiting. She is clinically jaundiced. Her biochemistry results show a raised bilirubin, abnormal liver enzymes, high uric acid and hypoglycaemia.

5. A 32-year-old woman of 38+4 gestation attends the antenatal day unit with pain in the suprapubic area that radiates to the upper thighs and perineum. It is worse on walking. Her urine dipstick showed a trace of protein, but no white cells, nitrites or blood.

Theme 7: Fetal presentation

Options

- A. Brow
- B. Extended breech
- C. Face
- D. Flexed breech
- E. Footling breech
- F. Left occipitoposterior
- G. Left occipitotransverse
- H. Occipitoanterior
- I. Occipitoposterior

For each of the following descriptions of examination, select the most appropriate mode of presentation. Each option may be used once, more than once or not at all.

As part of your obstetrics end-of-firm assessment, your tutor asks you to examine someone and comment on the likely fetal presentation:

1. On vaginal examination, the cervix is fully dilated and the head palpable. Anteriorly, you can feel a Y-shaped dip in the bones of the skull, with a straight suture leading to a diamond-shaped dip posteriorly.

2. On abdominal examination, you palpate a 37-week uterus with a longitudinal lie. The back is palpable on the left side. The head is three-fifths palpable.

3. On vaginal examination, the head is high. Anteriorly, the sagittal suture is palpable leading to the anterior fontanelle. The supraorbital ridges and bridge of the nose are also palpable.

4. On abdominal palpation, the lie feels longitudinal, although the back is not easily felt. The contour of the uterus is irregular. The head is two-fifths palpable and the fetal heart is difficult to locate. The anterior fontanelle is easily palpable on vaginal examination.

5. On abdominal examination, you palpate a 38-week uterus with a longitudinal lie. The presenting part at the lower uterine pole is difficult to assess for engagement. The fundal part is ballottable to the left of the midline, and the fetal heart is heard above the umbilicus. The presenting part is high on vaginal examination.

Theme 8: Diabetes in pregnancy

Options

    A. 0.5%
    B. 2–5%
    C. 25%
    D. 50%
    E. 60%
    F. 85%
    G. 98%

For each of the following statements, select the most appropriate response. Each option may be used once, more than once or not at all.

1. Diabetes complicates this proportion of pregnancies.

2. The proportion of babies born to diabetic mothers who are over the 50th percentile in weight.

3. The risk of major congenital malformation if the first maternal HbA_{1c} result is >10%.

4. The risk of recurrence of gestational diabetes in future pregnancies.

5. The proportion of women with gestational diabetes who will develop type 2 diabetes in the next 10 years.

Theme 9: Hormone replacement therapy

Options

- A. Bisphosphonates
- B. Continuous combined hormone replacement therapy
- C. Cyclical combined hormone replacement therapy
- D. Not suitable for hormone replacement
- E. Oestrogen cream/pessary
- F. Oestrogen-only hormone replacement
- G. Specialist referral

For each of the following scenarios, select the most appropriate choice for hormone replacement therapy. Each option may be used once, more than once or not at all.

1. A 52-year-old postmenopausal woman presents to her GP with symptoms of atrophic vaginitis. She denies any other symptoms related to her menopause.

2. A 51-year-old woman presents to the GP with infrequent bleeding per vagina. On further questioning, she admits to suffering from occasional hot flushes and night sweats. Her last menstrual period was 4 months ago.

3. A 56-year-old woman attends her primary care clinic complaining of bouts of hot flushes and a low mood. She had her last menstrual period 2 years ago.

4. A 50-year-old woman is requesting treatment for hot flushes and irritability – symptoms she attributes to her menopause. Her last menstrual period was 12 months ago. She has a history of breast cancer, for which she had a wide local excision.

5. A 64-year-old woman, who is postmenopausal, attends the emergency department following a fall on an outstretched hand. An X-ray confirms a Colles' fracture and a subsequent DXA scan shows evidence of marked osteoporosis. She has never suffered from menopausal symptoms or taken any form of hormone replacement.

Theme 10: Premature labour

Options

A. Atosiban
B. Betamethasone
C. Co-amoxiclav
D. Erythromycin
E. Gentamicin
F. Indometacin
G. Nifedipine
H. Ritodrine

For each of the following descriptions, select the most appropriate drug. Each option may be used once, more than once or not at all.

1. A β-agonist that is used to reduce uterine contractions.

2. An oxytocin receptor antagonist licensed for tocolysis.

3. A drug that is proven to reduce the risk of respiratory distress syndrome following preterm labour.

4. Clinical evidence recommends this to be used for infection prophylaxis in preterm rupture of membranes.

5. Use of this drug in preterm labour is associated with necrotizing enterocolitis.

Theme 1: Antenatal screening

1. C – Chorionic villus sampling

Chorionic villus sampling (CVS) is a diagnostic test: it will give a definite answer rather than the 'risk' of a condition being present. A chorionic villus (placental) biopsy is taken, either transabdominally or transcervically under ultrasound guidance, and the cells analysed. It is performed between 11 and 14 weeks (which is why it is appropriate for the couple in this question), and therefore a decision regarding possible termination can be made as early as possible before a pregnancy becomes easily visible 'under the clothes'. It is not performed before 9–11 weeks, as there is a risk of fetal limb abnormalities. The risk of miscarriage is around 2%. Results of CVS are ready in 48 hours. In a few cases, inconclusive results occur due to placental mosaicism (a variation in the chromosomal complements of the placenta that is not a reflection of the true genetics of the fetus); this would mean that amniocentesis would have to be performed later. There is also a possibility of maternal contamination, which would lead to false-negative results. Rhesus D-negative women must receive anti-D when undergoing CVS.

Mosaic, from Greek *mouseios* = artistic.

Chorionic villus, from Greek *khorion* = placenta + Latin *villus* = hair.

2. H – First-trimester ultrasound scan

The first-trimester ultrasound scan helps establish fetal viability and confirm gestation. It detects defects in gross anatomy and determines the chorionicity and amnionicity of multiple pregnancies. The second-trimester ultrasound scan detects abnormalities in structural anatomy, measures fetal growth and locates the site of the placenta. It can determine fetal sex with 99% accuracy.

3. A – Amniocentesis

Amniocentesis is a diagnostic test. A needle is inserted abdominally, under ultrasound guidance, into the uterus. Amniotic fluid, containing fetal cells shed from the gut and skin, is extracted and cultured for chromosome analysis. It takes up to 3 weeks for a full karyotype; however, laboratory techniques such as polymerase chain reaction (PCR) and fluorescence *in situ* hybridization (FISH) can provide a more rapid result for a number of conditions, including trisomies, triploidy and Turner's syndrome. Amniocentesis is performed from 15 weeks' gestation as there is increased risk of miscarriage and talipes if performed earlier. The risk of miscarriage is 0.5–1%. Amniocentesis can be used for chromosomal analysis (either for diagnosis following a positive Down's syndrome screening test or for pregnancies that are known to be at high risk of chromosomal disorders), DNA analysis for genetic diseases, enzyme assays for inborn errors of metabolism, diagnosis of fetal infection and information about rhesus iso-immunization. Anti-D is given to rhesus D-negative women undergoing amniocentesis. Amniocentesis is appropriate for the couple in this scenario, as they have already had a triple test and they are too far on in gestation to have CVS.

Amniocentesis, from Greek *amnion* = bowl + *kentesis* = puncture.

4. K – Serum 'triple test'

The triple test screens for Down's syndrome and spina bifida. A number of serum markers are used in combination with the age of the mother and confirmed gestation of the pregnancy to give a 'risk' of Down's syndrome. The serum markers used are α-fetoprotein (AFP), oestriol and the human chorionic gonadotropin β-subunit (βhCG), hence 'triple'. Triple testing is available from 14 to 20 weeks (optimal being 15–16 weeks), with results being ready in 2 weeks. A high βhCG, low AFP and low oestriol are associated with Down's syndrome. The false-positive rate is around 5%. Increasing maternal age is the strongest factor in the incidence of Down's syndrome. A 'risk' of the fetus having Down's syndrome is presented to the parents with a counsellor present so that the appropriate course of action can be taken. A 'positive' result is said to be anything above a risk of 1 in 250. In these cases, amniocentesis or chorionic villus sampling is offered. An incidental finding of raised AFP alone is associated with a break in fetal skin, often indicating neural tube defects such as spina bifida and anencephaly. As there is a large overlap with the normal and abnormal levels of AFP, further testing (imaging) is needed to confirm a diagnosis of spina bifida.

5. E – Fetal echocardiography

Echocardiography is used for women with a high risk of fetal cardiac abnormalities and is performed in the second trimester. Indications for echocardiography are mothers with congenital heart disease, diabetes or epilepsy, those with a previous child with congenital heart disease, abnormal or inadequate views of the heart at routine second-trimester scans, or a high-risk nuchal translucency result.

The *nuchal translucency (NT) test* is a screening tool for Down's syndrome and other abnormalities. It is used at 11–14 weeks when the crown–rump length is 45–84 mm. A measurement is made of the thickness of the skinfold over the neck of the fetus. This information is combined with the mother's age and the gestation of the pregnancy. A greater NT, i.e. oedema of the fetal neck, is associated with a higher risk of Down's syndrome. There is a false-positive rate of 5%. Increased NT is also seen in cardiac defects and other chromosomal abnormalities such as trisomies 18 and 13 and Turner's syndrome. Where there is increased NT but no chromosomal abnormality, an association with multiple structural abnormalities is seen (congenital heart disease, exomphalos, diaphragmatic hernia and skeletal defects).

Uterine artery Doppler ultrasound is used to measure the resistance in the maternal uterine arteries. If a high resistance is seen between 20 and 24 weeks, there is a high chance of pre-eclampsia, abruption and growth restriction; therefore such mothers require more careful monitoring.

Antenatal fetal blood sampling (FBS) is a diagnostic test performed transabdominally under ultrasound guidance. The target is blood from the umbilical cord (cordocentesis), fetal intrahepatic vessels or fetal heart. The risk of miscarriage is much greater than that with the other invasive diagnostic tests, so it is used only where blood is the only source of the information required (*in utero* transfusion in haemolytic disease or alloimmune thrombocytopenia, investigation of fetal infection such as parvovirus, and investigation of fetal hydrops). Anti-D must be given to rhesus D-negative women undergoing antenatal FBS.

Fetal tissue sampling is rarely performed to diagnose uncommon conditions that specifically require histological examination of the skin or assay of the enzymes restricted to the liver. It is performed under ultrasound guidance.

Theme 2: Chronic pelvic pain

1. D – Endometriosis

Endometriosis is a painful inflammatory condition where functioning endometrial tissue grows outside the uterine cavity. It responds to the cyclical hormonal changes and bleeds at menstruation, forming abdominal adhesions. Common sites of deposition are the ovaries, uterosacral ligaments and ovarian fossae, although endometriosis may be found further afield (bladder, rectum or lung). It is most common in 25–35 year olds, with a prevalence of 1%. The aetiology is unclear and likely to be multifactorial. Women present with cyclical abdominal pain due to bleeding at the affected sites with menstruation, dyspareunia, secondary dysmenorrhoea and subfertility. Bimanual palpation can reveal uterosacral nodules, endometriomas, uterine or ovarian enlargement, or adnexal tenderness. In advanced cases, the uterus is retroverted, retroflexed and immobile, with thickening of the cardinal or uterosacral ligaments. Ultrasound is useful to exclude other pathology, but is not diagnostic of endometriosis. Diagnosis is made by finding characteristic appearances on laparoscopy, such as brown spots ('powder burn'), adhesions and endometriomas ('chocolate cysts').

Treatment involves patient choice, and is dependent on age, fertility wishes and location of disease. Medical treatment includes analgesia, combined oral contraceptive pill (COCP), progestogens, gonadotropin-releasing hormone (GnRH) analogues and antiandrogens, and is useful for symptomatic relief. Medical management is not effective in improving underlying subfertility. Surgical treatment is used for patients where maintaining fertility is a requirement. Infertility is common even without visible tube blockage.

2. B – Chronic pelvic inflammatory disease (PID)

Chronic PID is where there are recurrent or untreated episodes of acute pelvic infection (see 'Acute pelvic pain' – Paper 4 Answers, Theme 5, page 104), which result in chronic inflammation of the pelvic organs and multiple adhesions, causing abdominal pain, dyspareunia and subfertility.

3. K – Renal calculus

This woman presents with spasmodic 'loin-to-groin' pain and haematuria, suggestive of underlying renal calculi. Calculi can be identified using ultrasound or an intravenous urogram. Management should be coordinated by a urologist.

4. L – Secondary dysmenorrhoea

Dysmenorrhoea describes a cyclical cramping pain that occurs before or during menstruation. It may be associated with malaise and gastrointestinal symptoms. Fifty per cent of women have some pain during periods, with 10% describing it as severe. Primary dysmenorrhoea begins at menarche and there is often no cause found. Secondary dysmenorrhoea has a later onset, and is often associated with pathology such as endometriosis, PID, fibroids or iatrogenic (intrauterine contraceptive device (IUCD) or cervical stenosis after LLETZ). Treatment includes hot water bottle use, transcutaneous electrical nerve stimulation (TENS), acupuncture and non-steroidal anti-inflammatory drugs (NSAIDs – especially mefenamic acid). Hormonal treatment includes COCP, depot progestogens and levonorgestrel. If these provide no relief, laparoscopic uterosacral nerve ablation can be considered.

5. F – Functional pain

Women must be informed at the beginning of investigation for pelvic pain that no cause may be found. This can reassure women and causes resolution of symptoms in some cases. If no pathology is found, then questions about sexual and social circumstances must be asked, as there may be an underlying problem, such as relationship difficulties, sexual abuse or other fears around sexuality or fertility.

Pain can be caused by *adhesions* from previous surgery or infection. Adhesiolysis (surgical removal of adhesions) is not proven, but is more likely to be effective if there are large adhesions and if it is done laparoscopically. However, there is significant risk of visceral damage and there is a chance of further adhesions developing. *Ovarian cysts* vary with regard to symptoms and investigation findings. A low-risk cyst is one with a normal CA-125, with ultrasound appearances of a simple, unilateral, unilocular cyst <5 cm. It can be managed conservatively if the patient is asymptomatic. They must be followed up in 3–4 months, and 50% resolve spontaneously. A high-risk cyst is one with an elevated CA-125 or with ultrasound appearances of a complex, bilateral, multinodular cyst that is >5 cm. High-risk and symptomatic cysts require surgical excision.

Fibroids rarely cause pain if uncomplicated. A fibroid may degenerate, or the uterus may attempt to expel an intracavity fibroid. Degeneration is initially managed conservatively with analgesia, fluids and antibiotics, but both examples may need surgery if pain is persistent or recurrent. Constipation is seen in many women with pelvic pain. A palpable loaded colon can be felt on examination. Diet modification is first-line treatment of constipation, with the use of laxatives and suppositories. Irritable bowel syndrome affects 20% of people in the UK. It is a diagnosis made clinically after exclusion of other pathology. Symptoms include constipation, diarrhoea, pelvic pain, passage of mucus with the stool and bloating. Symptoms are worse with eating, defecation, stress and in the premenstrual period. Treatment is symptomatic.

Theme 3: Cardiotocography

Cardiotocography (CTG) measures the fetal heart rate and uterine activity. It can be used confidently after 32 weeks' gestation to monitor the condition of a fetus in correlation with the clinical situation. Prior to this gestation, the autonomic nervous system is not sufficiently developed to produce the predictable responses of the more mature fetus. A normal CTG is reassuring, but an abnormal CTG is not always pathological.

Indications for CTG monitoring can be maternal (previous caesarean section, pre-eclampsia, diabetes or antepartum haemorrhage), fetal (intrauterine growth restriction (IUGR), prematurity, oligohydramnios, multiple pregnancy or breech) or intrapartum (oxytocin use, epidural use or induction of labour).

The use of CTG does not appear to improve long-term neonatal outcome.

1. J – Sustained tachycardia

2. H – Reduced variability

3. C – Early decelerations

4. A – Accelerations

5. K – Variable decelerations

A CTG tracing should be assessed as follows.

Baseline
The normal baseline fetal heart rate is the mean fetal heart rate over 5–10 min. The normal range is 110–160 beats/min. This represents a balance between sympathetic and parasympathetic systems. Sustained tachycardia may be due to prematurity, with the rate slowing physiologically with advancing gestational age. It is also seen in hypoxia, fetal distress and maternal pyrexia and with the use of exogenous β-agonists (e.g. salbutamol). Baseline bradycardia may suggest severe fetal distress, possibly due to placental abruption or uterine rupture, but occurs more commonly with hypotension, maternal sedation, postmaturity and hypoxia. A sustained baseline under 90 beats/min usually indicates impending fetal demise and should be acted on without delay.

Baseline variability
This describes the fluctuations in the fetal heart rate from one beat to the next. Variability is produced by the balance between the parasympathetic and sympathetic nervous systems. Minor fluctuations in the baseline fetal heart rate occur at 3–5 cycles/min. Baseline variability is calculated by measuring the distance between the highest peak and the lowest trough in a 1-minute segment of a CTG trace. Normal variability is between 5 and 25 beats/min and is a good indicator of fetal well-being. Reduced variability can be seen most commonly during phases of fetal sleep, which may safely last up to 40 minutes. It is also seen in early gestation (as the nervous system develops only later in pregnancy), and with certain drugs, particularly opiates or benzodiazepines. A prolonged reduced variability suggests acute fetal distress.

Accelerations and decelerations

Accelerations are defined as a rise in the fetal heart rate of at least 15 beats/min, for at least 15 s. Antenatally, you should expect at least two accelerations every 15 min. They are reassuring and often seen with contractions, although their absence in advanced labour is not uncommon. *Decelerations* are a fall in the fetal heart rate of at least 15 beats/min for more than 15 s. *Early decelerations* occur with contractions and return to normal by the end of the contraction. They are probably physiological and are thought to reflect increased vagal tone when fetal intracranial pressure increases during a contraction. They are uniform in depth, length and shape. *Late decelerations* occur during a contraction and return to baseline only after the contraction. They suggest fetal distress. Late contractions are more worrying if they are shallow and late. *Variable decelerations* vary in timing and shape in relation to uterine contraction. They suggest cord compression, especially in oligohydramnios. 'Shouldering' is a sign that the fetus is coping well with the compression: this is when there is a small acceleration before and after the deceleration. These may resolve if the mother's position is changed.

Sinusoidal trace

A *sinusoidal trace* is a smooth undulating sine-wave-like baseline with no variability. The pattern lasts over 10 minutes with an amplitude of 5–15 beats/min. A sinusoidal pattern may be physiological or can represent fetal anaemia/hypoxia, but *must* be considered serious until proven otherwise. Sinusoidal patterns should be distinguished from *pseudosinusoidal traces*, which are a benign, uniform, long-term pattern. They are less regular in shape and amplitude when compared with sinusoidal traces.

Sinusoidal, from Latin *sinus* = curve or hollow space.

Theme 4: Sexually transmitted infections 1

The presence of a sexually transmitted infection (STI) points towards the possibility of the affected person having further STIs; therefore all patients should be fully examined and investigated.

1. O – Reiter's syndrome

Reiter's syndrome, or reactive arthritis, is a triad of urethritis, seronegative (rheumatoid factor-negative) arthritis and conjunctivitis resulting from a pathological immune response to an infectious agent ('can't see, can't pee, can't climb a tree!'). Two other associated features of Reiter's syndrome are circinate balanitis (erythematous lesions on the penis) and keratoderma blenorrhagicum (hard nodules on the soles of the feet that are clinically and histologically indistinguishable from plantar psoriasis). There are two main subtypes of Reiter's syndrome: genitourinary infection (*chlamydial* infection or gonorrhoea) or gastrointestinal infection (*Salmonella, Shigella, Yersinia* or *Campylobacter* spp.). Reiter's syndrome is much commoner in males (25:1). Diagnosis is normally clinical, although the erythrocyte sedimentation rate (ESR) is raised and HLA-B27 is often present.

Hans Conrad Reiter, German military physician (1881–1969). Reiter was convicted of war crimes for his medical experiments on concentration camp detainees. Because of this association, it is becoming more preferable to use the term 'reactive arthritis'.

2. M – Molluscum contagiosum

Molluscum contagiosum is caused by a DNA poxvirus. Spread is by sexual contact, personal contact and fomites (an inanimate object that is contaminated with disease-causing microorganisms, such as a used towel). Hemispherical papules of 2–5 mm diameter that are pearly, raised and firm develop on the face, abdomen, buttocks and genitals. There is a latent period of 15–50 days. Spontaneous regression generally occurs, but lesions can be present for several months. Lesions can be extensive and persistent in immunocompromised patients, including those with HIV.

3. F – Genital candidiasis

Candidiasis (thrush) is caused by yeasts, particularly *Candida albicans* and *C. glabrata*, and produces vulval pruritis, burning, swelling and dyspareunia. White discharge and plaques are seen in the vagina, with redness of the vulva and labia minora. Candidiasis is seen more commonly with pregnancy, tissue maceration, diabetes mellitus, HIV infection, and use of antimicrobial agents and immunosuppressive drugs. Diagnosis is confirmed by culture, and treatment is with antifungals, e.g. topical imidazoles (Canesten) or oral fluconazole.

Candida, from Latin *candidus* = clear and white.

4. L – Lymphogranuloma venereum

Lymphogranuloma venereum (LGV) is an STI caused by serovars L1, L2 and L3 of *Chlamydia trachomatis*. It is mainly found in the tropics. Between 3 and 21 days after infection, one-third of people develop a small painless papule, which ulcerates and heals after days. The patients then develop lymphadenopathy, which is unilateral in two-thirds of cases. Inguinal abscesses (buboes) may form and develop a sinus. Acute ulcerative proctitis may develop when infection takes place via the rectal mucosa. Treatment is with appropriate antibiotics.

Bubo, from Greek *boubon* = groin or swollen groin. Also gives rise to the 'bubonic plague' and, allegedly, the American colloquial 'boo boo', used to describe little cuts and scrapes.

Venereal, from Latin *venereus* = desire (derived from Venus, the goddess of love).

5. Q – Syphilis (specifically neurosyphilis)

Syphilis is caused by the bacterium *Treponema pallidum* and is spread by sexual contact (it can also be acquired congenitally). There are many stages of syphilis infection:
- *Primary syphilis*: this occurs 10–90 days post-infection. A dull, red papule develops on the external genitalia and forms a single, well-

demarcated, painless ulcer associated with bilateral inguinal lymph node enlargement. This lesion heals within 8 weeks.

- *Secondary syphilis*: this develops 7–10 weeks after primary infection and involves malaise, mild fever, headache, a pruritic skin rash, hoarseness, swollen lymph nodes, patchy or diffuse hair loss, bone pain and arthralgia.
- *Latent syphilis*: here, there is no clinical evidence of disease, but it is still detectable by serological testing.
- *Gummatous syphilis*: this is a late stage of infection when the host resistance to the infection begins to fail. Areas of syphilitic granulation tissue develop on the scalp, upper aspect of the leg or sternoclavicular region. These so-called 'gummatous' lesions are copper in colour. Granulation can also occur internally, e.g. on heart valves and bone. At this stage, there is still a good response to treatment.
- *Neurosyphilis*: this is where disease is detectable in the cerebrospinal fluid. Patients complain of headache, cranial nerve palsies, general paralysis of the insane (psychosis with muscular reflex abnormality, dementia and seizures), tabes dorsalis (degeneration of the dorsal column of the spinal cord, resulting in poor coordination), trophic ulcers, Charcot's joints (a peripheral neuropathy resulting in excessive trauma to distal joints, with subsequent bony destruction) and Argyll Robertson pupils (bilateral small, irregular pupils that *do* accommodate but *do not* react to light).

Jean-Martin Charcot, French neurologist (1825–93).

Douglas Argyll Robertson, Scottish ophthalmologist (1837–1909).

Trichomoniasis

This is an STI caused by the flagellated protozoan *Trichomonas vaginalis,* which invades superficial epithelial cells of the vagina, urethra, glans penis, prostate and seminal vesicles. Affected females present with an offensive greeny-grey discharge, vulval soreness, dyspareunia, dysuria, vaginitis and vulvitis. On examination, the cervix may have a punctate erythematous (strawberry) appearance. Males are mostly asymptomatic. Treatment is with metronidazole.

Granuloma inguinale (donovanosis)

This is caused by the bacterium *Klebsiella granulomatis.* A flat-topped papule develops on the genitalia days to months post-infection, and then degenerates into a painless ulcer. The ulcer spreads along skinfolds and heals with scarring.

Gonorrhoea

This is caused by the Gram-negative diplococcus *Neisseria gonorrhoeae.* The majority of females are asymptomatic, but some complain of vaginal discharge and urethritis. Complications include Bartholin's abscess and gonococcal salpingitis with irreversible tube damage. Infected males present with dysuria, frequency and/or a mucopurulent discharge after 3–5 days, coupled with urethritis and meatal oedema. Disseminated gonococcal infection occurs in <1% cases and causes pyrexia, a vasculitic rash and polyarthritis.

'Crabs'

These are caused by the crab-louse *Phthirus pubis*, which mainly lives in the thic
hairs of the pubic and perianal areas. Most are transmitted by sexual contact,
but any close contact with an infected person can transmit the crabs. Clinically,
there is itching in the affected areas. The lice feed on blood and can leave spots
on the skin (pediculosis pubis).

Phthirus, from Greek *phtheir* = louse.

Theme 5: Hormones of menstruation

1. D – Luteinizing hormone

Luteinizing hormone (LH) is a glycoprotein produced by the anterior pituitary
gland. LH causes ovulation to occur and peaks 18 hours prior to release of
the ovum. It is regulated by gonadotropin-releasing hormone (GnRH) from the
hypothalamus. LH is initially inhibited by oestrogen from the ovary until the
level of circulating oestrogen becomes so high that it induces the pre-ovulatory
surge. Concentrations of LH are low in childhood, higher during puberty and
much higher in menopause.

Luteinizing, from Latin *luteus* = yellow (so called because this hormone stimulates
growth of the corpus luteum, or 'yellow body').

2. G – Progesterone

Progesterone is a steroid hormone produced by the corpus luteum (and by the
placenta during pregnancy). It creates secretory changes in the endometrium.
It stimulates production of thick cervical mucus, which is less penetrable by
sperm. Progesterone also decreases contractility of uterine smooth muscle and
inhibits lactation during pregnancy (hence a drop in progesterone facilitates the
onset of labour and the production of breast milk).

Progesterone, from PROGEstational STERoidal ketONE.

3. B – Follicle-stimulating hormone

Follicle-stimulating hormone (FSH) is a glycoprotein that is produced by the
anterior pituitary gland. Its function is to stimulate the growth of 6–12 primary
follicles each month; therefore it is low during childhood, increases with
puberty and is very high after the menopause (as there are no follicles left to
be released, so there is no negative-feedback mechanism). It is variable through
the menstrual cycle – at the onset of menstruation, there is a rise in FSH, which
eventually falls as oestrogen levels increase. GnRH from the hypothalamus
stimulates FSH production. The ovary is involved in the control of FSH via
oestrogen and inhibin (which both inhibit FSH production) and activin (which
stimulates FSH production). FSH production is also inhibited by high levels of
progesterone.

4. F – Estradiol

Estradiol is a steroid hormone that is mainly secreted by the ovary. It is maximal just before day 14 of menstruation. It stimulates proliferation of glandular and stromal elements of the endometrium and increases progesterone receptors in endometrial cells. It stimulates production of thin cervical mucus that is easily penetrable by sperm.

5. E – Luteinizing hormone and follicle-stimulating hormone

As mentioned above, LH and FSH are secreted by the anterior pituitary gland. Other hormones released by the anterior pituitary are growth hormone, prolactin, thyroid-stimulating hormone and adrenocorticotrophic hormone. The posterior pituitary gland secretes oxytocin and antidiuretic hormone.

Theme 6: Pain in pregnancy

1. F – HELLP syndrome

The HELLP syndrome presents with nausea and vomiting, together with epigastric pain/right upper quadrant pain due to haemorrhage with stretching of the liver capsule. Although HELLP syndrome and pre-eclampsia are related conditions, features often begin suddenly without any previous indication of pre-eclampsia. The biochemical findings are haemolysis, elevated liver enzymes and low platelets (HELLP). It has a high mortality and morbidity, often progressing to acute renal failure, disseminated intravascular coagulation (DIC) and an increased risk of abruption. Treatment includes haematological and biochemical monitoring and treatment of hypertension. Delivery is the only cure, but deterioration can still occur 48 hours after delivery.

Cholecystitis

The biliary stasis seen in pregnancy means that gallstones grow rapidly during pregnancy. The incidence of cholecystitis is 1 in 1000 pregnancies. The patient presents with sudden-onset right upper quadrant pain coupled with nausea, vomiting and fever (jaundice is rare). Differential diagnoses include severe pre-eclampsia, acute fatty liver, appendicitis and HELLP. Biochemical tests and an ultrasound scan are needed to confirm the diagnosis. Treatment includes antibiotics, analgesia and fluids. A cholecystectomy is generally postponed until after delivery.

2. B – Acute pyelonephritis

Ascending urinary tract infections (UTIs) are more common in pregnancy, thanks to dilatation of the urinary system by progesterone and obstructive uropathy with urinary stasis. They are seen in 1–2% of pregnancies. Patients typically present with fever and rigors, nausea and vomiting, abdominal and loin tenderness, and urinary frequency with dysuria. A positive culture from midstream urine (MSU) will be seen and there may be hydronephrosis on ultrasound scanning. Treatment includes analgesia, fluids and intravenous antibiotics. Uterine tightenings may be reported – do not confuse these with contractions. However, there is a risk of preterm labour with severe UTI and bacteraemia.

The incidence of UTIs in pregnancy is 1%. A short female urethra and a gravid uterus are predisposing features. Clinically, there is increased frequency, dysuria, offensive urine, suprapubic pain, fever, tachycardia and suprapubic tenderness. A dipstick and MSU culture are performed, with the most likely organism being *Escherichia coli*. Treatment is with oral cephradine or amoxicillin, which are both safe and effective in pregnancy. Recurrent UTIs need further investigations.

Labour is the most common cause of physiological pain in pregnancy. Pains are intermittent with uterine contractions. There is associated cervical dilatation and downward progression of the presenting part. It is important to remember that pathological causes of abdominal pain may also precipitate labour. *Braxton Hicks' contractions* ('false labour') describe when the uterus contracts intermittently from early pregnancy. As labour approaches, the frequency and amplitude of these contractions increase.

John Braxton Hicks, English obstetrician (1823–97).

3. E – Chorioamnionitis

Chorioamnionitis (inflammation of the amniotic sac) presents with abdominal pain, uterine tenderness and maternal pyrexia with a raised CRP and white cell count, meconium-stained or foul-smelling liquor, and fetal tachycardia. It is usually preceded by prelabour rupture of the membranes, but it can be present without membrane rupture. Chorioamnionitis is more likely if there is proven UTI or vaginal infection. It can result in overwhelming neonatal or maternal infection.

4. A – Acute fatty liver of pregnancy

Acute fatty liver of pregnancy is rare and occurs in only 1 in 10 000–15 000 pregnancies in the third trimester. It presents similarly to cholecystitis, with sudden-onset epigastric abdominal pain, anorexia, malaise, nausea, vomiting and diarrhoea, with the distinguishing features of jaundice, mild hypertension, proteinuria and fulminant liver failure. On biochemical testing, there is raised bilirubin with abnormal liver enzymes, leukocytosis, thrombocytopenia, hypoglycaemia and coagulation defects. Acute fatty liver of pregnancy is biochemically distinguished from HELLP syndrome by the hypoglycaemia and high uric acid. Diagnosis is clinical (computed tomography (CT) or magnetic resonance imaging (MRI) may help), but a liver biopsy may be needed. Management is by correction of fluid balance, coagulation and electrolyte disturbances with hasty delivery. Women may need admission to a specialist liver unit or intensive care unit. Maternal mortality rate is 20%.

Obstetric cholestasis only occurs after 30 weeks' gestation. Women present with severe pruritis of the limbs, trunk, palms and feet. There is no abdominal pain. It is more common in women with a family history. Impaired bile acid secretion causes the symptoms, and diagnosis is confirmed by finding an increased serum total bile acid concentration. Other causes of itching and abnormal liver function should be investigated if there are any other symptoms. There is an increased risk of preterm labour, intracranial haemorrhage, fetal distress and intrauterine fetal death. Delivery at 37–38 weeks reduces the risk of intrauterine death. There are no long-term maternal risks. Chlorphenamine is used for symptomatic relief of itching. Ursodeoxycholic acid can be used to reduce serum bile acids in more severe cases.

5. K – Symphysis pubis dysfunction

This common condition occurs in 3% of pregnancies, and women describe pain and discomfort in the pelvic area, which can radiate to the upper thighs or perineum. Pain is worse on walking and may be severe enough to limit mobility. Diagnosis is clinical, and can be confirmed by increased pain on pressure over the symphysis pubis or compression of the pelvis. Treatment is supportive, with analgesia, pelvic support braces and crutches.

The *round ligaments* are prone to stretching during pregnancy with the increasing size of the uterus. This presents with non-specific abdominal pain.

Theme 7: Fetal presentation

It is important to be proficient in abdominal and vaginal examination, as they can provide important information that affects the progress of labour. Do not forget the labour triad of the 'powers' of the uterus (contractions), the 'passages' (the birth canal) and the 'passenger' (the fetus).

Abdominal examination

First inspect for previous scars. The pregnant uterus is palpable from 12 weeks. By 20–22 weeks, it reaches the umbilicus and, by 36 weeks, it lies under the ribs. Palpation is subjective and often unreliable, especially when there is ample subcutaneous tissue, but can be an indicator of gestational age. You must determine the number of fetuses, the lie (longitudinal, oblique or transverse), the presentation (cephalic or breech) and the engagement. Engagement involves passage of the maximum presenting part through the pelvic inlet. 'Fifths palpable' states the proportion of the head palpable abdominally if the head was divided into fifths. Always watch the patient's face, as Pawlik's grip (examining the lower pole of the uterus with the thumb and finger of the right hand) can be very uncomfortable. Measure the symphysis–fundal height (SPH) from the symphysis pubis in centimetres (from 16 weeks, the SPH increases approximately 1 cm/week). Finally, auscultate the fetal heart (with a Doppler ultrasound from 12 weeks or a Pinard stethoscope from 24 weeks).

Vaginal examination

This can be uncomfortable and may be embarrassing, so a full explanation should be given and consent obtained. Speculum examination is used to assess the vagina and cervix. A speculum examination alone is appropriate in spontaneous rupture of membranes (SROM) or suspected SROM to avoid infection. Placenta praevia is an absolute contraindication to manual vaginal examination, as is an inability to rule out a placenta praevia without an ultrasound scan. The Bishop score is used to assess the favourability of the cervix (see 'Induction of labour' – Paper 2 Answers, Theme 10, page 54). An assessment of the presenting part is important to give information regarding the position of the fetal head, and to rule out malpresentation. Malpresentation includes breech, shoulder, face and brow presentations, in decreasing order of incidence.

Adolphe Pinard, French obstetrician (1844–1934).

1. H – Occipitoanterior

Occipitoanterior is the most preferable position of presentation. The 'attitude' of the fetal head refers to the degree of flexion/extension. In this case, the head is well flexed, allowing the smallest diameter to pass through the outlet first (occiput to anterior fontanelle). The fontanelles are junctions between the sutures of the skull bones. The anterior fontanelle is diamond shaped, and the posterior fontanelle is Y shaped or triangular. They allow the bones to 'mould' without affecting the brain in order to facilitate labour.

2. G – Left occipitotransverse

Of the options available with the back on the left side, occipitotransverse is more likely if the back is easily palpable. The shoulder will lie in the midline, above which the fetal heart is heard abdominally with Doppler ultrasound. Underlying causes of a transverse or oblique (diagonal) lie include multiparity, structural uterine abnormality, pelvic tumours, fetal prematurity, multiple pregnancy, fetal abnormality, placenta praevia and a fundal placenta.

3. A – Brow

This is the least common presentation, occurring in 1 in 2000 labours. For the brow to present, the neck is extended, which results in the largest diameter of the fetal head presenting (chin to occiput). This is often too large to pass through the pelvis, and if it persists can cause delay in the second stage of labour. Do not forget that the pelvic brim (inlet) is widest in transverse diameter, but the outlet is widest in anterior–posterior diameter, which requires the head to rotate.

Face presentation occurs in 1 in 500 cases and is due to full extension of the head. It can delay engagement and progress, possibly because the facial bones do not mould. These babies are at risk of facial oedema. This case is not a face presentation, as the sagittal suture and anterior fontanelle are palpable as well as some of the face.

4. I – Occipitoposterior

In the occipitoposterior position, the limbs are anterior, which may visibly affect the contour of the abdomen. An occipitoposterior position can result in relative cephalopelvic disproportion of the fetal head to the maternal pelvis (i.e. the diameter of the head in that particular position may be too big to fit through the mother's pelvis), particularly if the head becomes partially extended.

5. D – Flexed breech

There are several indicators of breech presentation here: the ballottable head at the fundus, the heart above the umbilicus and a high presenting part due to failure to engage. Breech presentation is not of concern until 37 weeks (except in preterm labour). The incidence of breech presentation at term is 3–4% of singleton pregnancies. Breech pregnancies must be considered high risk due to increased perinatal morbidity and mortality. Risk factors for breech presentation include grand multiparity, bony pelvic abnormalities, uterine abnormalities, fetal prematurity (insufficient time to rotate), multiple pregnancy, fetal abnormality, extended legs, oligo-/polyhydramnios and placenta praevia.

There are three types of breech presentation, from most to least common: extended (feet extended near head), flexed (feet next to bottom) and footling (foot presents at cervix). This case is a flexed breech, with the chin tucked into the chest, which leaves the head to the left of the midline. Management of a breech presentation at 37 weeks is planned in every case detected. External cephalic version (ECV) is initially offered. In this procedure, the fetus is manually rotated to a cephalic presentation, usually under ultrasound guidance. It is more difficult in primips with firm abdominal muscles, in overweight women, in those with fibroids and when the breech is engaged with the cervix. ECV is successful in two-thirds of attempted cases when performed by a senior obstetrician, provided that there are no contraindications (e.g. previous caesarean section, history of antepartum haemorrhage, multiple pregnancy, oligo-/polyhydramnios and placenta praevia). Complications of ECV include placental abruption, transplacental haemorrhage (possibly requiring anti-D in rhesus-negative women), fetal bradycardia and prelabour rupture of membranes (PROM). If ECV is declined, contraindicated or unsuccessful, then elective caesarean section is planned.

Theme 8: Diabetes in pregnancy

1. B – 2–5%

Among the 2–5% of pregnant diabetic women, 65% have gestational diabetes, 25% type 1 diabetes and 10% type 2 diabetes.

2. F – 85%

Around 85% of babies born to diabetic mothers are over the 50th percentile in weight.

There are several risks to both mother and baby with poorly controlled diabetes, including the following:

Mother:
* miscarriage
* pre-eclampsia
* stillbirth
* preterm labour

Baby:
* congenital malformations (e.g. cardiac, neural tube and skeletal defects)
* large for gestational age (this increases the risk of birth injuries, and the likelihood of induction of labour, operative delivery and caesarean section)
* perinatal mortality and morbidity requiring admission to neonatology, such as neonatal hypoglycaemia.

3. C – 25%

There is a 25% risk of major congenital malformation if the first HbA$_{1c}$ result is >10%. Good management of diabetes includes educating pregnant women and diabetic women who wish to conceive. It must be emphasized that good preconception glycaemic control can reduce the incidence of the above complications. Monthly HbA$_{1c}$ is advised in those wishing to conceive and, if levels are above 10%, contraception should be strongly recommended until better control is achieved. An HbA$_{1c}$ <6.1% is advised. Folic acid (5 mg daily) is given to reduce the incidence of neural tube defects (women without diabetes are advised to take 0.5 mg folic acid for the first 12 weeks of pregnancy). A urine test for ketonuria is encouraged if patients are hyperglycaemic or feeling unwell. Diabetic ketoacidosis in pregnancy must be managed in hospital, preferably in an HDU (high dependance unit) setting.

Blood sugar control during, and prior to, pregnancy should be strict and ideally between 3.5 and 5.9 mmol/L (fasting) or less than 7.8 mmol/L (1-hour postprandial). Women taking insulin must have hypo- and hyperglycaemic symptoms reinforced. A regular monitoring plan covering different times of the day is advised, as symptoms may go unnoticed in the first trimester. Nausea and vomiting can also affect diabetic control.

Gestational diabetes (i.e. diabetes developing in pregnancy) is more likely if:
- maternal BMI is >30 kg/m^2
- a previous baby weighed >4.5 kg
- there was previous gestational diabetes
- there is a family history of diabetes in a first-degree relative
- the patient is south Asian, African–Caribbean or Chinese (high-risk ethnic groups)

A 2-hour oral glucose tolerance test (OGTT) is undertaken at 24–28 weeks' gestation. If a positive diagnosis is made, conservative management is implemented, with advice on diet, weight loss (if BMI >27 kg/m^2) and gentle exercise. Dietary advice encourages unrefined carbohydrates (most wholegrain and wholemeal foods), and a balance of monounsaturated and polyunsaturated fat sources. If this advice is unsuccessful, a small number of patients require insulin therapy.

Pregnant women with diabetes should ideally be seen every 1–2 weeks by a joint diabetic and antenatal clinic to monitor glycaemic control. A regular regimen of short-acting insulin injections may be advised. Pregnancy can worsen diabetic retinopathy, so retinal checks are needed during pregnancy and annually thereafter. Renal function should also be monitored before and during pregnancy, with attention to glomerular filtration rate (GFR) and referral for nephrology input if necessary.

A detailed ultrasound scan of the heart chambers and outflow tracts is performed with the fetal normality scan at 18–20 weeks. Fetal growth and amniotic fluid volume are checked regularly, usually at 28, 32 and 36 weeks. If there are indications for induction, such as macrosomia, this should be planned from 36 weeks' gestation. Otherwise, diabetic women with normally growing babies are offered induction or elective caesarean section if indicated after 38 weeks.

During labour, blood sugars should be monitored hourly, and control maintained between 4 and 7 mmol/L. An insulin/ dextrose sliding scale may be helpful in this. It is essential that delivery occur where there are immediately available neonatal facilities. Babies born to diabetic mothers must be rigorously assessed for hypoglycaemia, respiratory distress, cardiac failure/dysfunction and jaundice. Insulin requirements after birth are usually greatly reduced, so monitoring is needed to establish the appropriate dose. Women are vulnerable to hypoglycaemia when breastfeeding.

4. E – 60%

At least 60% of gestational diabetic women have recurrence in future pregnancies. Gestational diabetic women are followed up with a fasting glucose measurement at 6 weeks. They are at greater risk of recurrence in future pregnancies, and so must be offered an early OGTT at 16–18 weeks. If this is normal, it is repeated at 28 weeks.

5. D – 50%

The risk of developing type 2 diabetes in the next 10 years after having gestational diabetes is 50%.

Theme 9: Hormone replacement therapy

The majority of symptoms associated with the menopause come from oestrogen-sensitive tissue, such as the skin, bladder, brain and uterus (see 'Perimenopausal hormones' – Paper 4 Answers, Theme 4, page 103). All women who are considered for hormone replacement therapy (HRT) should be assessed to consider the extent of their symptoms, the consequences on their daily life and the desired effect of treatment. The date of the last period must be established, as this will affect the management plan. The diagnosis of the menopause can be made by the finding of a low estradiol (<70 pmol/L) despite a high FSH and LH.

1. E – Oestrogen cream/pessary

The woman in this scenario has no typical menopausal symptoms and so is not in need of systemic hormone replacement. Systemic therapies are best avoided if possible, as raised blood levels of these preparations can cause endometrial hyperplasia (and possibly malignancy) if given for long periods of time. A preferable option would be topical oestrogen administration, in the form of a cream or a pessary.

2. C – Cyclical combined hormone replacement therapy

There are a huge number of hormone replacement options available on the market. Overall, the minimum effective dose should be used for the shortest duration. For the purposes of treatment, women should be divided into those with a uterus and those who have had a hysterectomy.

In women with a uterus who *have bled within the last year* (perimenopausal), low dose cyclical HRT is recommended, which gives progesterone on the last 12 out of 28 days. This results in a regular post-progesterone withdrawal bleed, which protects the endometrium. Prolonged use of cyclical HRT can increase the risk of endometrial cancer, so should be given for a maximum of 5 years. Higher doses are available for symptom control. Once the patient has been amenorrhoeic for 1 year or reaches age 54 (whichever is sooner), she should be transferred to continuous combined therapy.

3. B – Continuous combined hormone replacement therapy

In women with a uterus who *have not bled for 1 year* (postmenopausal), low-dose continuous combined HRT is the first-line option. This means that they are given continuous oestrogen and progesterone. Around 90% of women will experience symptomatic relief on a low dose. The combined preparation causes endometrial atrophy, so treated women should have no bleeding. The progesterone protects the endometrium from hyperplasia and reduces the risk of endometrial cancer; however, unwanted side-effects of progesterone include withdrawal bleeds and premenstrual-like symptoms.

Women who have had a hysterectomy can be given oestrogen-only preparations in doses titrated to their symptoms. They do not require progesterone, as they are not at risk of unopposed oestrogen-induced endometrial hyperplasia.

4. G – Specialist referral

Indications for HRT include menopausal-related symptoms, early menopause and prevention of osteoporosis. Contraindications to oestrogen replacement therapy are carcinoma of the endometrium, liver disease (e.g. active hepatitis), suspected pregnancy and inherited thrombophilias. Relative contraindications to HRT are hypertension and a previous personal or family history of thromboembolism or breast cancer. High blood pressure should be controlled prior to treatment. Those who have a history of thromboembolism or breast cancer should probably be referred to a specialist for close consideration of risk–benefit analysis. Other indications for specialist referral are menopause before the age of 40, a confirmed risk of osteoporosis and a high risk or a personal history of oestrogen-dependent cancers such as those of the breast or endometrium. Women should also be referred for specialist assessment if they have abnormal bleeding before the start of HRT, while using cyclical HRT or more than 6 months after the start of continuous combined HRT.

5. A – Bisphosphonates

Bisphosphonates are drugs that inhibit osteoclast-mediated bone resorption, and consequently prevent osteoporosis. Examples include pamidronate and alendronate. Oral calcium and vitamin D supplements are often given in addition to bisphosphonates for the prevention of osteoporosis. Tibolone is a synthetic steroid that has oestrogenic, progestogenic and some androgenic effects. It does not cause endometrial proliferation, but can still cause irregular bleeding within the first few months. Raloxifene is the first of the new class of selective oestrogen receptor modulators (SERMs). They selectively stimulate oestrogen receptors, so can prevent osteoporosis and have a beneficial effect upon the lipid profile. However, SERMs do not relieve the menopausal symptoms of oestrogen deficiency.

Benefits of hormone replacement include a 50% reduction in osteoporosis. It may also delay the onset of Alzheimer's disease (although it has no effect on established disease). Risks of HRT include a positive association with breast cancer and a threefold risk of venous thromboembolism. Recent data suggest that there may be an increased risk of cardiovascular disease with combined HRT preparations. Women on HRT should be followed up 6-monthly to assess symptomatic improvement and adverse effects. Note that the presence of postmenopausal bleeding (i.e. vaginal bleeding occurring 6–12 months after the menopause) is an indication for immediate referral for endometrial biopsy.

Theme 10: Premature labour

Prematurity is defined as delivery before 37 weeks' gestation, but the majority of morbidity and mortality occurs before 34 weeks. Premature labour may be preceded by premature prelabour rupture of membranes (PPROM), or can occur with intact membranes, with subsequent rupture of membranes and delivery. Preterm labour complicates 5–10% of pregnancies, and is responsible for 75% of all perinatal deaths. Survival rates are improving with advances in maternal and neonatal management. The management of each case must be adjusted to the individual. Although there is national evidence-based guidance, as with much of obstetrics there are always local protocols with which you must be familiar.

The biggest risk factor for preterm delivery is a previous preterm delivery. Other risk factors include maternal age <20 years, low socioeconomic class, multiparity, smoking, multiple pregnancy, fetal growth retardation and fetal congenital abnormality. Certain features of the current pregnancy can also increase the risk of preterm delivery, including antepartum haemorrhage, pre-eclampsia, polyhydramnios and infection (e.g. chorioamnionitis).

In reality, the diagnosis of premature labour can be difficult. A clear history and examination are required, and discussion with a registrar or consultant. A good history includes noting the strength, intensity and frequency of contractions, evidence of a 'show' (characteristic cervical mucus) or rupture of membranes, presence of fetal movements and additional symptoms, such as urinary symptoms, vaginal bleeding, discharge or systemic symptoms (fever, cough or shortness of breath).

Examination includes observations (temperature, blood pressure, pulse rate, and urine testing for protein, leucocytes and nitrites) and abdominal palpation (for tenderness, symphysiofundal height, fetal lie and position, and palpation for contractions). A *sterile* speculum examination will help assess the cervix and detect spontaneous rupture of membranes by looking for pooling of liquor in the speculum or leakage on coughing. Investigations include vaginal swabs, blood tests for inflammatory markers, a CTG (if >26 weeks) and a pelvic ultrasound (can provide information about fetal growth/presentation and an estimate of liquor volume, low amounts of which suggest rupture of membranes).

Do not perform a digital examination if rupture of membranes is suspected. There is a risk of transmission of infection from the vagina into the cervix, which can cause intrauterine infection, prostaglandin release and preterm labour.

1. H – Ritodrine

Tocolytics act by inhibiting smooth muscle contraction in the uterus in an attempt to delay labour. They must be used with caution in ruptured membranes. A variety of drugs has been used in clinical trials. Cases most likely to benefit are those that are very preterm, those requiring time for transfer to specialist units and those requiring time for corticosteroids. There is as yet no proven significant benefit of tocolytics on perinatal mortality.

Ritodrine, a β-agonist, is the most widely evaluated tocolytic, but it is being overtaken by other drugs due to its poor side-effect profile. Side-effects include tachycardia, headache, palpitations and impaired glucose tolerance. Because of these effects, it is avoided in cardiac disease and diabetes.

2. A – Atosiban

Atosiban is an oxytocin inhibitor that has been found to have some benefit in reducing delivery within a 48-hour period, and has a preferable side-effect profile compared with ritodrine. Nifedipine, a calcium channel blocker that is often used as a tocolytic, is easier and cheaper to administer than atosiban. It is, however, not yet licensed for use in the UK. Other tocolytics include magnesium sulphate and indometacin. Relative contraindications to tocolysis include rupture of membranes, fetal distress and intrauterine infection.

3. B – Betamethasone

Corticosteroids, such as betamethasone and dexamethasone, are indicated between 24 and 34 weeks' gestation in preterm labour in the absence of infection to promote pulmonary maturity and stimulate surfactant production. They have been proven to reduce the incidence of respiratory distress syndrome, intraventricular haemorrhage and necrotizing enterocolitis in the premature infant. One commonly used dosing regimen is two intramuscular injections of betamethasone 12 mg given 12 hours apart. The steroids take 24 hours to become effective. Delivery may then be delayed, by tocolysis if necessary, to occur after 24 hours and within 7 days of treatment.

4. D – Erythromycin

5. C – Co-amoxiclav

Antibiotics are indicated as infection prophylaxis in preterm rupture of membranes. Erythromycin is the antibiotic of choice following the diagnosis of PPROM. It is given as a 10-day course and has been found to reduce the incidence of delivery within 48 hours, and has a positive impact upon neonatal and maternal morbidity. If group B streptococci have been isolated, penicillin is given in addition. Co-amoxiclav (Augmentin) is not recommended, as it has been associated with an increased incidence of fetal necrotizing colitis. Gentamicin is not advised in pregnancy, as it has been associated with auditory or vestibular damage in the second and third trimesters.

Women with PPROM should be observed for signs of chorioamnionitis (infection of the chorion and amnion affecting fetal and maternal blood vessels), which include maternal pyrexia, offensive vaginal discharge and fetal tachycardia. If there is evidence of sepsis then delivery should be expedited and broad-spectrum antibiotics given intravenously after blood cultures and swabs are taken.

Theme 1: Antepartum haemorrhage

Options
- A. Bloody show
- B. Cervical ectropion
- C. Cervical polyp
- D. Placental abruption
- E. Placenta praevia
- F. Uterine rupture
- G. Vasa praevia

For each of the following scenarios, select the most likely cause of antepartum haemorrhage. Each option may be used once, more than once or not at all.

1. A 34-year-old woman is labouring well at term with an epidural *in situ*. She has reached 8 cm of cervical dilatation with good progression. Since insertion of the epidural, she has felt no contractions. Suddenly, she experiences severe lower abdominal pain associated with per vagina bleeding and tachycardia. The cardiotocograph (CTG) does not detect any contractions and shows signs of significant fetal distress. She has had three previous pregnancies, including two spontaneous vaginal births and one caesarean section for failure to progress.

2. A 42-year-old woman, who is 39 weeks' gestation with five previous normal deliveries, calls an ambulance as she is having heavy, unprovoked, painless vaginal bleeding. The midwife had mentioned on her previous visit that the baby was still high and free in the pelvis on abdominal palpation. She decided to have no scans in this pregnancy as she felt that there were no problems with her previous children.

3. A 32-year-old primigravida is being induced at term + 14 days and has an artificial rupture of membranes performed. The midwife confirms that there is no cord in the cervix, although she does note heavily bloodstained liquor. The mother is not complaining of pain, but the CTG demonstrates significant abnormalities.

4. A 33-year-old primigravida attends the antenatal day unit. She is very concerned as she had a mucus-like bloodstained loss vaginally earlier in the day, and this was associated with gradual-onset abdominal cramps approximately every 15–20 minutes.

5. A 24 year old at 38 weeks' gestation presents to the antenatal day unit with significant lower abdominal pain and back pain. She also admits to having some per vagina blood loss. On examination, the uterus is tender and hard. Maternal observations are pulse rate 115 beats/min and blood pressure 95/68 mmHg. The CTG shows fetal distress.

Theme 2: Menorrhagia

Options

   A. Antifibrinolytics (tranexamic acid)
   B. Combined oral contraceptive pill
   C. Danazol
   D. Endometrial ablation
   E. Gonadotropin-releasing hormone analogues
   F. Hysterectomy
   G. Hysteroscopic laser/resection of fibroids
   H. Intrauterine or systemic progestogens
   I. Myomectomy
   J. Polypectomy
   K. Non-steroidal anti-inflammatory drugs (mefanamic acid)
   L. Uterine artery embolization

For each of the following scenarios, select the most appropriate management option. Each option may be used once, more than once or not at all.

1. A 16-year-old girl, who is normally fit and well, attends her GP complaining of heavy and <u>painful</u> periods. She is requesting treatment for these complaints. She denies being sexually active.

2. A 43-year-old woman has suffered with heavy periods for many years, and has tried many medical treatments without success. She is constantly flooding and at times cannot leave her house due to heavy bleeding. She has completed her family of five children and her last blood test showed a haemoglobin level of 8.9 g/dL. She feels that she cannot cope with the bleeding anymore, and her husband is asking for a treatment that can guarantee success.

3. A 29-year-old woman presents to her GP with troublesome heavy periods. The medical treatments that she has tried have made little difference. She is known to have large uterine intramural fibroids. You confirm that she is currently trying for more children.

4. A 42-year-old overweight smoker attends with heavy periods. A scan reveals a normal uterus. She would like a long-term treatment with minimal side-effects that would offer treatment for the menorrhagia and provide contraception. She is unsure whether she would like more children. She is adamant that she does not want surgery, as she is terrified of the prospect.

5. A 41-year-old woman, who has completed her family, has suffered from extremely heavy periods for many years. No medical treatments have worked. She admits that she would rather avoid surgery. After discussion, you collectively decide on a procedure that would not require open surgery or a general anaesthetic.

Theme 3: Physiological changes in pregnancy

Options

- A. Decreases
- B. Increases
- C. Increases only in twins
- D. Increases only with female fetuses
- E. Increases only with male fetuses
- F. Stays the same

For each of the following, select the correct answer for what happens physiologically in pregnancy. Each option may be used once, more than once or not at all.

1. Respiratory rate.

2. Haemoglobin concentration.

3. Renal blood flow.

4. Albumin.

5. Heart rate.

Theme 4: Vaginal bleeding

Options

- A. Cervical cancer
- B. Cervical ectropion
- C. Cervical polyps
- D. Chlamydial infection
- E. Endometrial carcinoma
- F. Endometrial polyps
- G. Perimenopausal symptoms
- H. Pregnancy
- I. Uterine fibroids (leiomyomas)

For each of the following scenarios, select the most likely diagnosis. Each option may be used once, more than once or not at all.

1. A 59-year-old overweight woman says that she has had some irregular vaginal bleeding. Her regular menstrual periods stopped 7 years ago. She has suffered from an offensive discharge for the last 3 months. She is unmarried and has never had sexual intercourse.

2. A 45-year-old lawyer presents to you complaining of postcoital bleeding and some weight loss. She is a smoker. She admits to having a number of sexual partners from a young age, but says that she

used barrier protection for them all. She has not seen a healthcare professional for the last 10 years, as she feels that she has previously been healthy, and has consequently never had a smear test.

3. A 51-year-old woman presents to the clinic with one episode of light vaginal bleeding unrelated to sexual intercourse. She says that her regular periods stopped 3 months ago, and since then she has had a light, clear vaginal discharge. She has been feeling hot and sweaty at night and suffers a dryness of her vagina.

4. A 35-year-old woman presents with a long history of very heavy periods. She has visited you now as she cannot cope with the bleeding. On examination, you feel a bulky uterus equivalent to a pregnancy at 18 weeks; however, the patient states that she has not been sexually active for over 3 years.

5. A 19-year-old student attends your surgery concerned about postcoital bleeding. She has recently had a GUM clinic appointment, where they did a cervical smear. The patient reports that all her tests from this clinic returned as negative. She mentions that the GUM consultant said that she had a 'funny area of skin' on her cervix, and she is now very concerned about cancer.

Theme 5: Contraindications to contraception

Options

    A. A diabetic patient who smokes
    B. Any smoker
    C. Body mass index >39 kg/m^2
    D. Family history of thromboembolism in a first-degree relative under 45 years
    E. Hypertension
    F. Migraine controlled with 5-HT$_1$ agonist
    G. Migraine with a typical focal aura
    H. Migraine without focal aura
    I. Pelvic inflammatory disease

For each of the following descriptions, select the appropriate contraindication. Each option may be used once, more than once or not at all.

1. In a woman who suffers with migraines, this form is an absolute contraindication to using combined hormonal contraception.

2. With respect to venous thromboembolism, this is an absolute contraindication to using combined hormonal contraception.

3. With respect to arterial disease, this is an absolute contraindication to using combined oral contraception.

4. This is neither a caution nor a contraindication to using combined oral contraception.

5. With respect to venous thromboembolism, combined oral contraception should be used with caution in these patients.

Theme 6: Rhesus disease

Options

A. Give antenatal anti-D prophylaxis 250 iu
B. Give antenatal anti-D prophylaxis 500 iu
C. Give postnatal anti-D
D. Give routine antenatal anti-D prophylaxis 500 iu at 28 weeks
E. Give routine antenatal anti-D prophylaxis 500 iu at 34 weeks
F. No action needed

For each of the following scenarios, select the most appropriate course of action you would take on that day. Each option may be used once, more than once or not at all.

1. A 28-year-old rhesus D (RhD)-negative pregnant woman attends the emergency department with a per vagina bleed at 7 weeks' gestation.

2. A 34-year-old RhD-negative woman, having her second baby at 25 weeks' gestation, attends the antenatal clinic with a story that her son pushed his play trolley hard into her abdomen (accidently). The baby has been moving well since and there has been no bleeding per vagina. The fetal heart is heard and is regular.

3. A 25-year-old woman who is RhD negative attends the emergency department with a per vagina bleed at 25 weeks' gestation. She does not want any more children and the baby's father is known to be RhD negative.

4. A 30-year-old woman attends the antenatal clinic to have her routine antenatal anti-D prophylaxis at 28 weeks. She tells you that she has already had an anti-D injection due to bleeding earlier on in her pregnancy.

5. A 31-year-old RhD-negative woman has had both routine antenatal anti-D prophylaxis at 28 and 34 weeks, as well as an antenatal anti-D prophylaxis injection prior to this. She has just delivered an RhD-positive infant and is asking you what needs to be done.

Theme 7: Classification of ovarian tumours

Options

    A. Brenner's tumour
    B. Clear cell carcinoma
    C. Dysgerminoma
    D. Fibroma
    E. Krukenberg's tumour
    F. Mucinous adenocarcinoma
    G. Non-gestational choriocarcinomas
    H. Serous adenocarcinoma
    I. Sex cord tumour
    J. Teratoma

For each of the following descriptions, select the most appropriate ovarian tumour. Each option may be used once, more than once or not at all.

1. One of the commonest oestrogen-producing tumours.

2. This is the commonest of all ovarian malignancies.

3. The ovarian tumour that is associated with Meigs' syndrome.

4. Rupture of these large tumours can lead to pseudomyxoma peritonei.

5. These arise from germ cells and can contain ectodermal tissue.

Theme 8: Management of endometrial and cervical cancer

Options

    A. Chemotherapy and radiotherapy
    B. Cone biopsy
    C. Cryocautery
    D. Radical hysterectomy and bilateral salpingo-oophorectomy
    E. Radical trachelectomy
    F. Radiotherapy
    G. Reassurance
    H. Simple hysterectomy

For each of the following scenarios, select the most appropriate management plan. Each option may be used once, more than once or not at all.

1. A 34-year old woman attends her GP clinic for a routine smear test. An abnormal area is only partially visible at colposcopy, and histology is reported as CIN 2.

2. A 68-year-old woman undergoes a staging laparoscopy after being found to have an invasive cervical tumour. The cancer extends visibly onto the pelvic wall.

3. A 32-year-old woman has a 3 cm tumour that is confined to the cervix. She mentions that she still wishes to conceive.

4. A 31-year-old woman, who was admitted under gynaecology with abdominal pain and heavy periods, is found to have an endometrial sarcoma.

5. A 65-year-old woman has an operation for an endometrial adenocarcinoma. The tumour visibly extends beyond the uterus into the adnexae, but a hysterectomy is performed anyway.

Theme 9: Drug management of pre-eclampsia

Options
  A. Betamethasone
  B. Furosemide
  C. Hydralazine
  D. Labetalol
  E. Magnesium sulphate
  F. Methyldopa
  G. Misoprostol
  H. Nifedipine
  I. Phenytoin
  J. Ramipril

For each of the following descriptions, select the most appropriate drug. Each option may be used once, more than once or not at all.

1. An α- and β-blocker often commenced at a dose of 100 mg twice daily.

2. A calcium channel blocker often used for acute rises in blood pressure.

3. The most effective infusion used in pre-eclampsia for preventing convulsions.

4. A drug used for induction of labour.

5. An antihypertensive agent that is avoided in women with asthma.

Theme 10: Induction of labour

Options

A. Artificial rupture of membranes
B. Caesarean section
C. Observation alone
D. Prostaglandin
E. Twice-weekly cardiotocography
F. Twice-weekly ultrasound

For each of the following scenarios, select the most appropriate management. Each option may be used once, more than once or not at all.

1. A 30-year-old woman at 41 weeks and 6 days attends antenatal clinic. On vaginal examination, she has a 1–2 cm dilated, posterior, firm cervix that is 2 cm in length and 2 cm above the ischial spines (Bishop score 3).

2. A 28-year-old primigravida, who is 3 days overdue, presents following spontaneous rupture of membranes 48 hours ago associated with intermittent lower abdominal pain. Her cardiotocography is reassuring. She complains of a vaginal discharge and is keen to 'get it over with'. Her Bishop score is 2.

3. A 24-year-old woman at 42 weeks attends clinic. She declines induction of labour despite appropriate counselling.

4. An unbooked 31-year-old multiparous woman at term is referred by the emergency department. She is G6P4 (three vaginal deliveries, one emergency caesarean section and two miscarriages). She is experiencing palpable contractions every 15 minutes and palpation shows a transverse lie. Cardiotocography demonstrates variable (and a few late) decelerations with reduced variability.

5. You are called to see a 25-year-old primigravida after her second dose of Prostin. She is having irregular contractions. Her cardiotocography is reassuring. The midwife tells you that her Bishop score is 8, and that her dilatation has improved from 2 to 4 cm in 4 hours.

Theme 1: Antepartum haemorrhage

Antepartum haemorrhage is bleeding from the genital tract after 24 weeks' gestation and before birth of the infant. Around 3% of women suffer antepartum haemorrhage. Bleeding can be maternal, fetal or placental. The patient with antepartum haemorrhage is at increased risk of postpartum haemorrhage.

1. F – Uterine rupture

Uterine rupture, where the uterine wall tears, is very rare. It generally occurs only in patients who have had previous surgery to the uterus, such as myomectomy or caesarean section, but can rarely occur in cases of excessive oxytocin use, in obstructed labour and in women of high parity. Pain is the principal feature (although a good epidural can mask this pain), with associated maternal shock, sudden termination of contractions and CTG abnormalities. A laparotomy must be performed immediately to deliver the baby and control maternal haemorrhage.

2. E – Placenta praevia

Placenta praevia is where the placenta lies in the lower segment of the uterus and can lie over the internal cervical os. It occurs in 1% of pregnancies and is more common in older women, multiparous women, previous caesarean section, smokers, and women with previous placenta praevia. It is usually detected on the 20-week ultrasound scan. However, because the placenta can move away from the internal os with uterine growth as the pregnancy progresses, a rescan is done at 34 weeks. Only 3% of women with placenta praevia at the 20-week scan have one at term. Placenta praevia is classified according to its proximity to the internal os, as marginal (placenta in lower segment, but not over os) or major (placenta partially or completely over os).

Clinically, there is unprovoked (or postcoital), intermittent, fresh, painless bleeding per vagina. The lack of pain excludes placental abruption. On abdominal examination, there is a soft, non-tender uterus with a high head or malpresentation (as the placenta blocks passage of the presenting part into the pelvis). Vaginal examination is contraindicated in suspected placenta praevia, as it can precipitate massive bleeding. The clinical condition of the mother correlates with the visible blood loss (unlike placental abruption – see below). Because only the maternal blood is lost, there is little risk to the fetus unless the mother becomes extremely hypovolaemic. Women with bleeding placenta praevia should be admitted and the baby delivered by elective caesarean section at 39 weeks. Massive haemorrhage requires maternal resuscitation and immediate delivery.

Placenta, from Greek *plakous* = flat cake.

Praevia, from Latin *prae* = ahead of + *via* = road (i.e. 'in the way').

3. G – Vasa praevia

In vasa praevia, the umbilical cord vessels traverse the membranes and overlie the internal cervical os. It occurs in 1 in 3000 pregnancies. The risk of vessels tearing is greatest when cervical dilatation occurs and at rupture of membranes. There is a small amount (<500 mL) of painless blood loss with associated CTG abnormalities, particularly following rupture of membranes. Because it is fetal blood that is lost in vasa praevia, fetal mortality rate is very high (35–95%), whereas there is little risk to the mother. A caesarean section must be performed immediately and the neonate transfused. There is no specific investigation for vasa praevia, so the diagnosis is clinical.

Vasa, plural of Latin *vas* = vessel.

4. A – Bloody show

The 'show' is a bloody, mucus-like vaginal loss that is associated with contractions and the initial stages of early labour.

5. D – Placental abruption

In placental abruption, the placental bed bleeds and a haematoma forms behind it, lifting the placenta away from the uterus. Risk factors are hypertension, pre-eclampsia, sudden decompression after membrane rupture in polyhydramnios or multiple pregnancies, previous abruption (10% recurrence), trauma to the abdomen, and tobacco or cocaine abuse (although the cause is unknown in many cases). The incidence is 0.5–2%. A mild abruption presents with a small amount of pain or bleeding with little effect to fetus or mother. Major abruptions present as variable amounts of darker vaginal bleeding coupled with sudden-onset, constant, sharp, severe lower abdominal or back pains and maternal shock. The uterus is irritable and tender and may become 'woody' hard due to tonic contraction. It is therefore difficult to palpate the fetal parts. There is often loss of fetal movements with fetal distress. The volume of vaginal bleeding is a poor indicator of grade of abruption or maternal blood loss (unlike placenta praevia), as bleeding can be contained behind the placenta (concealed abruption). Intrauterine death from hypoxia is common, as there is a sudden reduction in the blood available for placental gas exchange.

The *cervical ectropion* is the most common cervical lesion that accounts for antepartum haemorrhage. It is diagnosed by appearance on speculum examination (only after placenta praevia has been excluded). The ectropion can resolve during the puerperium, and cauterization should be avoided in pregnancy. *Cervical polyps* are occasionally found in pregnancy and should be managed expectantly. Avulsion should be considered only if bleeding from polyps is uncontrolled, as haemostasis is much harder to maintain due to the greater cervical vascularity in pregnancy. A hysteroscopy can be performed postnatally if there is concern about uterine polyps.

Theme 2: Menorrhagia

Menorrhagia means heavy periods and should not be confused with dysmenorrhoea (painful periods), although both often occur simultaneously. Menorrhagia is defined as menstrual blood loss >80 mL per period. This value represents two standard deviations above the mean period blood loss (40 mL).

Menorrhagia, from Greek *meniaios* = monthly + *rhoia* = flowing.

1. K – Non-steroidal anti-inflammatory drugs (mefenamic acid)

This girl is suffering from subjective menorrhagia (heavy cyclical menstrual bleeding over several consecutive cycles) and dysmenorrhoea. The first-line treatment of menorrhagia is with NSAIDs, such as mefenamic acid and ibuprofen. NSAIDs act as inhibitors of prostaglandin synthesis. They can reduce blood loss by 25%. They also are helpful with dysmenorrhoea. Side-effects of NSAIDs are mainly gastrointestinal. Other medical interventions for heavy bleeding include antifibrinolytic agents, such as tranexamic acid. These reduce fibrinolytic activity by inhibiting plasminogen activator (i.e. they stop activation of plasminogen to plasmin). Clot formation is subsequently increased in the spiral arteries, which reduces menstrual loss. Antifibrinolytics must not be used by women with a predisposition to thromboembolism. These drugs can reduce blood loss by 50%.

Gonadotropin-releasing hormone analogues are a treatment for fibroids and simple menorrhagia. These cause amenorrhoea by downregulation of the pituitary, which leads to inhibition of ovarian activity. There are consequences of the hypo-oestrogenic state, including hot flushes and vaginal dryness. Loss of bone mineral density is also a problem when these drugs are used for longer than 6 months; therefore they should be used only short term. Danazol is a synthetic androgen that has antioestrogen and antiprogestogen activity, leading to a significant reduction in blood loss. Its use is limited by significant androgenic side-effects, including hirsutism, acne, weight gain and breast atrophy.

2. F – Hysterectomy

This woman is clearly at the end of her tether and requires treatment. A hysterectomy is the best option, as this is the only treatment that will ensure amenorrhoea, and the patient has finished her family. The surgical approach is either vaginal or abdominal. Risks of this procedure are bleeding, infection, pain, damage to the bowel/urinary tracts, postoperative thromboembolism and vaginal prolapse in later life.

3. I – Myomectomy

Myomectomy allows conservation of a patient's fertility. This is either an abdominal or a laparoscopic procedure. The pseudocapsules of the fibroids are incised, the bulk of the tumour enucleated and the resulting defect sealed. Risks of this procedure include uncontrolled bleeding requiring hysterectomy, adhesion formation (leading to reduced fertility) and recurrence of fibroids. Hysteroscopic resection is not an option in this case, as this woman's fibroids are too large and are intramural. Hysteroscopic resection is possible only with small, submucosal fibroids.

4. H – Intrauterine or systemic progestogens

Progestogen administration is the most appropriate treatment in this woman, who does not wish to have surgery. This treatment offers her both contraception and a reduction in bleeding. She can use either a systemic formulation (progesterone-only pill) or a Mirena coil (an intrauterine device impregnated with progestogen, licensed for 5 years' use in the treatment of menorrhagia). This would be her personal choice. Because of the risk of thromboembolism (weight, age and smoking habits), she is not suitable for the combined oral contraceptive pill.

5. L – Uterine artery embolization

Uterine artery embolization is performed by radiologists. A catheter is inserted, via the femoral artery, and is fed up to the uterine artery, where a coil or piece of foam is deposited to occlude the blood supply to the fibroid. This can cause fibroids to shrink by 50%. Healthy myometrium is unaffected, as there is collateral circulation via the ovarian and vaginal vessels. Risks of this procedure include pain, bleeding, infection, fibroid expulsion and damage to the ovaries secondary to ionizing radiation. It is not recommended for patients wishing to remain fertile.

Endometrial ablation can improve menorrhagia by destroying the endometrium. Hysteroscopic procedures include laser ablation, resection or coagulation using an electric roller-ball, microwave ablation, heat ablation and electrocautery. Pregnancy is contraindicated after ablation.

Theme 3: Physiological changes in pregnancy

1. F – Stays the same

2. A – Decreases

3. B – Increases

4. A – Decreases

5. B – Increases

The physiological changes in pregnancy are summarized as follows.

	Increase	Unchanged	Decrease
Respiratory	Tidal volume: +200 mL Inspiratory capacity: +100 mL	Respiratory rate	Total lung capacity: −200 mL Residual volume: −200 mL Expiratory reserve: −100 mL Inspiratory reserve: −100 mL Functional residual capacity: −300 mL

Cardiovascular system	Plasma volume: 45% by 32 weeks
	Red cell mass: 25%
	Cardiac output: 40%
	Heart rate: 10%
	Stroke volume: 30%
	Blood flow:
	  Uterus: 400 mL
	  Skin: 500 mL
	  Renal: 300 mL
		Mean arterial pressure
		Central venous pressure
		Pulmonary wedge pressure
			Haematocrit
			Haemoglobin concentration
			Midtrimester blood pressure

Haematology	Mean cell volume Plasma volume: 50% White cell count Total iron-binding capacity	Mean cell haemoglobin concentration	Haemoglobin concentration Haematocrit Platelet count Serum ferritin, iron
Gastrointestinal	Weight: 10 kg Insulin Nutritional requirements Gastric reflux Gallstones		Fasting glucose Glucose tolerance Gastrointestinal tract motility Stomach pH
Liver	Alkaline phosphatase (placental) Plasma cholesterol Triglycerides	Aspartate transaminase, alanine transaminase, bilirubin	Albumin
Immunology	Erythrocyte sedimentation rate C3, C4 complement	C-reactive protein	Circulating immune complexes
Endocrinology	Total triiodothyronine (T_3) + thyroxine (T_4) Thyroid-binding globulin Adrenocorticotropic hormone, corticotropin-releasing hormone, cortisol Prolactin 1,25-Dihydroxyvitamin-D_3	Free T_3 + T_4 Tetracosactide (Synacthen), adrenaline, noradrenaline Calcitonin, free ionized calcium	Thyroid-stimulating hormone Total serum calcium, albumin, parathyroid hormone
Renal	Renal blood flow: 25% Creatinine clearance: 40% Kidney length: 1–1.5 cm Bladder capacity Renin, angiotensin II	Daily voided volume Plasma Na^+, K^+, Cl^-	Plasma urea, creatinine, phosphorus

Theme 4: Vaginal bleeding

1. E – Endometrial carcinoma

Presentation of endometrial carcinoma is often with postmenopausal bleeding. In rare cases that present prior to the menopause, there is abnormal bleeding, discharge or pyometra (pus in the uterus). Endometrial tumours are oestrogen dependent and are therefore linked with long-term unopposed oestrogen administration and tumours of the ovary. There is a higher risk in obese women (as adiposity increases oestrogen levels) and in nulliparous women with a late menopause. Investigations include prompt ultrasound or MRI, hysteroscopy and endometrial sampling. Prior to surgery, a chest X-ray and liver function tests should be performed to assess spread. Endometrial tumours are locally invasive, spreading through the endometrial cavity and cervix, along the fallopian tubes to the ovaries and peritoneal cavity. Endometrial carcinoma is less common than ovarian and cervical tumours.

2. A – Cervical cancer

Cervical cancer is the second most common malignancy in women in the world. There are two peaks of diagnosis: at 35–39 years and 60–64 years. There is an association with early sexual activity, multiple partners and smoking. Human papillomaviruses (HPVs) 16 and 18 are associated with invasive tumours. The vast majority of women diagnosed with invasive carcinoma have not had screening, and there are a small number of women who are diagnosed with early cervical cancer from smear tests. Most (80%) are symptomatic, complaining of abnormal per vagina bleeding (postcoital, intermenstrual or postmenopausal) or a chronic vaginal discharge, with or without odour. Pain, haematuria, malaise and weight loss generally occur only in late disease.

3. G – Perimenopausal symptoms

The average age of the menopause is 50.5 years. This is the cessation of periods due to ovarian failure following depletion of oocytes. As oestrogen production falls, the production of follicle-stimulating hormone rises. Absolute cessation of periods is often preceded by irregular bleeding. Persistent irregular bleeding or vaginal bleeding 6 months to 1 year following the menopause warrants endometrial investigation for possible carcinoma. Irregular bleeding before this point can be considered normal, if there are no other concerning features.

4. I – Uterine fibroids (leiomyomas)

Fibroids are whorls of smooth muscle cells interspersed with collagen. They are benign tumours of the myometrium. Fibroids are present in 20% of women of reproductive age and are largely asymptomatic. They are more common in nulliparous and African–Caribbean women. Fibroids can be intramural (within the uterine wall), subserous (beneath the serosal surface of the uterus) or submucosal (beneath the mucosal surface of the uterus). They can be multiple and vary widely in size. Presentation depends on the size and location of fibroids, as some are microscopic and others have been known to be 40 kg! The most common presentation is menorrhagia with intermenstrual bleeding and abdominal swelling. Pressure on the bladder can lead to frequency of micturition or hydronephrosis, due to ureteric compression. Other presenting features include infertility, miscarriage, dyspareunia and pelvic discomfort.

Treatment is not required if fibroids are asymptomatic. Medical treatment includes progesterone tablets and gonadotropin releasing hormone analogues. Surgical options include myomectomy (abdominally, laparoscopically or hysteroscopically), uterine artery embolization and hysterectomy.

Leiomyomas, from Greek *leios* = smooth + *myos* = muscle + *oma* = tumour.

5. B – Cervical ectropion

Cervical ectropion describes a florid appearance of the lower cervical canal. It is caused by hormonal changes during puberty, pregnancy and oral contraceptive pill use. Ectropion is usually asymptomatic, but may cause persistent vaginal discharge or postcoital bleeding. If the patient has had a normal smear test, it can be treated by diathermy or cryocautery.

Endometrial polyps are very common. Usually, they are multiple in premenopausal women, but single in postmenopausal women. They are found in the body of the uterus and are adenomatous in histology. Polyps present with menstrual irregularities. They can cause dysmenorrhoea or postcoital bleeding if they protrude through the cervix. If found, they should be excised and the tissue sent for histology.

Cervical polyps are the most common benign growth of the cervix. They are usually pedunculated and arise from the endocervical mucosa. Cervical polyps often protrude through the external cervical os and look like bright-red growths. They can be inflammatory in origin and can be up to a few centimetres in diameter. Most are asymptomatic and are found incidentally during smear tests, whilst some cause chronic discharge or postcoital or intermenstrual bleeding. Cervical polyps should be avulsed, and the base cauterized with diathermy, due to the risk of malignancy (1 in 6000).

Theme 5: Contraindications to contraception

1. **G – Migraine with a typical focal aura**

2. **C – Body mass index (BMI) >39 kg/m²**

3. **A – A diabetic patient who smokes**

4. **I – Pelvic inflammatory disease**

5. **D – Family history of thromboembolism in a first-degree relative under 45 years**

Combined hormonal contraceptives (combined oral contraceptive pills: COCP) contain two hormones – oestrogen and progesterone – which prevent ovulation, thicken cervical mucus to prevent sperm reaching an egg and thin the lining of the womb to prevent ovum implantation. They are over 99% effective if taken appropriately, and are widely used as first-line contraception. Advantages are a reduction in bleeding, period pains and premenstrual symptoms. They protect against cancer of the ovary, uterus and colon, as well as some pelvic infections. Fertility quickly returns to normal when the medication is discontinued. The disadvantages include temporary minor side-effects such as headaches, mood changes and breast tenderness, and there is a slightly increased risk of venous thrombosis, breast cancer and cervical cancer. Missed pills, some drugs, vomiting or severe long-lasting diarrhoea can make combined oral contraception less effective.

There are many contraindications to combined oral contraceptives: thromboembolism (below), heart/arterial disease (below), migraine (below), transient ischaemic attacks, liver disease, infective hepatitis, systemic lupus erythematosus, porphyria, liver adenoma, gallstones, post-evacuation of hydatidiform mole, haemolytic uraemic syndrome, history during pregnancy of pruritis, cholestatic jaundice, chorea or pemphigoid gestations, breast or genital carcinoma, undiagnosed vaginal bleeding, breastfeeding and pregnancy.

A personal *history of venous or arterial thrombosis* is a contraindication to the COCP. They should be used with caution if one of the following is present, but must be avoided if two or more are present:
- family history of thromboembolism in a first-degree relative under 45 years
- obesity: BMI >30 kg/m^2 (avoid if BMI >39 kg/m^2)
- long-term immobilization, e.g. wheelchair-bound (avoid if leg in plaster/ bedbound)
- varicose veins

With respect to *arterial disease*, use the COCP with caution if one of the following is present (avoid if two or more are present):
- family history of arterial disease in a first-degree relative under 45 years
- diabetes mellitus
- hypertension
- smoking
- age over 35 years
- obesity

With respect to *migraines*, contraindications to the COCP are:
- migraine with typical focal aura
- severe migraine regularly lasting >72 hours despite treatment
- migraine treated with ergot derivatives (e.g. dihydroergotamine)

Use with caution in women who have:
- migraine without focal aura
- migraine controlled with 5-HT$_1$ agonist (e.g. sumatriptan)

Theme 6: Rhesus disease

1. F – No action needed

2. B – Give antenatal anti-D prophylaxis 500 iu

3. F – No action needed

4. D – Give routine antenatal anti-D prophylaxis 500 iu at 28 weeks

5. C – Give postnatal anti-D

At booking, all women have their bloods taken to screen for infection and to determine maternal blood group. Around 15% of women are rhesus-negative (RhD–ve), which means that their red blood cells do not carry the RhD antigen. Women who are rhesus-positive (RhD+ve) do carry the D antigen on their red blood cells. These antigens are inherited. Rhesus status should be documented, as it can have serious consequences for the fetus if there is any mixing of fetal blood into the maternal circulation.

RhD–ve women are at risk of developing anti-D antibodies to a RhD+ve fetus. If a RhD–ve woman is carrying a RhD+ve fetus and any fetal blood cells cross into the maternal circulation (a sensitizing event) she will react to the 'foreign' D antigens on the red blood cells of the fetus and produce antibodies against them. This will not cause a problem in the current pregnancy, but in later pregnancies the antibodies from the mother can cross the placenta and destroy the blood cells of a subsequent RhD+ve fetus. This is known as haemolytic disease of the newborn. Anti-D prophylaxis prevents women producing antibodies against RhD+ve blood cells by providing anti-D immunoglobulins either routinely or following sensitizing events. Haemolytic disease of the newborn can vary from very mild disease, which is detectable only by laboratory testing, to severe disability or stillbirth.

Royal College Guidelines for use of rhesus D prophylaxis

All women who are RhD–ve are offered routine antenatal anti-D prophylaxis at 28 and 34 weeks *regardless* of any sensitizing events. If, on testing the baby's blood after birth, it is found to be RhD+ve, the mother is offered further postnatal anti-D prophylaxis. If a sensitizing event occurs during pregnancy, the RhD–ve mother is offered antenatal anti-D prophylaxis at that time (as described below). A sensitizing event is defined as an event when fetal blood could pass into the maternal circulation. The doses of anti-D are 250 iu before 20 weeks' gestation and 500 iu after 20 weeks' gestation. The anti-D immunoglobulin is given intramuscularly as soon after the sensitizing event as possible (ideally within 72 hours). However, there is some evidence that it still provides some protection if given within 10 days.

Prophylaxis following abortion

Therapeutic termination of pregnancy: anti-D prophylaxis should be given to all non-sensitized RhD–ve women having therapeutic termination of pregnancy, whether it is medical or surgical, regardless of gestational age. *Ectopic pregnancy*:

anti-D prophylaxis should be given to all non-sensitized RhD–ve women who have ectopic pregnancy. *Spontaneous miscarriage*: anti-D prophylaxis should be given to all non-sensitized RhD–ve women who have spontaneous complete or incomplete abortion after 12 weeks' gestation. In RhD–ve women with spontaneous complete or incomplete miscarriage of fewer than 12 weeks' gestation, anti-D prophylaxis is not required unless uterine evacuation is performed. *Threatened miscarriage*: anti-D prophylaxis should be given to all RhD–ve women after 12 weeks' gestation.

Prophylaxis following sensitizing events before delivery

Anti-D prophylaxis should be given to all RhD–ve women after the following sensitizing events during pregnancy:
- antepartum haemorrhage
- closed abdominal injury
- external cephalic version of fetus
- invasive prenatal diagnosis (amniocentesis, villus sampling or fetal blood sampling)
- other intrauterine procedures (insertion of shunts or embryo reduction)
- intrauterine death

Postnatal prophylaxis

If a RhD–ve woman gives birth to a RhD+ve infant, 500 iu of anti-D immunoglobulin should be administered within 72 hours.

The rhesus system is named after the rhesus Macaque (the 'rhesus monkey'), which were first shown to possess the antigens. The five main rhesus antigens are C, c, D, E and e.

Theme 7: Classification of ovarian tumours

Ovarian cancer is the commonest gynaecological cancer in England and Wales (whereas endometrial cancer predominates worldwide). The incidence of ovarian cancer is around 1 in 2500 women aged over 55 years, and it is seven times commoner in western countries. One per cent of those affected have familial disease, and having two close relatives affected (i.e. mother or sister) increases the risk up to 40%. Other risk factors include early menarche, late menopause and nulliparity, as continuous ovulation is thought to be contributory. The combined oral contraceptive pill (COCP) is thought to be protective. The Lynch II syndrome, an autosomal dominant condition, predisposes to ovarian, endometrial, breast and colon cancer. Most (70%) women with ovarian tumours have no presenting symptoms, but those who do describe vague abdominal discomfort and distension, a 'dragging' sensation, urinary frequency (due to pressure effects), weight loss and occasionally menstrual changes such as bleeding. Because of the chance of spread, work-up of these patients includes abdominal examination, palpation for enlarged supraclavicular lymph nodes, examination of the breast and chest, and rectal and vaginal examination. Features suggestive of malignancy include rapid growth, size >5 cm and ascites.

Staging of ovarian tumours is as follows:

- Stage I: disease is macroscopically confined to the ovaries
- Stage II: disease is beyond the ovaries, but confined to the pelvis
- Stage III: disease is beyond the pelvis, but confined to the abdomen
- Stage IV: disease is beyond the abdomen

Because of a lack of specific symptoms, ovarian tumours tend to present as advanced disease (stage III or stage IV). Ovarian tumours may be primary (94%) or secondary (6%). Sites of spread include breast, stomach, colon and lung.

Ovarian cancer is staged at the time of laparotomy. Serum CA-125 is a useful tumour marker in 80% of cases, which can be used to assess response to treatment. Pelvic and abdominal ultrasound and CT scans may be useful in addition. Staging laparotomy includes pelvic washings, total abdominal hysterectomy with bilateral salpingo-oophorectomy and omentectomy for tissue diagnosis. Radiotherapy may be used for remaining disease not removed in theatre, and may be useful for palliative symptom control to reduce tumour bulk or metastases. Adjuvant chemotherapy is given more commonly than radiotherapy, and is used when disease has spread further than stage I.

Henry Lynch, American physician (b1928).

Lynch I syndrome describes a familial predisposition to colorectal carcinoma alone.

1. F – Mucinous adenocarcinoma

Around 85% of primary ovarian tumours are surface epithelial adenocarcinomas, including serous and mucinous types. Those remaining include sex cord tumours (6%) and germ cell tumours (2%). Surface epithelial tumours are further divided into benign, borderline and malignant forms (where 'borderline' describes increased epithelial proliferation without stromal invasion).

Mucinous carcinomas are the commonest oestrogen-producing tumours, and can be very large and multilocular. They are most frequent in younger women (20–30 years). The stromal cells secrete oestrogen, and such tumours often present with bleeding per vagina.

2. H – Serous adenocarcinoma

These are the most common type of ovarian cancer. The peak incidence occurs at 30–40 years. Thirty per cent are bilateral. Thirty per cent are malignant.

3. D – Fibroma

Meigs' syndrome describes the simultaneous presence of a benign ovarian fibroma, ascites and a transudative pleural effusion (more commonly on the right side). The effusions are benign, and often resolve after removal of the offending tumour.

Joe Vincent Meigs, American gynaecologist (1892–1963).

4. F – Mucinous adenocarcinoma

Pseudomyxoma peritonei (also known as 'jelly belly') is the rupture and dissemination of jelly-like mucus in the pelvis from mucinous ovarian tumours or, rarely, mucinous appendiceal tumours. If left untreated, the mucus can eventually build up enough to cause compression damage to the surrounding organs.

5. J – Teratoma

Teratomas arise from primitive germ cells. Over 95% of germ cell tumours are benign dermoid cysts, which can contain well-differentiated ectodermal tissue including hair and teeth. Teratomas are the commonest benign tumour, especially in premenopausal females. Dysgerminomas are also germ cell tumours, the equivalent of testicular seminomas, which usually occur in adolescence and early adulthood. Germ cell tumours are usually treated by salpingo-oophorectomy and may respond to chemotherapy or radiotherapy. The 5-year survival rate is in the region of 90%.

Other ovarian tumours include non-gestational choriocarcinomas, a rare form of germ cell tumour that secretes the β-subunit of human chorionic gonadotropin (βhCG) and can therefore mimic pregnancy. Yolk sac tumours and malignant teratomas secrete α-fetoprotein (AFP). Sex cord carcinomas are rare and arise from the gonadal stroma. Granulosa cell tumours and thecomas are both examples of sex cord tumours. They both secrete oestrogen, and can result in precocious puberty, endometrial hyperplasia and endometrial carcinoma. Endometroid carcinomas may occur in patients with endometriosis. Clear cell carcinomas are also associated with endometriosis and are frequently malignant.

Brenner's tumours are rare, small, benign ovarian tumours of uroepithelial origin. *Krukenberg's tumours* are secondary ovarian tumours that have arisen from peritoneal spread of gastrointestinal tumours.

Friedrich Ernst Krukenberg, German physician (1871–1946).

Theme 8: Management of endometrial and cervical cancer

1. B – Cone biopsy

Cervical intraepithelial neoplasia (CIN) describes the presence of atypical cells in the squamous epithelium of the cervix. It is graded from 1 to 3, depending on histology: CIN 1 (mild dysplasia, atypical cells found only in the lower third of the epithelium); CIN 2 (moderate dysplasia, atypical cells in the lower two-thirds); and CIN 3 (severe dysplasia. atypical cells located across the full thickness of the epithelium). CIN 3 is described as carcinoma *in situ*, i.e. it has a malignant appearance but there is no invasion of the basement membrane.

CIN 1 can progress to CIN 2 or 3, but many cases regress spontaneously, so a watch-and-wait approach is employed. However, one-third of women with CIN 2 or 3 will develop cervical cancer in the next 10 years if untreated, so

Get Ahead EMQ.s

①

1) C ✱ A J E   2) D B K L E

3) J U C A D   4) O M F G K

5) F G B D U   6) F B E A K

7) U F C A E   8) B G C D A D

9) E B B G A   10) B A B D C

②

1) F E G A D   2) U F G B C

3) B A B B B   4) E A G I B

5) G C A I D   6) F A B D C

7)   8) B D C A G

9) C U E G D   10) B D E B C

intervention is required. The management options for microinvasive cervical cancer can be classified as either local ablation (e.g. diathermy or cryocautery) or excision techniques (e.g. cone biopsy or large loop excision of transformation zone). Local ablation techniques are suitable only when dysplastic areas are completely visible. In this scenario, the abnormality is only partially visible, so an excision technique is required, of which cone biopsy (where a cone of tissue is removed with the aim of eliminating all dysplastic tissue) is the only option.

2. A – Chemotherapy and radiotherapy

Cervical tumours are staged as follows:
- Stage 0: carcinoma *in situ*
- Stage I: lesions confined to cervix
- Stage II: invasion into upper vagina but not pelvic wall
- Stage III: invasion of lower vagina/pelvic wall, or causing ureteric obstruction
- Stage IV: invasion of bladder or rectal mucosa

Stage I is further divided into IA1 (tumour <3 mm deep and <7 mm across), IA2 (<5 mm deep and <7 mm across), IB1 (tumour <4 cm) and IB2 (tumour >4 cm). Stage II is divided into IIA (invasion of upper two-thirds of vagina but not parametrium) and IIB (invasion of parametrium).

Management depends on the stage of the tumour. Stage IA1 can be treated with cone biopsy or simple hysterectomy. All other stage I and stage IIA disease requires radical abdominal hysterectomy (Wertheim's procedure). This operation involves a hysterectomy with the additional removal of the upper third of the vagina, parametrium and pelvic lymph nodes (and the ovaries if the patient is not a young woman). Cervical tumours that are stage IIB and beyond, and less invasive tumours in women who are unfit for surgery, are treated with radiotherapy and chemotherapy, without hysterectomy. The cervical malignancy in this scenario invades the pelvic wall, and is thus a stage III tumour. Management is therefore by chemotherapy and radiotherapy. Platinum-based chemotherapy has been shown particularly to reduce mortality from cervical cancer.

Ernst Wertheim, Austrian gynaecologist (1864–1920).

Parametrium, from Greek *para* = beside + *metra* = womb. This term describes the connective tissue found immediately alongside the body of the uterus.

3. E – Radical trachelectomy

This young woman has a stage I cervical tumour, specifically stage IB1. Although this is normally managed with radical hysterectomy, a radical trachelectomy provides a less invasive alternative for women who wish to remain fertile. Radical trachelectomy involves removal of the upper 2–3 cm of the vagina, 80% of the cervix (up to the internal os) and the parametrial tissue, including pelvic lymph nodes. This can preserve fertility by maintaining cervical competence.

Trachelectomy; from Greek *trachelos* = neck; the cervix essentially being the neck of the uterus.

4. D – Radical hysterectomy and bilateral salpingo-oophorectomy

Endometrial sarcomas are rare tumours and account for <4% of uterine tumours (around 150 cases per year in the UK). A recognized risk factor is pelvic irradiation. There are three types: leiomyosarcomas (malignant fibroids), endometrial stromal tumours and mixed müllerian tumours (derived from embryological remnants of the uterus). Management is by radical hysterectomy, with or without lymphadenectomy. Surgery can be curative if the tumour is confined to the uterus; however, sarcomas are highly malignant and have a poor response to chemoradiotherapy. Less than 0.1% of fibroids become malignant, but leiomyosarcoma should be considered if a fibroid grows quickly.

5. A – Chemotherapy and radiotherapy

Endometrial cancer is the commonest cancer of the female genital tract, occurring most commonly in the over-65s. The majority of tumours are adenocarcinomas (>90%). Risk factors include those related to unopposed oestrogen exposure (e.g. oestrogen-only oral contraceptive pill use, nulliparity, late menopause). The COCP and pregnancy are protective. Affected women present with postmenopausal bleeding (in postmenopausals) and irregular/ intermenstrual bleeding or menorrhagia (in premenopausals).

Endometrial tumours spread directly through the myometrium to the cervix and upper vagina. Staging is as follows:
- Stage I: lesion confined to uterus
- Stage II: lesion confined to uterus and cervix
- Stage III: tumour invades through cervix/uterus
- Stage IV: bowel/bladder involvement or distant metastases

Endometrial biopsy (e.g. using a pipelle) helps confirm a diagnosis. Stage I and II tumours are treated with radical hysterectomy and bilateral salpingo-oophorectomy, with or without lymphadenectomy. Adjuvant radiotherapy is used in addition if there is a high risk of recurrence. Stage III disease (as in this scenario) requires surgical debulking before proceeding with radiotherapy and chemotherapy. Stage IV tumours are incurable and are managed palliatively.

Radiotherapy has many side-effects, which are easily divided into acute and chronic problems. Acute issues include skin irradiation, dysuria and diarrhoea. More chronic side-effects are urinary frequency, vaginal dryness and dyspareunia.

Theme 9: Drug management of pre-eclampsia

Pre-eclampsia is a pregnancy-specific condition, characterized by high blood pressure and proteinuria, which occurs after the 20th week of pregnancy. In rare cases, it can terminate in eclampsia. Eclampsia is fitting due to brain hypoxia, which occurs as a result of oedema and vasospasm. Pre-eclampsia occurs in 5–7% of pregnancies. It is the most important cause of intrauterine growth restriction in singletons without congenital malformations. It has two peaks of incidence: mothers under 20 years and those over 35 years. Risk factors include nulliparity, multiple gestation, diabetes, thyroid disease, chronic hypertension, renal disease and a family history of pre-eclampsia. The aetiology of pre-eclampsia is unknown. One theory is that vascular endothelial injury reduces production of prostacyclin (a prostaglandin), which is a potent vasodilator and inhibitor of platelet aggregation. This, along with increased intravascular pressure, moves fluid into extravascular spaces, including the brain, retinas, liver and subcutaneous tissues, causing oedema.

Symptoms of pre-eclampsia include headache, blurred vision and epigastric pain (although most cases are asymptomatic). Clinical signs are high blood pressure, hyperreflexia, proteinuria, vomiting, hepatic tenderness, oliguria and spontaneous bleeding. Classification of pre-eclampsia is as follows: mild (blood pressure >140/90 mmHg with proteinuria of >0.3 g in 24 hours), moderate (diastolic blood pressure 100–110 mmHg with proteinuria) and severe (blood pressure >160 mmHg systolic or >110 mmHg diastolic, with proteinuria). The blood pressure readings must be taken with the patient resting, with at least two readings 6 hours apart. Indicators of severe disease are cerebral or visual disturbances, abdominal pain, fetal growth restriction, oliguria (urine output <500 mL in 24 hours), impaired liver function tests and thrombocytopenia.

1. D – Labetalol

The best treatment of pre-eclampsia for the mother is delivery. This obviously may not be in the best interests of the fetus, so safe measures are used to prolong pregnancy. The decision to induce labour or consider emergency caesarean section is made by a consultant. Factors to consider include severity of disease, fetal maturity, maternal and fetal condition, and cervical status.

Mild disease presenting before 37 weeks usually warrants admission for observation for 48 hours with baseline investigations. If blood pressure settles, subsequent management is with regular outpatient attendance to the antenatal day unit, or blood pressure and urine checks at home. Corticosteroids are administered in gestations under 34 weeks to improve pulmonary maturity. There is a low threshold for considering induction in women with pre-eclampsia of 37–40 weeks' gestation with a favourable cervix. There is evidence that blood pressure less than 160/110 mmHg does not require immediate antihypertensive treatment; however, other signs of severe disease, such as large proteinuria, necessitate treatment. Severe disease requires hospitalization to stabilize the patient. Intravenous infusions of antihypertensives and anticonvulsants are given. Blood pressure and cardiotocography are continuously monitored. Reflexes are checked every 4 hours, as hyperreflexia can suggest imminent eclampsia.

Antihypertensive medication is indicated to reduce blood pressure in order to protect cerebral circulation. There are a number of options. Labetalol is an α- and β-adrenergic blocker, available as 100, 200 and 300 mg tablets. Labetalol causes vasodilatation and bradycardia, and reduces myometrial activity.

2. H – Nifedipine

Nifedipine is a calcium channel blocker and vasodilator. This is commonly used to manage acute rises in blood pressure in pre-eclampsia. Slow-release preparations are preferred for maintenance therapy.

3. E – Magnesium sulphate

An infusion of magnesium sulphate is indicated in those at high risk of an eclamptic seizure. Regular assessment is required of patients on magnesium sulphate, including details of urine output, respiratory rate and reflexes. Infusions must be continued for at least 24 hours after delivery, as women are still at high risk of seizures at this time.

Fitting in pregnancy requires protection of the airway if necessary, and an ABC approach. Fits are terminated with intravenous diazepam or magnesium sulphate. Blood pressure is controlled with intravenous antihypertensives. If the fetus is still *in utero*, the mother is stabilized and delivery is expedited with emergency caesarean section. Intensive monitoring is continued for 48 hours.

4. G – Misoprostol

Misoprostol is a synthetic prostaglandin E analogue that induces labour by causing uterine contraction and effacement of the cervix. It is also used as part of medical abortions in conjunction with mifepristone. The mifepristone (an antiprogesterone steroid) causes degeneration of the lining of the uterus, and the misoprostol expels the detached material, including the fetus, from the uterus.

5. D – Labetalol

Labetalol blocks both α- and β-adrenergic receptors. Remember that β-blocking agents can cause bronchospasm in asthmatic patients.

Methyldopa is a centrally acting antihypertensive that stimulates β-adrenergic receptors and decreases total peripheral vascular resistance. Hydralazine acts through an unknown mechanism to vasodilate arterioles and reduce blood pressure. Angiotensin-converting enzyme (ACE) inhibitors (ramipril) and diuretics (furosemide) are avoided in pre-eclampsia.

Theme 10: Induction of labour

1. D – Prostaglandin

Induction of labour (IOL) describes the artificial initiation of labour before its spontaneous onset. Around 15–25% of pregnancies in the UK end in IOL. IOL is considered when the risks to the baby/mother in continuing the pregnancy outweigh the risks of induction. The commonest indication is prolonged pregnancy, 12 days or more beyond the estimated delivery date. Research has shown that the risk of stillbirth trebles between 37 and 42 weeks' gestation, to 1 in 1000 pregnancies. Other risks of prolonged pregnancy are fetal compromise in labour, meconium aspiration and mechanical problems during delivery.

Women are seen in clinic post term to discuss and offer induction at term + 12 days (42 weeks). They are also offered a 'stretch and sweep' at this time, where a midwife/doctor tries to release the membranes manually from the lower segment with a gloved finger. This is thought to release prostaglandins to cause spontaneous onset of labour in 50% of patients.

Bishop observed a natural change in the cervix at the time of labour. In 1964, he devised a scoring system to assess the 'favourability' of the cervix, to assist in predicting whether IOL would be required. A higher score is associated with an easier, shorter induction that is less likely to fail.

Bishop score	0	1	2	3
Dilatation (cm)	0	1 or 2	3 or 4	≥5
Consistency	Firm	Medium	Soft	–
Length of canal (cm)	>2	1–2	0.5–1	<0.5
Position	Posterior	Central	Anterior	–
Station of presenting part (related to ischial spines)	–3	–2	–1 or 0	Below spines

Total score (out of 13): 0–5 unfavourable, 6–13 favourable.

Women with an unfavourable cervix require one to three doses of prostaglandin (gel or tablets) inserted vaginally into the posterior fornix, 4–6 hours apart. This can be done whether or not membranes have ruptured. Nulliparous patients can have a maximum of 4 mg; a multiparous woman has a 3 mg maximum. Fetal well-being must always be confirmed with a cardiotocograph (CTG) before induction, and for 2 hours following induction.

2. D – Prostaglandin

Another common indication for IOL is spontaneous prelabour rupture of membranes (PROM), which occurs in 6–19% of term pregnancies. Most women will go into spontaneous labour within 24 hours of PROM. IOL is advised 24–72 hours after membranes rupture due to increasing risks of fetal and maternal infection, but opinions vary. Women with spontaneous rupture of membranes beyond 37 weeks with a normal CTG can go home for up to 72 hours and return for an antenatal check and CTG prior to augmentation on the delivery suite as soon as possible. The woman's discharge in this scenario could be an early sign of chorioamnionitis. This is an ascending infection from the vagina, caused by *Escherichia coli* or group B streptococci. She should be screened for infection and considered for intravenous antibiotics.

3. E – Twice-weekly cardiotocography

These patients must be counselled thoroughly about the risks of post-term labour. Beyond term +12, they must return to the antenatal clinic for twice-weekly CTG and weekly ultrasound scan to check that liquor (amniotic fluid) volume is over 3 cm at the deepest pool. A reduced liquor volume is indicative of placental insufficiency.

4. B – Caesarean section

This does happen! The patient has several factors that increase the risk of obstetric complication: she is unbooked, so has not had blood tests, blood pressure checks or midwife contact. She has also had a previous caesarean section, which usually requires assessment and counselling for vaginal birth after caesarean section (VBAC). She is having some uterine activity, and the CTG is showing signs of fetal distress. In addition, the baby is in a transverse lie, which is a contraindication to IOL. The safest option here is therefore caesarean section.

5. A – Artificial rupture of membranes

This patient should be transferred to the delivery suite for artificial rupture of membranes (ARM), as she has had slow progress following two doses of Prostin (a prostaglandin). ARM is considered when patients have a favourable cervix (Bishop score >5) and some uterine activity. ARM is performed under aseptic conditions with an amnihook or Kocher's forceps, and the membranes should be swept back to induce prostaglandin release. After ARM, some women will spontaneously commence labour, but most require augmentation with an oxytocin infusion to ensure progress of 1 cm/h, on the instruction of medical staff. High-risk patients, such as those with previous caesarean sections, should be discussed with the registrar or consultant.

Complications of induction and augmentation of labour include the following:
- Failure of induction – this requires operative delivery.
- Uterine hyperstimulation (>7 contractions/15 min) – this can cause maternal and fetal distress. An oxytocin infusion must be stopped, and continuous monitoring is needed. Tocolysis (suppression of contractions) can be used, but, if there is suspicion of fetal compromise, delivery is needed as soon as possible.
- Nausea, vomiting and diarrhoea – these are systemic side-effects of prostaglandins.
- Water intoxication – as oxytocin is infused with fluid.
- Uterine rupture.

Toco-, from Greek *tokos* = childbirth.

Theme 1: Infection in pregnancy

Options

    A. Bacterial vaginosis
    B. Chickenpox
    C. Cytomegalovirus
    D. Group B streptococci
    E. *Listeria* spp.
    F. Parvovirus
    G. Rubella
    H. *Salmonella* spp.
    I. Toxoplasmosis

For each of the following scenarios, select the most likely underlying infection. Each option may be used once, more than once or not at all.

1. A 34-year-old woman tells you that she had a flu-like illness with a macular rash at around 20 weeks' gestation. She has a child with learning difficulties who is deaf. When he was a baby, he underwent a heart operation.

2. A 24-year-old woman is very concerned that she had severe gastroenteritis in the 28th week of her pregnancy, which she attributed to uncooked eggs. She has delivered what appears to be a healthy baby.

3. A 27-year-old woman of 32 weeks' gestation was admitted to hospital 4 weeks ago with fever, headache and abdominal pain. She has just delivered a stillborn baby. On further questioning, she admitted to eating soft cheese 6 weeks ago.

4. A 32-year-old woman is in labour. She is receiving antibiotics to treat an infection that was picked up on swabs she had taken during an admission 4 weeks previously. The antibiotics, she has been told, are for the benefit of the baby.

5. A baby is in special care with dermatomal skin scarring, neurological defects, limb hypoplasia and eye defects. The mother reports having had a vesicular rash over her trunk and legs at 16 weeks' gestation.

Theme 2: Female anatomy

Options

  A. Ampulla
  B. Ascending colon
  C. Bladder
  D. Broad ligament
  E. Cervix
  F. Fimbriae
  G. Hepatic vein
  H. Inferior vena cava
  I. Infundibulum
  J. Ligament of the ovary
  K. Pouch of Douglas
  L. Right renal vein
  M. Round ligament of the uterus
  N. Suspensory ligament of the ovary
  O. Uterine vein

For each of the following descriptions, select the most appropriate anatomical structure. Each option may be used once, more than once or not at all.

1. The venous drainage of the right ovary.

2. A relation of the posterior vagina.

3. This is made up of, in part, the mesovarium.

4. This is the longest and broadest part of the fallopian tube.

5. This ligament attaches to the medial side of the ovary and passes to the lateral side of the uterus posteroinferior to the uterotubular junction.

Theme 3 Obstetric emergencies

Options

    A. Cervical shock
    B. Cord prolapse
    C. Deep vein thrombosis
    D. Disseminated intravascular coagulation
    E. Shoulder dystocia
    F. Uterine inversion
    G. Uterine rupture

For each of the following scenarios, select the most appropriate obstetric emergency that the mother is at risk of. Each option may be used once, more than once or not at all.

1. A 32-year-old woman, who is 34 weeks pregnant, presents to the emergency department with lower abdominal pain associated with constant per vagina blood loss. On examination, the uterus feels firm to palpation. Observations include a heart rate of 128 beats/min and a blood pressure of 104/60 mmHg.

2. A 28-year-old woman attends the antenatal clinic for a routine ultrasound scan. The midwife informs her that she has a fundal placenta.

3. A 35-year-old woman, who has a history of diabetes, attends the antenatal clinic for a routine ultrasound scan. To her dismay, she is told that her baby is 'large'.

4. A 24-year-old woman has an artificial rupture of membranes for failure of progression of labour.

5. A 25-year-old woman is having an oxytocin infusion in conjunction with a vaginal delivery. She has a previous child born by caesarean section.

Theme 4: Contraception

Options

   A. Ampicillin
   B. Cerazette (progesterone-only pill)
   C. Depo-Provera (medroxyprogesterone acetate)
   D. Implanon
   E. Levonelle (levonorgestrel)
   F. Lisinopril
   G. Microgynon (levonorgestrel, ethinylestradiol)
   H. Mirena
   I. Noristerat (norethisterone enantate)
   J. Rifampicin

For each of the following scenarios, select the most appropriate medication. Each option may be used once, more than once or not at all.

1. A 25-year-old woman attends the early morning GP clinic. She had unprotected intercourse the night before last and is requesting a tablet to stop her from becoming pregnant.

2. A 29-year-old woman is requesting long-term injection contraception as she does not like the idea of having a coil fitted and she will not remember to take the pill. She works full-time and finds it hard to get to the clinic, so she wants the longest-acting injection.

3. A 37-year-old smoker is requesting pill contraception. She has no significant past medical history.

4. When counselling patients on using combined oral contraception, you must inform them that this drug decreases the effectiveness of both combined and progesterone-only oral contraceptives by hepatic enzyme induction.

5. When counselling patients on using combined oral contraception, you must inform them that this drug decreases the effectiveness of combined oral contraceptives by impairing the bacterial flora responsible for recycling ethinylestradiol from the large bowel.

Theme 5: Postpartum haemorrhage

Options

- A. Atonic uterus
- B. Cervical tear
- C. Disseminated intravascular coagulation
- D. High vaginal tear
- E. Infection
- F. Perineal trauma
- G. Retained placental fragments

For each of the following descriptions, select the most appropriate answer. Each option may be used once, more than once or not at all.

1. This is the most common cause of primary postpartum haemorrhage.

2. This is the most common cause of secondary postpartum haemorrhage.

3. Carboprost can be used in the management of this condition.

4. A B-lynch brace suture can be used in the management of this condition.

5. Preterm labour is a risk factor for this condition.

Theme 6: Cervical screening

Options

A. Colposcopy
B. Hysterectomy
C. Repeat in 6 months
D. Repeat in 4 months
E. Repeat in 1 year
F. Repeat in 3 years
G. Repeat in 5 years
H. Urgent colposcopy

For each of the following scenarios, select the most appropriate management plan. Each option may be used once, more than once or not at all.

1. A 30-year-old woman attends her GP for a smear test. Histology returns as showing mild dyskaryosis. Her previous smear 6 months ago gave similar results.

2. A 30-year-old woman attends her GP for a smear test. Histology returns as showing moderate dyskaryosis.

3. A 30-year-old woman, who is HIV-positive, attends her GP for a smear test. Histology confirms a normal smear.

4. A 30-year-old woman attends her GP for a smear test. She has no significant medical history. Histology confirms no dyskaryosis.

5. A 30-year-old woman, who is positive for HPV, attends her GP for a smear test. Histology shows mild dyskaryosis.

Theme 7: Mechanisms of labour

Options

    A. Descent
    B. Effacement
    C. Engagement
    D. Extension
    E. External rotation
    F. Flexion
    G. Internal rotation
    H. Resolution
    I. Restitution

For each of the following descriptions, select the most appropriate term. Each option may be used once, more than once or not at all.

1. This term refers to when the maximum diameter of the head has passed through the pelvic brim.

2. This is required for easy passage into the mid-cavity.

3. The levator ani muscle helps the head move into an occipitoanterior position by this movement.

4. This movement causes 'crowning' of the head.

5. This term describes the way that the head moves into alignment with the shoulders before they are delivered.

Theme 8: Complications of caesarean section

Options

A. Aspiration pneumonia
B. Aspiration pneumonitis
C. Endometritis
D. Fetal head compression
E. Pleurisy
F. Pulmonary embolism
G. Retained products of conception
H. Spontaneous pneumothorax
I. Urinary tract infection
J. Urinary tract injury
K. Uterine rupture

For each of the following scenarios, select the most appropriate diagnosis. Each option may be used once, more than once or not at all.

1. A 37-year-old woman had an elective lower segment caesarean section (LSCS) 1 day ago. You are called to see her as she becomes short of breath with left-sided chest pain and a cough. She has had three other children, two of these born by LSCS. On examination, she has reduced air entry at both lung bases. Her observations include saturations 92% in air, blood pressure 105/84 mmHg, pulse 120 beats/min and temperature 37.2°C.

2. You are called to see a 20-year-old 2 hours post-LSCS. She has not passed urine since her operation. She denies any urinary symptoms preoperatively. On examination, she appears unwell, with a temperature of 37.5°C, blood pressure 94/73 mmHg, pulse 116 beats/min and saturations 97% in air. Her abdomen is distended, with tenderness in the left flank and suprapubic region. Bowel sounds are not audible.

3. A 25 year old had an LSCS 24 hours ago for fetal distress. She now complains of intermittent vaginal bleeding. Observations include saturations 98% in air, blood pressure 124/82 mmHg, pulse 84 beats/min and temperature 37.8°C. The midwife tells you that she had a retained placenta, which required manual removal in the operating theatre.

4. A 28-year-old woman at 39+4 gestation is in labour. She develops abdominal pain and a heart rate of 125 beats/min. Blood pressure is 100/42 mmHg, temperature 37.2°C and saturations 99% in air. On examination, her lower abdomen is exquisitely tender. The CTG, which was previously normal, now shows reduced variability, and a late deceleration develops with slow recovery. She has had one previous LSCS for a breech baby.

5. The woman in case 4 becomes acutely short of breath in the recovery bay and is coughing after a general anaesthetic. On auscultation, she has reduced air entry at the right lung base and diffuse wheeze. Observations include a heart rate of 88 beats/min, blood pressure 112/76 mmHg, temperature 37.8°C and saturations 91% in air.

Theme 9: Gynaecological malignancies

Options

A. Cervix
B. Endometrium
C. Fallopian tube
D. Ovary
E. Vagina
F. Vulva

For each of the following descriptions, select the most appropriate site of the malignancy. Each option may be used once, more than once or not at all.

1. Lichen sclerosis is considered a predisposing factor of this malignancy.

2. This is the commonest cause of gynaecological cancer death in the UK.

3. There has been a recent increase in the incidence if this tumour in the 20- to 35-year-old age group.

4. Diabetes is a risk factor for this malignancy.

5. Presentation of this tumour characteristically includes intermittent abdominal pain, which is relieved following a sudden watery discharge.

Theme 10: The infertility clinic

Options

A. Anorexia nervosa
B. Asherman's syndrome
C. Hyperprolactinaemia
D. Hypogonadotropic hypogonadism
E. Iatrogenic amenorrhoea
F. Mayer–Rokitansky–Küster–Hauser syndrome
G. Polycystic ovary syndrome
H. Premature ovarian failure
I. Primary ovarian failure
J. Sheehan's syndrome
K. Turner's syndrome

For each of the following presentations at the infertility clinic, select the most appropriate underlying diagnosis. Each option may be used once, more than once or not at all.

For reference ranges, see Answers.

1. An Asian woman, who is 35 years old, presents with difficulty conceiving. Unfortunately, her first child died due to extreme prematurity. Since then, she has had a 35-day menstrual cycle, and her last period was 6 months ago. She has had no recent change in weight and no previous surgery, and is having regular intercourse. Her blood tests show FSH 35, LH 15.1, estradiol 102, SHBG 42 and TSH 3.2. A pregnancy test is negative.

2. A 34-year-old Caucasian female is referred with secondary infertility. She has tried to have another baby with her husband for 2 years. She had regular periods prior to starting her family, and now has a cycle interval of 35 days, and bleeds for 5 days. Her body mass index is 39. She has no other symptoms. She has had one normal delivery. Blood tests show FSH 9, LH 20, testosterone 1.3, estradiol 358, SHBG 15 and TSH 3.2.

3. A 36-year-old Asian barrister attends the infertility clinic with her partner. She complains of 'deep' pelvic pain on intercourse and a failure to conceive in the last 2 years. She has a history of two previous miscarriages, and an operation under anaesthetic for per vagina spotting 10 years ago. She has had only one normal period in the last 9 months and two episodes of per vagina spotting. Her last smear was normal. Blood tests show FSH 3.1, LH 12, estradiol 305 and progesterone 25 on day 21 of her cycle.

4. A 32-year-old Caucasian woman attends a follow-up appointment for oligomenorrhoea. She is obviously hirsute, with scarring from acne on her face. She has a 7-year-old son, delivered with forceps following a failed induction for gestational diabetes. Her BMI is 30.

5. A 27-year-old nulliparous Caucasian woman is concerned about her periods. She has always had irregular periods, the last being 8 months ago. Her BMI is 20, and a pregnancy test is negative. She informs you that she has never enjoyed intercourse, finding it painful. Blood tests show FSH 1.2, LH 3 and estradiol 94.

Practice Paper 3: Answers

Theme 1: Infection in pregnancy

1. G – Rubella

Rubella is a viral infection spread by person-to-person contact. It has an incubation period of 14–21 days. Rubella is rare nowadays thanks to immunization (MMR vaccine). Women develop a non-specific, flu-like illness with a macular rash covering their trunk (20–50% of infections are asymptomatic). Diagnosis is confirmed by serological antibody testing. There is an 80% risk of infection to the fetus if rubella develops in the first trimester, dropping to 25% at the end of the second trimester. Teratogenic effects are worse at earlier gestations. The characteristic abnormalities from maternal rubella infection are sensorineural deafness, cataracts, congenital heart disease, learning difficulties, hepatosplenomegaly and microcephaly.

Rubella is also known as German measles because the first three reported cases were described by German physicians, who all thought that the condition was a variant of measles.

2. H – *Salmonella* spp.

This Gram-negative bacterium is found in raw or partially cooked eggs, raw meat and chicken. Incubation time is 12–72 hours. Pregnancy increases the incidence and severity of symptoms of gastroenteritis. There are no adverse effects of maternal gastroenteritis on the fetus as long as the mother remains well hydrated.

3. E – *Listeria* spp.

The Gram-positive coccus *Listeria monocytogenes* is found in soil, animal faeces, pâté and unpasteurized dairy products such as soft cheese. The incubation period is 3–70 days. The incidence and severity of infection are increased in pregnancy. Symptoms include fever, headache, malaise, backache, abdominal pain, pharyngitis and conjunctivitis. Diagnosis is by blood cultures or placental/neonatal swabs. Treatment is with high-dose penicillin. Listeria infection during pregnancy can lead to miscarriage, stillbirth, preterm delivery and neonatal listeriosis, which carries a 50% mortality rate.

4. D – Group B streptococci

One-quarter of women have group B streptococcal vaginal colonization at some stage of their pregnancy. It is asymptomatic to the mother and generally only picked up incidentally on vaginal swabs taken for other reasons. It results in 1 in 65 of all neonatal deaths by causing overwhelming neonatal infection. If group B streptococcal infection is picked up on routine swabs, antibiotics must be given during labour to reduce neonatal infection. There is currently no national screening programme for group B streptococci.

5. B – Chickenpox

Chickenpox, caused by the varicella-zoster virus (human herpesvirus 3), is spread via the airborne route. It has an incubation period of 3–21 days. Around 3 in 1000 pregnancies are affected. Ninety per cent of women are immune due to previous infection, which is checked at booking. The mother develops a prodromal malaise and fever, followed by an itchy vesicular rash. The sequelae of maternal infection are more serious in pregnant women, with a 10% risk of pneumonia and 1% mortality rate. Diagnosis is clinical and treatment supportive, with advice to avoid other pregnant women. The fetus is at risk of developing fetal varicella syndrome, particularly if infection occurs before 16 weeks, which involves dermatomal skin scarring, neurological defects, limb hypoplasia and eye defects.

Toxoplasmosis

Toxoplasma gondii is a parasite that comes from unwashed fruit and vegetables, raw/cured/poorly cooked meat, unpasteurized goats' milk, or contamination from soil or cat faeces. The incidence is 2 in 1000 pregnancies. Thirty per cent of women are immune due to previous infection. It is rare for mothers to display clinical features, although some develop flu-like symptoms. Treatment is with spiramycin. Fetal infection occurs in 40% cases, with the majority occurring at higher gestations (severity is greatest at lower gestations). Fetal effects of toxoplasmal infection are miscarriage, stillbirth, hydrocephalus, deafness and blindness. Fetal infection can be diagnosed by amniocentesis or cordocentesis.

Cytomegalovirus

Cytomegalovirus affects 3 in 1000 live births. It is transmitted through urine, saliva and other bodily products. Maternal infection is usually asymptomatic, after a 3- to 12-week incubation period. Maternal primary infection can be confirmed by immunoglobulin M (IgM) in the blood, and maternal immunity is revealed by detecting IgG. There is no treatment and therefore there is no benefit to screening. Fetal infection can be diagnosed using amniocentesis or cordocentesis. Around 10–15% of infected fetuses develop symptoms. Eighty per cent of infected fetuses develop symptoms later in life, such as learning difficulties, visual impairment, progressive hearing loss or psychomotor retardation, with only 10–20% showing signs of infection at birth (hydrops, intrauterine growth restriction, microcephaly, hydrocephalus, hepatosplenomegaly and thrombocytopenia).

Parvovirus

Parvovirus B19 infection is spread by respiratory droplets, with an incubation period of 18 days. It is often seen in outbreaks at schools and manifests in children as erythema infectiosum – a 'slapped-cheek' appearance. Erythema infectiosum is also known as fifth disease – so called because it is the fifth of the six classic childhood skin rashes (the others being measles, chickenpox, rubella, scarlet fever and roseola infantum). In adults, parvovirus infection presents with fever, malaise and arthralgia. Among pregnant women with parvovirus infection, fetal death is seen in 9%. The second trimester holds the highest risk of fetal infection. The fetal sequelae are non-immune hydrops due to chronic haemolytic anaemia and myocarditis. *In utero* blood transfusion of hydropic fetuses may prevent demise. There are no long-term sequelae among survivors.

Parvovirus B19 is so called since it was first discovered in well B19 (row B, column 19) of a large series of Petri dishes.

Theme 2: Female anatomy

1. H – Inferior vena cava

Venous drainage of the ovaries starts with the pampiniform plexus – a mass of veins in the broad ligament in close proximity to the ovary. The pampiniform plexus drains into a single ovarian vein, which leaves the pelvic cavity to journey upwards alongside the ovarian artery. The right ovarian vein drains directly into the vena cava. The left ovarian vein drains into the left renal vein and ultimately into the vena cava.

The ovarian arteries arise directly from the abdominal aorta, descend along the posterior abdominal wall, cross the external iliac arteries at the pelvic brim and enter the suspensory ligament of the ovary.

Pampiniform, from Latin *pampinus* = tendril (a threadlike structure of climbing plants used for support and attachment).

2. K – Pouch of Douglas

The relations of the vagina are as follows:
- posteriorly (superior to inferior): pouch of Douglas, rectum, anal canal
- laterally: levator ani, visceral pelvic fascia, ureters
- anteriorly: base of the bladder, urethra

James Douglas, Scottish anatomist and physician (1675–1742).

3. D – Broad ligament

The broad ligament, rather than being a thin tube-like structure, is instead a double layer of peritoneum (continuous with the abdominal peritoneum), which hangs suspended by the uterus, fallopian tube, ovary and other ligaments. The organs by which it is suspended divide the broad ligament up into its different sections:
- uterus: mesometrium (the major part of the broad ligament)
- uterine tube: mesosalpinx
- ovary: mesovarium

The broad ligament also covers the ligament of the ovary, the suspensory ligament of the ovary and the round ligament of the uterus. It extends from the sides of the uterus to the lateral walls and floor of the pelvis, and assists in keeping the uterus in position.

4. A – Ampulla

Starting laterally, the parts of the fallopian tube are as follows: the infundibulum, ampulla, isthmus and uterine part. The infundibulum is the funnel-shaped distal end of the tube. It opens into the peritoneal cavity through a 2 mm gap at its base (the abdominal ostium). Fimbriae are finger-like projections at the end of the infundibulum, which spread over the medial surface of the ovary. The superior pole of the ovary has attached to it one large 'ovarian fimbria'. The ampulla is the longest and widest part – this is where fertilization occurs. The isthmus enters the uterine horn and is thick walled. Finally, the uterine part of the fallopian tube passes through the uterine wall (intramural) and terminates in the uterine ostium to enter the uterine cavity.

Infundibulum, from Latin *infundibulum* = funnel.

Ampulla, from Latin *ampulla* = flask.

Isthmus, from Greek *isthmus* = a connecting band (often used to describe a narrow strip of land that connects two larger land masses, like the Isthmus of Panama connecting the Americas).

5. J – Ligament of the ovary

The ligament of the ovary attaches to the medial aspect of the ovary and passes to the lateral edge of the uterus, posteroinferior to the uterotubular junction. It lies posterosuperiorly between the layers of the broad ligament to form the medial part of the mesovarium.

The *round ligament* of the uterus is a fibromuscular cord. This attaches anteroinferiorly to the uterotubular junction, lies anteroinferiorly between the layers of the broad ligament and travels to the lateral pelvic wall. It crosses the external iliac vessels and is transmitted, via the inguinal canal, to the subcutaneous tissue of the labium majus. The round ligament is the remnant of the fetal gubernaculum. The *suspensory ligament* of the ovary is part of the broad ligament (lateral part of the mesovarium). It connects the distal end of the ovary to the lateral wall of the pelvis and contains the ovarian vessels, lymphatics and nerves that run to and from the ovary.

Theme 3: Obstetric emergencies

1. D – Disseminated intravascular coagulation

This woman has presented with placental abruption, a complication that occurs in 1% of pregnancies. Placental abruption is when all or part of the placenta separates from the uterus before delivery, resulting in bleeding. Abruption can be described as 'revealed' (visible per vagina blood loss) or 'concealed' (blood remains behind placenta). Features include painful antepartum haemorrhage, a tender, 'woody-hard' uterus, maternal shock and fetal distress. Management includes ABC and urgent caesarean section if there is fetal distress. If abruption is minor and there is no evidence of fetal distress, the mother can be observed for 3–5 days and discharged. Complications of abruption include fetal death, postpartum haemorrhage and DIC.

DIC can develop after any severe haemorrhage. It is a secondary event that involves pathological activation of coagulation pathways, producing thrombin. This results in a bleeding diathesis, platelet aggregation, consumption of coagulation factors and fibrin deposition causing ischaemic organ damage. The commonest obstetric conditions associated with DIC are amniotic fluid embolism, pre-eclampsia/eclampsia, antepartum/postpartum haemorrhage, placental abruption and the HELLP syndrome. Clinical findings may include generalized bleeding, purpura and thromboembolism. Investigations may reveal fever, hypotension, proteinuria and hypoxia, with low platelets, increased prothrombin and activated partial thromboplastin times (PT and APTT), and reduced fibrinogen. Fibrinogen correlates most with the severity of the event. Management is initially supportive. Platelets are replaced in active bleeding with a platelet count of <50 000/μL or prophylactically if levels are 20–30 000/μL. Low-dose heparin is effective in treating the intravascular clotting process without affecting activated clotting factors. Most cases of obstetric DIC will improve with delivery of the fetus or evacuation of the uterus.

2. F – Uterine inversion

A fundal placenta is one that occurs on the anterior wall of the uterus (i.e. at the top of the 'bump'). It is a risk factor for uterine inversion. Uterine inversion is a rare but serious complication of mismanagement of the third stage of labour. It occurs when the uterine fundus has prolapsed into the uterine cavity (incomplete inversion) or even through the cervix/vulva (complete inversion), and often results from excessive cord traction or rapid decompression of the uterus. Patients suffer extreme abdominal pain with associated haemorrhage and circulatory collapse. Fluid resuscitation via two large-bore cannulae is necessary, and transfusion may be required. If manual removal of the placenta is required, it is done in theatre. Johnson's manoeuvre is performed – this is where the fundus is cupped in the hand and pressure is applied in the direction of the posterior fornix to replace its position, and is held in place until a contraction occurs. Intravenous oxytocin can then help to maintain uterine contraction and the cervix to reform. If manual methods fail, a laparotomy is required.

3. E – Shoulder dystocia

'Large for gestational age' (LGA) refers to babies above the 90th centile for weight at any gestational age. Macrosomia refers to fetuses with a weight of >4500 g. Factors predisposing to macrosomia include diabetes (gestational or type 1 (insulin dependent)), obesity, multiparity, previous LGA baby, male fetus and large maternal stature. In diabetic mothers, high levels of glucose can cross the placenta and lead to macrosomia.

Delivery complications of macrosomic babies are failure to progress (with a higher requirement for caesarean section) and shoulder dystocia. This happens when the shoulders of the large baby become impacted on the symphysis pubis in the anteroposterior diameter. The baby is unable to breathe due to compression of the thorax, so immediate action is required before the baby dies of asphyxia. A warning sign is when delivery of the chin is delayed or it appears to recede. The woman is put into the MacRobert's position (knees to shoulders), a large episiotomy is performed, and suprapubic pressure is applied. These actions are usually successful, but, if not, attempts can be made to deliver the posterior arm first in a diagonal diameter. Other alternatives are to break the baby's clavicles, or perform a symphysiotomy by incising the symphysis pubis under local anaesthetic. Trauma to the baby is common, including Erb's palsy.

4. B – Cord prolapse

Cord prolapse is when the umbilical cord descends below the presenting part after the membranes rupture. Cord prolapse usually occurs when the presenting part is high, allowing the cord to pass below it. Most cases are associated with artificial rupture of membranes. The diagnosis is made when there are signs of fetal distress and the cord can be palpated vaginally. Management is by asking the mother to sit on 'all-fours' and pushing the presenting part upwards with two fingers of the examining hand, to relieve compression of the cord and to prevent cord spasm (both of which compromise fetal oxygen supply). If significant delay is expected (e.g. in the community), 500 mL fluid and a catheter can be inserted into the bladder to aim for the same effect. Emergency caesarean section is performed in almost all cases.

5. G – Uterine rupture

Uterine rupture in planned vaginal birth after caesarean section is 35 per 10 000, compared with 12 per 10 000 in those with a planned repeat section. The use of oxytocin to induce labour in a woman with a previous section increases the risk to 80 per 10 000, and prostaglandin administration increases the risk to 240 per 10 000. For more details on uterine rupture, see 'Complications of caesarean section', Theme 8, Page 80.

Theme 4: Contraception

1. E – Levonelle (levonorgestrel)

This is the 'morning-after pill'. It is most effective when taken as soon as possible after sexual intercourse, but can be used up to 72 hours later. The patient must be told to return if she vomits within 3 hours of taking the tablet, that the next period may be early or late, that she must use barrier protection until the next period, and to seek medical attention if she experiences symptoms of an ectopic pregnancy (as there is a failure rate). The only contraindication is porphyria. Side-effects are menstrual irregularities, nausea, lower abdominal pain, fatigue, headache, dizziness, breast tenderness and vomiting.

2. C – Depo-Provera (medroxyprogesterone acetate)

Depo-Provera is a long-acting progesterone, given by intramuscular injection, which lasts for 12 weeks. It is used for long-term contraception and is over 99% effective. It stops ovulation, thickens cervical mucus to prevent sperm reaching an egg and thins out the lining of the womb to prevent embryo implantation. It may protect against endometrial cancer and offers some protection from pelvic inflammatory disease. Depo-Provera is not affected by other medicines, and patients do not have to remember contraception for as long as the injection lasts. The injection cannot be removed from the body, so side-effects (irregular periods, weight gain, headaches, spotty skin, mood changes and breast tenderness) cannot be stopped. Also, menstruation and normal fertility may take some time to return after stopping the injections. Cautions and contraindications are the same as for oral progesterones.

Noristerat is very similar to Depo-Provera but lasts for only 8 weeks. It is generally used only for shorter-term contraception.

3. B – Cerazette

Cerazette is a progesterone-only pill (POP) and is suitable for patients where combined pills are contraindicated, such as this woman (see 'Contraindications to contraception' – Paper 2 Answers, Theme 5, page 45). However, it may be less effective in women who weigh over 70 kg. The progestogen in the pill thickens cervical mucus to prevent passage of sperm, thins out the lining of the womb to prevent implantation and stops ovulation in some women. It is 99% effective if taken correctly. The advantages are possible cessation of periods, although they can become irregular, and quick return of fertility on stopping the POP. Disadvantages include mild side-effects and an increased risk of ectopic pregnancy if it fails. POPs are not effective if taken over 3 hours late (12 hours for Cerazette), or after vomiting or severe diarrhoea. Contraindications to POP use include undiagnosed vaginal bleeding, severe arterial disease, liver adenoma, porphyria, immediately post-evacuation of a hydatiform mole, a history of breast cancer and pregnancy.

Implanon

Implanon is a small, flexible rod inserted below the skin of the upper arm that releases progestogens ($\rightarrow$ stops ovulation, thickens cervical mucus and thins uterine lining). It is over 99% effective and works for up to 3 years. The Implanon can be removed at any time with a resumption of normal fertility. The advantage is that the patient does not have to remember to take contraception. Disadvantages include mood changes, breast tenderness, acne and irregular periods. Cautions and contraindications are the same as for oral progesterones.

Intrauterine device

The IUD is a small plastic or copper device, with no embedded hormones, that is inserted into the uterus. It stops sperm reaching an egg, and stops fertilized ova implanting in the endometrium. It is 99% effective. Advantages are that the woman does not have to remember to take contraception and, when the device is removed, fertility returns to normal. IUDs can remain *in situ* for 3–10 years depending on type, but can be removed at any time. They are not affected by other medicines. The disadvantages are that periods may be heavier, longer and more painful, and there is an increased risk of ectopic pregnancy if the IUD fails. Infection risk is increased during the first 3 weeks post-insertion and IUD insertion should be covered by antibacterial prophylaxis. Screening for existing infection is advised before an IUD insertion. Contraindications for IUDs are severe anaemia, recent sexually transmitted infection, unexplained uterine bleeding, a distorted or small uterine cavity, genital malignancy, active trophoblastic disease, pelvic inflammatory disease, immunosuppression and pregnancy. Contraindications that are specific to copper IUDs are copper allergy, Wilson's disease and medical diathermy. IUDs can be used as emergency contraception and are more effective than hormonal methods. They can be used up to 120 hours after unprotected intercourse.

Mirena

The Mirena coil is a progesterone-only plastic intrauterine system that is inserted into the uterus. It releases progestogen. It is over 99% effective and works for 5 years, but can be taken out at any time with resumption of normal fertility. Mirena is licensed for contraception, treatment of primary menorrhagia and prevention of endometrial hyperplasia during oestrogen replacement. Advantages are that the patient does not have to remember to take contraception and, as the hormone is locally acting, progestogenic side-effects and drug interactions are less likely. Periods will be much lighter and shorter, usually less painful and may stop completely, although irregular bleeding or spotting is common. The risk of ectopic pregnancy is lower than with older IUDs. The disadvantages are that some women report having mood changes, spotty skin and breast tenderness, and there is often irregular bleeding on insertion of the coil (and for 6 months after). There is a minimal risk of infection during the first 3 weeks after insertion. Contraindications are the same as for other IUDs.

4. J – Rifampicin

Hepatic enzyme inducers may considerably reduce the effectiveness of combined oral contraceptive and POPs, so additional contraception should be used. Examples of hepatic enzyme inducers include rifampicin, rifabutin, carbamazepine, griseofulvin, modafinil, nelfinavir, nevirapine, oxcarbazepine, phenytoin, phenobarbital, primidone, ritonavir and topiramate. This is an important list to know.

5. A – Ampicillin

The efficacy of combined oral contraceptives may be reduced by some antibacterials that do not induce liver enzymes, such as ampicillin and doxycycline. These drugs instead impair the bacterial flora responsible for recycling ethinylestradiol (the synthetic oestrogen derivative used in the pill) from the large bowel. If women are using such antibiotics, additional contraceptive measures should be implemented. Other occasions when additional contraception should be used include missed pills, diarrhoea and vomiting.

Oestrogens antagonize the hypotensive effect of angiotensin-converting enzyme (ACE) inhibitors, so drugs such as lisinopril or ramipril may not be effective in women taking the combined pill.

Theme 5: Postpartum haemorrhage

Postpartum haemorrhage (PPH) is defined as over 500 mL blood loss from the genital tract, or less than 500 mL if associated with haemodynamic changes in the mother. Normal blood loss during delivery is 200–300 mL. Primary PPH occurs within 24 hours after birth, and secondary PPH ranges from 24 hours to 6 weeks post partum. PPH is reported to occur in 5% of deliveries, although blood loss is often underestimated, so it is probably more common. Life-threatening PPH occurs in 1 in 1000 deliveries. Management includes anticipating risk so that preventive measures can be initiated. Resuscitation of the patient must be initiated while identifying the cause of the bleeding. Resuscitation includes ABC and aggressive fluid or blood replacement. If coagulopathy develops, a haematologist must be involved.

Causes of primary PPH include atonic uterus, cervical tear, high vaginal tear, perineal trauma, retained placenta or placental fragments, clotting disorders, uterine inversion and uterine rupture. Risk factors include antepartum haemorrhage, previous history of PPH, over-enlarged uterus due to multiple pregnancy, polyhydramnios, macrosomic fetus, fibroids, placenta praevia, prolonged labour, grand multiparity, uterine fibroids, chorioamnionitis and bleeding diathesis.

1. A – Atonic uterus

Ninety per cent of PPHs are caused by an atonic uterus. During the third stage of labour, the uterus compresses the intramyometrial blood vessels to stop any bleeding. However, in some cases, this does not happen (hence the uterus is described as being atonic). It is more common if there is a retained placenta, as its physical presence prevents contraction of the uterus.

2. E – Infection

Infection is the commonest cause of secondary PPH, and is often due to retained products of conception. Investigations include a high vaginal swab. Antibiotics are the first-line treatment, and may settle the bleeding. If there is significant bleeding, evacuation of retained products of conception is required.

3. A – Atonic uterus

Initial management of PPH (prior to surgical measures) includes emptying the bladder and rubbing up uterine contractions, while initiating oxytocics to contract the uterus. To 'rub up a contraction', the uterus is massaged through the abdominal wall, or directly if the abdomen is open in theatre. In an otherwise uncomplicated labour and pregnancy, the oxytocics used are a bolus of intravenous ergometrine followed by an infusion of oxytocin. If bleeding persists, bimanual compression can be employed. For further persistent bleeding, carboprost (15-methylprostaglandin/Haemobate) can be given intramuscularly into the thigh or the myometrium.

4. A – Atonic uterus

Following exhaustion of medical management of PPH, surgical options are attempted. A B-lynch suture is a uterine compression stitch that opposes the anterior and posterior walls to apply continuing compression. Other surgical approaches include under-sewing the placental bed, uterine artery or internal iliac artery ligation, or hysterectomy as a last resort.

5. G – Retained placental fragments

Following delivery, the placenta should be examined for completeness. If retained products are suspected, and there is significant bleeding, manual removal of the placenta or its fragments is required. If this is suspected in a secondary PPH, an ultrasound scan can be used to confirm the diagnosis.

Injury to the genital tract accounts for 7% of PPH. These can be soft tissue injuries, such as episiotomy, or cervical and vaginal lacerations. If there is profuse bleeding, vessels can be clamped or packed while definitive repair is achieved. Genital tract injuries are more common after instrumental delivery.

Theme 6: Cervical screening

Cervical smears, which are used to screen for cervical cancer, are performed on all women over 20 years (or after first intercourse if later), and are repeated every 3 years until the age of 64. Three-yearly smears reduce the incidence of cervical cancer by 90%. Smears are performed by scraping an Aylesbury spatula or cytobrush 360° around the cervical os in order to retrieve the loose cells around the transitional zone. At colposcopy, areas of cervical intraepithelial neoplasia (CIN) appear as a white area with a well-defined edge on application of 5% acetic acid solution.

1. A – Colposcopy

A summary of the management of abnormal smears is as follows:

Cervical intraepithelial neoplasia (CIN)	Action
Normal smear	Repeat in 3 years
1 (mild dysplasia)	Repeat in 4–6 months
1 on two occasions	Colposcopy
2 (moderate dysplasia)	Colposcopy
3 (severe dysplasia/carcinoma *in situ*)	Urgent colposcopy
Glandular dysplasia	Urgent colposcopy/hysterectomy

2. A – Colposcopy

If untreated, one-third of women with CIN 2 or 3 will develop cervical cancer in the next 10 years. CIN 1 may progress to CIN 2 or 3, but commonly regresses spontaneously.

3. E – Repeat in 1 year

Annual screening is recommended in immunosuppressed patients. There is evidence to show that they are at increased risk of false-negative cytology.

4. F – Repeat in 3 years

Since this woman has a normal result, she does not need another smear for 3 years.

5. A – Colposcopy

Human papillomavirus (HPV) is a sexually transmitted DNA virus, of which more than 80 types exist. Types 6 and 11 are associated with genital warts; types 16 and 18 are associated with a predisposition to cancer. There is now a vaccine for HPV (Gardasil). It is licensed for use in children of both sexes between 9 and 15 years, and females between 16 and 26 years, to assist in prevention of cervical and vulval dysplasias and genital warts. These patients still require cervical screening to cover for infection prior to vaccination. Three injections are given, at 0, 2 and 6 months, and immunity lasts for at least 5 years. Immunocompromised patients may still be re-infected despite a completed course.

Women with mild dyskaryosis and a positive test for HPV are at higher risk of developing cervical cancer than HPV-negative patients, and are therefore recommended for colposcopy. It is thought that this secondary screening for HPV will reduce the number of referrals to colposcopy with CIN 1.

Cervical cancer is the second most common malignancy in women in the world (after breast cancer). It is commonest in the 40- to 44-year and 70- to 74-year age groups. Cervical cancer occurs mainly in the squamous epithelium, with 90% being squamous cell carcinomas and the remainder adenocarcinomas (which have a worse prognosis). Patients present with postcoital bleeding, offensive discharge and intermenstrual/postmenstrual bleeding. Spread can occur to the pelvic side wall (involving the ureters, bladder or rectum), or via lymphatics to the pelvic nodes. Blood-borne metastases are rare. For more details on the staging and management of cervical tumours, see 'Management of endometrial and cervical cancer' (Paper 2 Answers, Theme 8, page 50).

Theme 7: Mechanisms of labour

In order to answer this question, it is important to understand the three stages of labour. A normal spontaneous labour should occur within 12 hours, which is to reduce the complications related to its duration.

The *first stage* of labour starts with the onset of regular uterine contractions associated with cervical change, and ends with full dilatation of the cervix (10 cm). The cervix is said to be 'fully effaced' when it shortens and becomes incorporated into the lower segment of the uterus. The *second stage* is the time between full dilatation and delivery of the baby. This is initially passive, then active when the woman begins to push, as the fetal head descends towards the perineum. Finally, the *third stage* is from delivery of the baby to delivery of the placenta. During the second stage of labour, the relationship of the fetal head and body to the maternal pelvis changes to allow ease of passage. The ideal mechanism is with the presentation of a well-flexed fetal head, rotating into an occipitoanterior, vertex presentation for delivery. The vertex refers to the area of skull between the two fontanelles.

1. C – Engagement

This occurs when the largest part of the fetal head enters the brim of the pelvis, which is usually in the occipitotransverse diameter. Do not forget that the pelvic inlet is widest in the transverse diameter, and the outlet in the anterior–posterior diameter. Engagement can occur before labour in nulliparous women, but rarely in the multiparous. On abdominal examination, engagement is measured as 'fifths' of the head palpable.

Descent is encouraged by uterine contractions, which accelerates when the membranes rupture.

2. F – Flexion

Flexion of the fetal head occurs passively throughout labour. With full flexion, the posterior fontanelle becomes palpable.

3. G – Internal rotation

The sloping inclination of the levator ani muscle encourages internal rotation of the head at the level of the ischial spines. This brings the sagittal suture of the head into the anterior–posterior plane of the pelvis, and the occiput rotates anteriorly towards the symphysis. If resistance occurs at this stage, the head may become engaged in the unfavourable occipito-posterior position. The head may later rotate 180° into a preferable occipito-anterior position. However, if the head remains occipito-posterior, there is extension of the neck, which can cause obstruction requiring an instrumental delivery.

4. D – Extension

The occiput extends as it passes underneath the symphysis pubis and becomes visible at the vulva, otherwise known as 'crowning'. Tearing of the perineum can occur at this stage, which can be prevented by shorter, smaller, active pushes at this time.

5. I – Restitution

Once the head is delivered, restitution is the reversal of the twist of internal rotation. This aligns the head with the shoulders, which descend in an oblique position. The shoulders externally rotate into the widest anterior–posterior diameter, with the anterior shoulder delivered first under the symphysis pubis, sometimes with gentle downwards traction, followed by upwards traction for the other shoulder to be delivered.

Midwives complete a *partogram*, which must be kept accurately to assess progress in labour. Data include demographics (name, date of birth), fetal heart rate, liquor colour, dilatation of the cervix, descent of the head, oxytocin infusion rate, contractions per minute, drugs and intravenous fluids, blood pressure and pulse, urinalysis and temperature. A cardiotocogram (CTG) is also recorded to assess fetal well-being. This documentation can quickly illustrate poor progress in labour, primary dysfunctional labour (poor progress in the active phase of labour with slow cervical dilatation) and secondary arrest (when the active phase stops or slows). Early recognition of these events and their complications are crucial. Presumed fetal compromise in labour is the commonest reason for medical intervention, and may be indicated by thick meconium liquor or an abnormal CTG.

A *fetal blood sample* can confirm fetal distress. Here, an amnioscope is used to visualize the fetal scalp, a small cut is made and the resulting blood is collected in a microtube. The results give a pH and are a guide to management:
- normal (pH >7.25): labour can continue
- borderline (pH 7.20–7.25): repeat pH is needed in 30–60 minutes
- abnormal (pH <7.20): confirms fetal compromise – needs delivery

Theme 8: Complications of caesarean section

Caesarean sections account for 15% of births in the UK. The lower segment caesarean section (LSCS) has overtaken the classic midline uterine incision because of a lower complication rate. Indications for LSCS can be maternal (two previous LSCSs, placenta praevia, maternal disease or maternal request) or fetal (breech, twin pregnancy if the first twin is not cephalic, fetal distress, cord prolapse or delayed first stage of labour). Complications include haemorrhage, gastric aspiration, infection and thromboembolic disease. LSCS can be performed under general or local anaesthetic. The patient is positioned supine and tilted 15° to the left, to minimise aortocaval compression. Access to the uterus is via a transverse suprapubic (Pfannenstiel's) incision.

Hermann Johannes Pfannenstiel, German gynaecologist (1862–1909).

1. F – Pulmonary embolism

This patient is likely to have been immobile for several days. She has a number of risk factors for thromboembolism that put her at moderate risk of a pulmonary embolism (PE) after LSCS. Risk factors for PE in obstetrics include age >35 years, obesity (>80 kg), parity >4, pre-eclampsia, having an emergency LSCS in labour, >4 days prior immobility, major current illness and current infection. A PE is the more likely explanation for her hypoxia on air, low pyrexia and lack of focal chest signs. A confirmed deep vein thrombosis or PE requires 6 weeks of thromboprophylaxis post partum.

Do not forget that thromboembolism is a leading cause of maternal mortality. The risk in pregnancy is six times higher than in the general population. This is thought to be due to normal homeostatic changes that reduce the risk of haemorrhage at delivery, including increased clotting factor concentration and reduced fibrinolysis. Guidance to reduce the incidence of thromboembolic events includes the use of compression stockings and heparin prophylaxis for those with risk factors, with early mobilization where possible. Patients who are at high risk (past history or family history of thrombosis, extended surgery (e.g. hysterectomy) or with antiphospholipid syndrome) should all receive postoperative heparin for 5 days, or until mobile.

2. J – Urinary tract injury

The close proximity of the urological tract to the uterus makes injury during caesarean section occasional but possible. Ureteral injury must be suspected in this scenario because of flank pain, abdominal distension and clinical suspicion of an ileus (absent bowel sounds). Resuscitation should involve oxygen, fluid resuscitation and catheterization with strict fluid balance. Investigations may include a renal ultrasound scan and an intravenous urogram (IVU) to detect hydronephrosis or hydroureter. If ureteral ligation or transection is suspected, surgical exploration and repair are essential.

3. C – Endometritis

Endometritis should be suspected above retained products of conception after an LSCS with irregular vaginal bleeding, particularly when a manual evacuation has been performed. Examination should include a speculum for high vaginal and cervical swabs, blood cultures and blood tests for inflammatory markers. Intravenous antibiotics should be administered until pyrexia settles for 24 hours. Antibiotic options could include a combination of cephalosporins with anaerobic cover (e.g. metronidazole).

4. K – Uterine rupture

Uterine rupture is an obstetric emergency that requires resuscitation of the mother and immediate delivery of the baby. The incidence of uterine rupture in vaginal birth after previous caesarean section is 35 in 10 000. Uterine rupture is usually associated with scar dehiscence from previous caesarean section (as in this scenario), but primary rupture can occur with obstructed labour, overzealous use of oxytocin, previous perforation during operative procedures and traumatic instrumental deliveries. The main symptoms are pain (abdominal, or at the shoulder tip due to peritonism), fetal distress (seen on the CTG as late decelerations), shock, vaginal bleeding or cessation of contractions. After delivery, the uterus is repaired or hysterectomy is performed, depending upon the site and extent of rupture, the woman's condition and parity.

Of note, fetal head compression is associated with early decelerations on the CTG.

5. B – Aspiration pneumonitis

Aspiration pneumonitis (Mendelson's syndrome) describes an acute lung injury that ensues after sterile gastric contents are inhaled into the lung. By contrast, aspiration pneumonia is an infectious process caused by the inhalation of pharyngeal secretions that are colonized by pathogenic bacteria (this will take longer to develop). Aspiration pneumonitis occurs in 1 in 3000 cases where general anaesthetic is used and causes 10–30% of anaesthetic deaths. Risk factors include absence of the gag reflex, difficult intubation, an inadequately emptied stomach, poor oesophageal sphincter tone, sedation and the pregnancy itself. Aspiration, as opposed to pulmonary embolism, is suggested by the findings at the right base and wheeze. To reduce the risk of aspiration pneumonitis, patients are offered drugs to reduce gastric volume (prokinetics, e.g. metoclopramide) and acidity (proton pump inhibitors, e.g. omeprazole) prior to caesarean section.

Curtis Lester Mendelson, American obstetrician and cardiologist (b1913).

Theme 9: Gynaecological malignancies

1. F – Vulva

Lichen sclerosis is an autoimmune loss of vulval collagen, leading to a thin epithelium. It is commonest in postmenopausal women. Affected lesions appear shiny, white and tight, and may be itchy or painful. Areas of lichen sclerosis should be biopsied, as there is a 5% risk of progression to vulval intraepithelial neoplasia (VIN) (and eventually vulval squamous cell carcinoma). VIN has less malignant potential than CIN, so lesions tend to undergo observation. The exception is symptomatic VIN 3, which is treated with laser therapy or topical chemotherapy.

Vulval cancer accounts for 5% of gynaecological cancers, with a wide presenting age range. Ninety per cent are squamous carcinomas, with rarer forms including Bartholin's gland adenocarcinomas and Paget's disease of the vulva (a well-defined scaly, erythematous lesion caused by malignant change in the cells of the epidermal layer). Vulval carcinomas can present with pruritus, bleeding, pain/dyspareunia or a mass. Lesions spread slowly to local tissues, with lymphatic spread to femoral nodes. Treatment varies from wide local excision to radical vulvectomy with bilateral node dissection. Local or systemic chemotherapy may also be effective.

2. D – Ovarian

Ovarian cancer is the commonest cause of gynaecological cancer *death* in westernized society. This is mainly due to its late, and often advanced, presentation and no current population screening. Endometrial cancer is the commonest malignancy of the female genital tract.

3. A – Cervical

There has been a recent rise in the incidence of cervical cancer among younger females. Some people blame increased promiscuity, and thus more widespread infection with human papillomaviruses, for this change. The younger age group has a worse prognosis.

4. B – Endometrial

Endometrial tumours are oestrogen dependent – hence many risk factors involve unopposed oestrogen exposure. Risk factors include exogenous oestrogen use (oestrogen-containing contraceptive pills), obesity (androgens are converted to oestrogens in the peripheral fat), nulliparity, late menopause, diabetes (independent of obesity) and pelvic irradiation for cervical cancer.

5. C – Fallopian tube

Fallopian tube cancer is rare, accounting for <0.3% of gynaecological cancers. These tumours are similar in presentation to ovarian cancers, with 70% being serous carcinomas. 'Hydrops tubae profluens' occurs in 10% of fallopian tube malignancies, where intermittent colicky pain settles with a sudden vaginal discharge of watery fluid. Spread is local, via the peritoneum and lymphatics, with metastases being present in around 50% of cases. The treatment options are much the same as for ovarian cancer.

Theme 10: The infertility clinic

Reference ranges for females in the luteal phase

Follicle-stimulating hormone (FSH)	1.2–9 u/L
Luteinizing hormone (LH)	<14.7 u/L
Day 21 progesterone	>20 nmol/L suggests ovulation
Prolactin	53–360 u/L
Thyroid-stimulating hormone (TSH)	0 –5.7 mu/L
Sex hormone-binding globulin (SHBG)	26–110 nmol/L
Estradiol	101–905 pmol/L
Testosterone	0.2–2.9 nmol/L

A couple are said to be subfertile if conception has not occurred within 1 year of unprotected sex. Subfertility affects one in seven couples, and those who do not conceive within 2 years should be investigated. Subfertility can be primary (where the woman has never conceived) or secondary (where she has previously conceived).

1. H – Premature ovarian failure

This woman has a low–normal estradiol despite a high LH and FSH. These results suggest premature ovarian failure (POF). Although the average age for the menopause in the UK is 50.5 years, a diagnosis of POF is made only in women less than 40 years. (If a girl never begins menstruating, it is termed primary ovarian failure.) By the age of 40 years, the prevalence of POF is 1%. Most cases of POF are idiopathic, although a small proportion of patients have underlying disorders such as Turner's syndrome and fragile X syndrome. POF occurs as a result of reduced follicle development or increased follicle atresia, and it causes amenorrhoea as well as other menopausal symptoms. Assisted reproductive techniques are the definitive management. The woman in this scenario may also need hormone replacement therapy for oestrogen deficiency to protect against osteoporosis.

2. G – Polycystic ovary syndrome

Polycystic ovary syndrome (PCOS – also known as Stein–Leventhal syndrome) is a common gynaecological disorder associated with menstrual disturbance and hyperandrogenism. It includes a range of clinical symptoms, such as oligomenorrhoea/amenorrhoea, subfertility, dyspareunia, acne and hirsutism. Remember that not all women with PCOS have polycystic ovaries, and up to 30% of patients can have a *regular* cycle (as in this scenario). Obesity in PCOS causes hypersecretion of insulin, which increases ovarian release of androgens and predisposes to diabetes. (Clinically, this has caused her subfertility.) Excess insulin causes increased LH production in the pituitary in response to gonadotropin-releasing hormone (GnRH). This increases the bioactivity of androgens, causing less SHBG to be produced by the liver. Because this patient is keen to conceive, weight loss and clomiphene are the first management options. Clomiphene is an antioestrogen that occupies oestrogen receptors in the hypothalamus. This induces ovulation by increasing FSH production. Ovulation is confirmed by a raised day-21 progesterone level. There is a risk of multiple pregnancy with clomiphene.

Michael Leo Leventhal, American gynaecologist (1901–71).

Irving Freiler Stein, American gynaecologist (1887–1976).

3. B – Asherman's syndrome

Asherman's syndrome is caused by intrauterine adhesions following dilatation and curettage (D&C). This was previously performed in this scenario to investigate the patient's intermenstrual bleeding, and has now largely been replaced by outpatient hysteroscopy and endometrial sampling. Hysteroscopy and dissection of scar tissue may be helpful in Asherman's syndrome.

Joseph G Asherman, Israeli gynaecologist (b. 1889).

4. G – Polycystic ovarian syndrome

This patient has more severe symptoms of PCOS, with acne, hirsutism and amenorrhoea. Patients with PCOS are more susceptible to diabetes, endometrial cancer and dyslipidaemia (↓ high-density lipoproteins (HDL), ↑ triglycerides and ↑ low-density lipoproteins (LDL)).

5. D – Hypogonadotropic hypogonadism

Hypogonadotropic hypogonadism is a rare condition caused by failure of the anterior pituitary to secrete the gonadotropins LH and FSH in order to stimulate ovulation. This is a form of secondary hypogonadism, as the fault is not from the gonads themselves, which may be functioning normally. Hypogonadotropic hypogonadism can be differentiated from premature ovarian failure, which has high gonadotropin levels. The woman in this scenario has the typical hypo-oestrogenic symptoms of reduced libido and vaginal dryness.

Secondary amenorrhoea is defined as the absence of menses for 6 months in previously menstruating women. Causes can be divided into:
- gonadal failure (premature ovarian failure)
- pituitary dysfunction (pituitary tumour)
- psychological causes (stress, travel and weight changes can reduce GnRH)
- endocrine dysfunction (hypothyroidism)
- oestrogen metabolism dysfunction (anorexia nervosa)

The commonest pituitary tumours are benign adenomas, such as the prolactinoma. The excess prolactin secreted by these tumours inhibits gonadotropin release. Diagnosis of prolactinoma is by MRI, and this tumour responds to dopamine agonists such as bromocriptine. Hypothyroidism should be screened for in all women with irregular menses. Low thyroxine (T_4) levels reduce negative feedback on the hypothalamic–pituitary axis, resulting in elevated prolactin and thyroid-stimulating hormone (TSH) levels. In anorexia nervosa, there is less adipose tissue for androgens to be converted to oestrogens, resulting in lower circulating levels of the active metabolite estradiol.

Women can present with primary amenorrhoea as a cause of infertility. *Turner's syndrome* (45XO) is one of the more common genetic conditions, with an incidence of 1 in 2500 girls. The lack of one X chromosome gives rise to characteristic signs, including short stature and webbing of the neck. The ovaries in Turner's syndrome do not respond to gonadotropic hormones, and patients are almost universally infertile. Woman who present with primary amenorrhoea and infertility, and who have high levels of FSH, should be karyotyped to exclude Turner's syndrome.

Mayer–Rokitansky–Küster–Hauser syndrome (or müllerian agenesis) occurs in 1 in 4500 women and describes a failure of development of the embryonic müllerian ducts. It is characterized by congenital absence of the uterus, cervix and the upper two-thirds of the vagina. Women can have normal external genitalia, a 46XX karyotype and normal secondary sexual characteristics, as the ovaries are intact. These women need psychological support, and surgery can create a 'neovagina' to allow intercourse.

Theme 1: Methods of delivery

Options

A. Elective caesarean section
B. Emergency caesarean section
C. External cephalic version
D. Kielland's forceps
E. Neville-Barnes forceps
F. Normal delivery

For each of the following scenarios, select the most appropriate method of delivery. Each option may be used once, more than once or not at all.

1. A 30-year-old primigravida, with an epidural *in situ* and a delayed second stage, has been pushing for 1½ hours and is now exhausted. On examination, the fetus is felt in the occipitoanterior position at 'station plus one'. The cardiotocogram is normal.

2. A 26-year-old woman is at 39 weeks' gestation. She has had a previous classic caesarean section.

3. A 27-year-old woman who is in labour is fully dilated. On examination, a face presentation is seen, with the chin posteriorly.

4. A 32-year-old woman has been fully dilated for an hour, but her labour is not progressing despite good maternal effort. On examination, the baby is in vertex presentation with an occipitoposterior position.

5. A 29-year-old woman is dilated at 10 cm. On examination, there is an occipitoanterior presentation with a flexed head. She has had one previous lower segment caesarean section.

Theme 2: Urogynaecology

Options

A. Abdominal colposuspension
B. Anterior repair
C. Hormone replacement therapy
D. Indwelling catheter
E. Intermittent self-catheterization
F. Oxybutynin
G. Periurethral injectables
H. Physiotherapy
I. Total abdominal hysterectomy
J. Transvaginal tape

For each of the following scenarios, select the next most appropriate management option. Each option may be used once, more than once or not at all.

1. A 70-year-old retired chef complains of urinary frequency. She visits the toilet every hour, and sometimes 'doesn't make it'. She has incontinence when climbing stairs and nocturia three times per night. She has had five normal deliveries, one with forceps. Past medical history includes two previous myocardial infarctions and insulin-controlled diabetes. Examination reveals an episiotomy scar, a cystocele with cervical descent when using a Sims speculum, and loss of urine on coughing.

2. A 55-year-old senior office manager suffers incontinence on coughing and laughing. She also has frequency and occasional dysuria. Her last period was 18 months ago. She has had three normal deliveries and a caesarean section, followed by a total abdominal hysterectomy 6 years ago. She smokes 15 cigarettes a day. On examination, she is slim with a caesarean section scar. Examination with Cuscoe's speculum is painful and shows an atrophic vagina. Vaginal examination reveals no masses. She has incontinence on a Valsalva manoeuvre.

3. A 59-year-old secretary complains of occasional incontinence. She has nocturia four times a night and passes urine hourly. She has tried physiotherapy without improvement. She has had two normal deliveries, and her menopause was 4 years ago. She has had a previous anterior repair. Apart from some scarring on the anterior vaginal wall, examination is unremarkable.

4. An 85 year old with severe rheumatoid arthritis has urinary frequency and incontinence on standing. After she passes water, she often 'needs' to go again although it takes her a while to 'get going'. She has had two recent episodes of vaginal bleeding and is undergoing investigation for a possible ovarian carcinoma. On examination, she has a non-tender suprapubic mass and a vague 'fullness' in the left iliac fossa. A bladder scan shows a residual volume of 700 mL.

5. A 50-year-old full-time mother is referred with nocturia of three times per night and frequency. She is sometimes unable to get to the

toilet on time, which she finds embarrassing, and is 'at her wits' end'. She also has leakage on coughing. Her past medical history includes hypertension and constipation. Abdominal examination reveals a large fibroid uterus and vaginal examination shows a large cystocele and significant cervical descent. Cystometry shows a positive cough stress test. She has finished a course of physiotherapy and is desperate for something to be done to get rid of her symptoms.

Theme 3: Drugs in pregnancy

Options

A. Carbimazole
B. Codeine phosphate
C. Diclofenac
D. Doxycyline
E. Erythromycin
F. Gabapentin
G. Iodine-131
H. Ondansetron
I. Paracetamol
J. Promethazine
K. Propylthiouracil
L. Thalidomide
M. Ursodeoxycholic acid

For each of the following scenarios, select the most appropriate drug. Each option may be used once, more than once or not at all.

1. A 32-year-old pregnant woman is diagnosed with Graves' disease. She expresses to her GP that she wishes to breastfeed and asks if there is any medication safe for her to take.

2. A 24-year-old woman who is 16 weeks pregnant sees her GP complaining of persistent vomiting. She is requesting medication.

3. A 24-year-old woman, who has been complaining of a persistent itch, is diagnosed with obstetric cholestasis.

4. A 28-year-old pregnant woman is found to have pelvic inflammatory disease. The GP is wary that this commonly used antibiotic is contraindicated.

5. A 31-year-old breastfeeding woman requires analgesia following caesarean section. Choose a suitable analgesic that is normally avoided during pregnancy.

Theme 4: Perimenopausal hormones

Options

    A. 17β-Estradiol
    B. Androstenedione
    C. Follicle-stimulating hormone
    D. Luteinizing hormone
    E. Oestrone
    F. Progesterone

For each of the following descriptions, select the most appropriate hormone. Each option may be used once, more than once or not at all.

1. There is reduced secretion of this hormone by the ovaries during the menopause.

2. This hormone is produced in peripheral adipose tissue after the menopause.

3. The hormone oestrone is produced from this.

4. Measurement of this hormone can confirm ovulation.

5. Menorrhagia or dysmenorrhoea during the perimenopausal period is attributed to a lack of this hormone.

Theme 5: Acute pelvic pain

Options

    A. Acute appendicitis
    B. Appendix abscess
    C. Complete miscarriage
    D. Corpus luteum cyst
    E. Ectopic pregnancy
    F. Incomplete miscarriage
    G. Inevitable miscarriage
    H. Missed miscarriage
    I. Mittelschmerz
    J. Pelvic inflammatory disease
    K. Threatened miscarriage
    L. Torsion of ovarian cyst

For each of the following scenarios, select the most appropriate diagnosis. Each option may be used once, more than once or not at all.

1. A 35-year-old woman presents to the emergency department with sudden-onset colicky pain, focused around the left iliac fossa, and vomiting. She admits to experiencing intermittent pain in this area over the last few months. Observations include heart rate 112 beats/min and blood pressure 96/64 mmHg. Speculum examination reveals no per vagina bleeding, although there is left adnexal tenderness. A urinary pregnancy test is negative.

2. A 19-year-old student attends the emergency department with generalized abdominal pain and malaise. She complains of increased urinary frequency and pain on passing water. She also admits to a purulent per vagina discharge and pain on intercourse. On examination, her temperature is 38.2°C and there is cervical excitation. A urinary pregnancy test has been requested.

3. A 26-year-old woman presents to the emergency department with generalized cramping pains in her lower abdomen and amenorrhoea for 7 weeks. She feels very faint and complains of heavy bleeding per vagina. She has also noticed some tissue mixed with the blood. Examination reveals a tender lower abdomen. The cervical os is open and active bleeding is seen. Observations include pulse rate 110 beats/min and blood pressure 96/64 mmHg. A urinary βhCG test is positive. An ultrasound scan demonstrates some material in the uterus.

4. A 25-year-old woman presents with right iliac fossa and shoulder-tip pain that has caused her to collapse. She is sexually active and is using the copper intrauterine device for contraception. On examination, she has an abdominal mass in the right iliac fossa. There is guarding in this area, but no rebound tenderness. Cervical excitation is present. Observations include pulse rate 125 beats/min and blood pressure 86/48 mmHg. A urinary pregnancy test result is awaited.

5. A 32-year-old woman complains of central vague abdominal tenderness that has localized to the right iliac fossa. She is sexually active and uses the combined oral contraceptive pill for contraception. Abdominal examination reveals tenderness in the right iliac fossa. No abnormality is found on vaginal examination. Observations include pulse rate 110 beats/min, blood pressure 132/84 mmHg and temperature 37.8°C. A urinary pregnancy test result is awaited.

Theme 6: Gametogenesis

Options

A. Mature oocyte
B. Oogonia
C. Polar body
D. Primary oocyte
E. Primary spermatocyte
F. Primordial germ cell
G. Secondary oocyte
H. Secondary spermatocyte
I. Spermatid
J. Spermatogonia
K. Spermatozoa

For each of the following descriptions, select the correct term. Each option may be used once, more than once or not at all.

1. This cell is the starting point of both male and female gametogenesis.

2. This is the end-product of spermatogenesis that is involved in fertilization.

3. A male cell that contains 23 single chromosomes prior to spermiogenesis.

4. A male cell that contains 46 double-structured chromosomes.

5. This is the by-product of female gametogenesis.

Theme 7: Sexually transmitted infections 2

Options

- A. Bacterial vaginosis
- B. Cervical cancer
- C. Chancroid
- D. Chlamydia
- E. Epstein–Barr virus
- F. Genital candidiasis
- G. Genital herpes
- H. Genital warts
- I. Gonorrhoea
- J. Granuloma inguinale (donovanosis)
- K. HIV
- L. Lymphogranuloma venereum
- M. Molluscum contagiosum
- N. Phthiriasis
- O. Reiter's syndrome
- P. Scabies
- Q. Syphilis
- R. Trichomoniasis

For each of the following scenarios, select the most appropriate diagnosis. Each option may be used once, more than once or not at all.

1. A 42-year-old man has developed multiple painful ulcers on his penis, with an associated phimosis. On examination, there is inguinal lymph node enlargement and a discharging sinus. A culture demonstrates *Haemophilus ducreyi*.

2. A 23-year-old female student presents with abdominal pain in the right upper quadrant. She has had multiple sexual partners with whom she used no barrier protection. When questioned further, she describes a vague history of dysuria and increased urinary frequency.

3. A 36-year-old woman attends the GP with a grey–white vaginal discharge that she says has a 'fishy' odour.

4. A 34-year-old woman attends the GP complaining of feeling generally unwell. She says that she is tired and mildly feverish, with headaches and an itchy diffuse skin rash. She also complains of pains in her joints. She noticed a painless ulcer on her labia that healed about 5 weeks previously. The last time she was sexually active was 2 months ago.

5. A couple in their 30s visit the GP. The woman works in a nursing home and is complaining of itching on her fingers and wrists, especially at night. Her partner says he developed a similar pattern of itching 3 weeks later, which has now spread to his penis.

Theme 8: Twins

Options

    A. Dizygotic dichorionic diamniotic
    B. Dizygotic dichorionic monoamniotic
    C. Dizygotic monochorionic monoamniotic
    D. Monozygotic dichorionic diamniotic
    E. Monozygotic monochorionic diamniotic
    F. Monozygotic monochorionic monoamniotic

For each of the following descriptions, select the most appropriate terminology. Each option may be used once, more than once or not at all.

1. These are the most common type of twins.

2. These twins share the same amniotic sac.

3. These twins occur if division occurs at day 5 post-fertilization.

4. If twins are of the opposite sex, they must be this type.

5. These are identical twins with a separate chorion, amnion and placenta.

Theme 9: Ectopic pregnancy

Options

A. Laparoscopy ± salpingectomy
B. Laparoscopy ± salpingotomy
C. Methotrexate injection
D. Repeat ±hCG in 48 hours
E. Repeat ±hCG in 72 hours
F. Repeat pelvic ultrasound in 48 hours
G. Urgent laparotomy

For each of the following scenarios, select the most appropriate management decision. Each option may be used once, more than once or not at all.

1. A 32-year-old woman, who had her last menstrual period (LMP) 8 weeks ago, returns for review. She presented 2 days ago with a light per vagina bleed, but denied pain. A pelvic ultrasound scan showed an empty uterus and a 2 cm × 1.6 cm echogenic mass around the left ovary. No free fluid was seen. Her βhCG was 625 iu/L 48 hours ago. On examination today, she is non-tender with blood pressure 116/68 mmHg and pulse 80 beats/min. A repeat βhCG is 642 iu/L.

2. A 31-year-old woman presents with a 2-day history of sharp right iliac fossa pain and one episode of per vagina spotting. She is unsure of her LMP, but had a positive pregnancy test 1 month ago. Her past obstetric history is G5P3+1 (three children born by normal vaginal delivery and one left-sided ectopic 3 years ago). On examination, she has right adnexial tenderness, with blood pressure 95/55 mmHg and pulse 76 beats/min. An ultrasound scan shows an empty uterus, free fluid in the pouch of Douglas and a 4 cm dilated right fallopian tube. She has no desire to have more children.

3. A 29-year-old woman is referred from the emergency department with severe left iliac fossa pain. Her LMP was 8 weeks ago and she has a positive pregnancy test. Past obstetric history is G1P1 (normal vaginal delivery). On examination, she appears unwell, with a blood pressure of 80/42 mmHg and pulse 120 beats/min. She has left iliac fossa tenderness and cervical tenderness on vaginal examination. Pelvic ultrasound shows a left adnexal mass, obscured by free fluid, demonstrating a fetal heartbeat.

4. The 32-year-old woman in question 1 returns 4 days later. She has had some cramping lower abdominal pain with no bleeding. Blood pressure is 110/83 mmHg and pulse 75 beats/min. A repeat βhCG is 587 iu/L.

5. A 25-year-old woman presents to the emergency department with 3 days of heavy per vagina bleeding, which is now settling, and left-sided lower abdominal pain. Her LMP was 6 weeks ago. Blood pressure is 124/80 mmHg and pulse 84 beats/min. Pelvic ultrasound showed no gestational sac or pole. The βhCG was 841 iu/L initially and 631 iu/L 48 hours later.

Theme 10: Ultrasound scanning in pregnancy

Options

A. Abdominal circumference
B. Amniotic fluid volume
C. Biophysical profile
D. Biparietal diameter
E. Crown–rump length
F. Femur length
G. Nuchal translucency

For each of the following scenarios, select the most appropriate measurement. Each option may be used once, more than once or not at all.

1. The most accurate parameter for assessment of gestational age in the first trimester.

2. From 13 weeks, this is the most reliable indicator of gestational age.

3. The most sensitive parameter to assess fetal growth and detect intrauterine growth restriction.

4. An abnormality on this test may suggest poorly functioning kidneys.

5. This can provide information regarding fetal neurological status and tone.

Theme 1: Methods of delivery

There is only limited information given in these scenarios. In real situations on the labour ward, many other factors are taken into consideration, including the views and skills of the obstetrician performing the delivery.

1. E – Neville-Barnes forceps

Forceps are used to aid pushing, and are likely to be successful in this case as the baby is in a good position but the mother is tired. Forceps have two interlocking blades with a cephalic curve that fit around a baby's head. When correctly applied, they should lock together easily and not be forced. With all instrumental deliveries, a maximum of three contractions should be used to deliver the baby. If it requires more than this, then a caesarean section should be performed. The patient should have adequate analgesia (ideally a spinal or epidural), but, if this is not possible, a pudendal nerve block or local anaesthetic infiltration at the perineum can be used for non-rotational forceps. Risks of all forceps deliveries include failure to deliver (requiring caesarean section), vaginal tears and fetal trauma, including facial bruising or abrasions.

Neville-Barnes forceps have both a cephalic curve, to fit the baby's head, and a pelvic curve that follows the contours of the sacral hollow. These are used to aid delivery when rotation is not required, such as in this case where the baby is almost delivered at the occipitoanterior position but needs extra assistance.

Robert Barnes, English obstetrician (1817–1907).

2. A – Elective caesarean section

Elective caesarean sections are planned to occur before the onset of labour, but are generally not performed before 39 weeks. An elective section should be offered in certain conditions, including previous classic caesarean section, breech presentations with failed external cephalic version (see below), placenta praevia that is partially or completely obstructing the cervical os, multiple pregnancies if the first twin is not cephalic, and for reducing the risk of infection transmission from mother to child (including HIV and primary genital herpes simplex). There is no evidence that caesarean section reduces the risk of transmission of hepatitis B or C. Maternal request is not an outright indication for caesarean section: a clinician may refuse a maternal request, but must instead refer her care to another healthcare provider.

A lower segment caesarean section (LSCS) is the most common type of section, where the incision is made in the lower uterine segment following reflection of the bladder. Classic caesarean sections, where a vertical incision is made in the upper segment of the uterus, are uncommon, as there is a higher postoperative morbidity and risk of scar rupture in subsequent pregnancies.

3. B – Emergency caesarean section

Emergency caesarean sections are performed for either fetal or maternal emergencies. A decision-to-delivery time of 30 minutes has been accepted as an audit standard for response to emergencies within maternity services. It is performed for failure to progress, fetal compromise or malposition (such as in this case).

4. D – Kielland's forceps

Kielland's forceps are rotational forceps and do not have a pelvic curve, as this would damage maternal soft tissue during rotation. In this instance, rotation would be used to turn the baby to the occipitoanterior position followed by traction to deliver the baby. Such procedures are usually done in theatre so that a caesarean section could be undertaken if needed. Rotation of a baby can also be achieved manually or using a ventouse.

In ventouse deliveries, a suction cap is attached to the baby's head at a specific point before traction is commenced. A combination of traction and maternal effort can rotate the baby to an occipitoanterior position (if not in this position initially). There is an element of operator choice when determining whether forceps or ventouse is used.

Christian Kielland, Norwegian obstetrician (1871–1941).

5. F – Normal delivery

An occipitoanterior position with a flexed head is a normal presentation of a presenting part, which should deliver with no complications or additional help being needed. Vaginal delivery is not contraindicated following one section, and is known as VBAC – vaginal birth after caesarean.

External cephalic version (ECV) is where a breech fetus is manually coaxed into a cephalic presentation through the maternal abdomen. Fifty per cent of ECVs are successful, and this is dependent on race, parity, uterine tone, liquor volume, engagement of the breech and whether or not the head is palpable. ECV should be offered to nulliparous women with breech presentations from 36 weeks and multiparous women from 37 weeks. Rarely, there are complications such as placental abruption, uterine rupture and fetomaternal haemorrhage, so ECV should be performed only where monitoring facilities and immediate delivery are available. Absolute contraindications are antepartum haemorrhage in the last 7 days, an abnormal cardiotocogram (CTG), major uterine abnormality, ruptured membranes and multiple pregnancy. Relative contraindications are small-for-gestational-age babies, proteinuric pre-eclampsia, oligohydramnios, major fetal anomalies, scarred uterus and unstable lie. Rhesus anti-D antibodies are given to all rhesus-negative women. Labours with a cephalic presentation following ECV are more likely to need obstetric intervention than cephalic ones without prior ECV.

Perianal tears can happen in normal deliveries, but can be more severe with operative delivery. Often, an episiotomy (a mediolateral cut through the perineum) is performed if a tear is likely.

Tears are graded as follows:
- first degree: injury to perineal skin only
- second-degree: injury to perineum involving muscles but not the anal sphincter
- third-degree: injury to perineum involving the anal sphincter complex
  - 3a: less than 50% EAS (external anal sphincter) thickness torn
  - 3b: more than 50% EAS thickness torn
  - 3c: both EAS and IAS (internal anal sphincter) torn
- fourth-degree: injury to perineum involving anal sphincter and anal epithelium

Third- and fourth-degree tears can lead to faecal incontinence. Obstetric anal injury is seen in 1% of vaginal deliveries. Risk factors include high birth weight (>4 kg), persistent occipitoposterior position, nulliparity, induction of labour, epidural, prolonged second stage (>1 hour), shoulder dystocia, midline episiotomy and forceps delivery.

Theme 2: Urogynaecology

1. H – Physiotherapy

This woman has mixed stress incontinence and detrusor instability, illustrated by the presence of both stress (leakage on exertion) and urge (frequency and urgency) symptoms. There are many risk factors in this scenario; she is postmenopausal and has had at least one traumatic birth causing weakness of pelvic floor muscles. Her episiotomy suggests a prolonged second stage of labour. She has several comorbidities that may make her unsuitable for the general anaesthetic for colposuspension. Conservative options are therefore preferable in the first instance. The physiotherapist will introduce the patient to a bladder drill, to gradually increase the time between voids with training. A ring pessary may also be appropriate to support the anterior vaginal wall prolapse. It is best to treat detrusor instability before considering surgery, as this can further worsen stress symptoms.

James Marion Sims, American gynaecologist (1813–83).

2. C – Hormone replacement therapy

This woman has genuine stress incontinence (GSI), which accounts for 50% of cases of incontinence in females. Stress incontinence is an involuntary loss of urine that occurs when the bladder pressure exceeds the minimum urethral pressure in the absence of detrusor muscle contraction (e.g. when coughing and laughing). Stress incontinence can be diagnosed confidently only once detrusor instability has been excluded by cystometry. On examination, a cystocele or urethrocele may be noted. Factors that weaken the pelvic floor and lead to GSI include pregnancy, vaginal delivery (especially prolonged labour or forceps use), multiparity, prolapse and previous pelvic floor surgery. GSI also becomes more common after the menopause as the supportive connective tissue around the pelvic floor begins to atrophy with the hypo-oestrogenic state. Topical vaginal preparations of hormone replacement, such as oestrogen cream, or a pessary may help.

Cystometry is an investigation used to measure detrusor pressures as the bladder is filled and 'provoked' with coughing. Transducers are placed in the rectum (to measure abdominal pressure) and the bladder (to measure intravesical pressure). Detrusor activity is calculated by subtracting the abdominal pressure from the bladder pressure. Normally, detrusor activity should not alter with filling or provocation. Involuntary detrusor contraction suggests detrusor instability. If leakage occurs in the absence of detrusor contraction, GSI is diagnosed. It is important to note that both GSI and detrusor instability can cause urgency followed by incontinence – only cystometry can distinguish between the two.

3. F – Oxybutynin

Detrusor instability (or urge incontinence) occurs as an involuntary loss of urine caused by uninhibited detrusor contractions. It accounts for 35% of female incontinence. Risk factors include previous surgery, multiple sclerosis and advancing age, although most cases are idiopathic. A urinary tract infection must be excluded. The diagnosis of detrusor instability is made by cystometry, which shows detrusor contraction on filling or provocation. Conservative management is the mainstay of treatment. Physiotherapists can educate patients about urgency control and relaxation strategies. In those who do not find this effective, anticholinergic drugs may prove effective (by causing relaxation of the bladder smooth muscle). Examples of anticholinergics include oxybutynin, solifenacin and tolteridone. Side-effects of anticholinergics include headache and a dry mouth. Desmopressin is a synthetic antidiuretic hormone that reduces urine production and is particularly useful for nocturnal symptoms.

4. D – Indwelling catheter

Overflow incontinence is characterized by frequent involuntary loss of small volumes of urine precipitated by a change in posture. Symptoms of hesitancy and sensation of incomplete emptying are common. Leakage occurs when intravesical pressure exceeds intraurethral pressure. Examination shows evidence of chronic urinary retention and suspicion of a pelvic mass (which may be the underlying cause of the retention). A catheter should be inserted to empty the bladder, and a long-term catheter may be needed if a trial without catheter fails. The woman in this scenario is not a candidate for intermittent self-catheterization (ISC), as she would struggle with the intricacy of the procedure (being elderly with severe arthritis). Compared with a long-term indwelling catheter, ISC has a lower risk of infection, bladder spasm and erosion, and is used when the cause of chronic retention is irreversible, e.g. neurological disease, diabetes or stroke.

5. I – Total abdominal hysterectomy

This woman has severe symptoms of stress incontinence and has not benefited from conservative measures. Because she also has fibroids and is desperate for intervention, it is appropriate to book her in for a hysterectomy (after appropriate counselling). Consent for the operation should discuss pain, bleeding, infection, thromboembolism and damage to the internal organs requiring repair. She may even be suitable for vaginal hysterectomy, which reduces hospital stay and associated morbidity.

There are many interventions available to help manage genuine stress incontinence. Transvaginal tape is a minimally invasive procedure performed under general or spinal anaesthetic for stress incontinence. A midurethral 'sling', or mesh tape, is inserted to limit urethral descent, provide support to the pubourethral ligaments and reinforce the anterior vaginal wall. An anterior repair is used to treat a cystocele by removing excess tissue from the anterior wall of the vaginal. It is a good operation for repair of symptoms associated with the cystocele, but has a high failure rate for genuine stress incontinence. Colposuspension is an abdominal procedure performed under general anaesthetic. Sutures are placed lateral to the bladder neck and are then sutured to the iliopectineal ligament, or the symphysis pubis. This acts to 'hitch up' the sagging bladder neck to improve continence. Periurethral injectables are injected paraurethrally to bulk up the sphincter and prevent involuntary urinary loss. They are done under local anaesthetic and require 'booster' injections. Short-term benefit rates of periurethral injectables are good.

Theme 3: Drugs in pregnancy

1. K – Propylthiouracil

The incidence of maternal hyperthyroidism is approximately 1 in 500 pregnancies. It usually predates pregnancy and 90% of cases are secondary to Graves' disease. Other causes include toxic nodular goitres and a hydatidiform mole. Graves' disease is an autoimmune disorder due to circulating thyroid-stimulating antibodies. The diagnosis in pregnancy is difficult, as many symptoms frequently occur in pregnancy, such as tachycardia, heat intolerance and a cardiac flow murmur. High levels of thyroid-stimulating antibodies can cross the placenta, causing fetal thyrotoxicosis; however, this is rare as IgG transfer is limited. Thyrotoxicosis in pregnancy can cause atrial fibrillation, abdominal pain, vomiting, diarrhoea and psychosis. There is a higher risk of pre-eclampsia, miscarriage, preterm labour and low birth weight.

The treatment of choice is either carbimazole or propylthiouracil (of the two, propylthiouracil is preferred, as it passes into breast milk less readily). These can be continued into pregnancy at the lowest dose required to keep free thyroxine (T_4) levels at the upper limit of normal, and to reduce the risk of fetal hypothyroidism as a side-effect. Women who remain euthyroid for 4 weeks can sometimes stop medication under close monitoring. However, some remain unstable and require hospital admission. Serial ultrasound scans are performed to assess fetal growth. Radioactive iodine is contraindicated in pregnancy.

2. J – Promethazine

Eighty per cent of women suffer vomiting during pregnancy, but less than 2% of women go on to develop hyperemesis gravidarum. Hyperemesis gravidarum describes intractable vomiting that can lead to severe dehydration, metabolic disturbance and electrolyte imbalance, including hyponatraemia, hypokalaemia, ketonuria, raised transaminases and transient thyrotoxicosis.

First-line management includes oral antiemetics, such as promethazine (an antihistamine), reducing fatty or spicy food intake and temporarily stopping iron supplements. However, when there is evidence of dehydration due to intolerance of oral fluids or significant ketonuria, hospital admission is required. Patients should remain nil-by-mouth until vomiting settles, while intravenous fluid resuscitation is given with additional antiemetics, e.g. metoclopramide (dopamine antagonist) and ondansetron (a 5-HT$_3$ receptor antagonist), on discussion with a senior. Thiamine (vitamin B$_1$) supplements are also given to reduce the risk of Wernicke's encephalopathy.

Thalidomide was prescribed for morning sickness in the late 1950s and early 1960s, until it was found to be associated with severe birth anomalies. The most characteristic deformity associated with maternal thalidomide use is phocomelia, a shortening or absence of the long bones. In the most extreme cases, all four limbs are affected, so the hands and feet appear directly attached to the body (tetraphocomelia).

Phocomelia, from Greek *phoco* = seal + *melos* = limb.

Hyperemesis gravidarum, from Greek *hyper* = excessive + *emeticos* = vomit and Latin *gravida* = pregnant.

Carl Wernicke, German neurologist (1848–1905).

3. M – Ursodeoxycholic acid

Pruritus in pregnancy is common (around 20% of pregnancies), but the prevalence of itching due to abnormal liver function tests (LFTs) is less than 1%. In obstetric cholestasis, bile acids accumulate in the blood, causing jaundice and pruritus. There is a 90% recurrence rate in pregnancy, and 35% have a positive family history. Itching typically involves the palms and soles, but can affect the whole body. It is important to rule out other causes of jaundice and pruritus, including hepatitis and gallstones. Screening blood tests include LFTs, bile acids, clotting screen, anti-smooth muscle antibody, anti-mitochondrial antibody and viral serology (hepatitis viruses, Epstein–Barr virus and cytomegalovirus). In obstetric cholestasis, transaminases, bile acids, alkaline phosphatase and bilirubin may all be raised.

Treatment includes chlorphenamine (an antihistamine) for pruritus and topical emollients. The lack of bile salts in the gut results in malabsorption of fat-soluble vitamins, including vitamin K, increasing the risk of postpartum haemorrhage and fetal intracranial bleeds. Oral vitamin K supplements are therefore required. Ursodeoxycholic acid, although not licensed for use in pregnancy, has been found to reduce accumulation of bile acids and relieve pruritus. It is important to treat obstetric cholestasis, as there is a risk of premature birth (60%), fetal distress (30%) and intrauterine death by acute anoxia (2%).

4. D – Doxycycline

Doxycycline is not safe in pregnancy. It is one of the tetracyclines, which are known to deposit in bones and teeth, delaying their growth. Breastfeeding mothers should also avoid doxycyline, as there is the additional side-effect of staining the baby's teeth. Erythromycin, a macrolide, is a suitable alternative for pregnant or breastfeeding women. It is also the antibiotic of choice in premature rupture of membranes, as there is evidence that it may delay delivery and reduce maternal and neonatal infective morbidity.

5. C – Diclofenac

Diclofenac, a non-steroidal anti-inflammatory drug, is often very effective for the pain experienced after a caesarean section. It should be avoided in late pregnancy, as it may cause premature closure of the ductus arteriosus. Diclofenac is the second-line analgesic after paracetamol, which is safe to administer during pregnancy. Codeine has recently been withdrawn from use in breastfeeding women due to cases of neonatal respiratory depression.

Theme 4: Perimenopausal hormones

The menopause is defined as the permanent cessation of menstruation due to failure of ovarian follicular development in the presence of adequate gonadotropin stimulation. The diagnosis is made retrospectively after 12 months of amenorrhoea. The average age of the menopause in the UK is 50.5 years. Premature menopause is diagnosed in those below 40 years, and can be a result of oophorectomy or radiotherapy. The perimenopausal period, or climacteric, is of variable duration as the menstrual cycle lengthens and anovulation ensues.

The symptoms attributed to the menopause are largely due to oestrogen deficiency. Immediate effects of the menopause include vasomotor symptoms (hot flushes, night sweats, sleep disturbance, palpitations and dizziness) and psychological symptoms (low mood, irritability, poor memory and loss of libido). Intermediate effects, which take a couple of years to develop, are atrophy of the vagina and vulva ($\rightarrow$ atrophic vaginitis, manifesting in dryness, itching and dyspareunia), of pelvic tissues ($\rightarrow$ prolapse) and of the urethral epithelium ($\rightarrow$ dysuria, frequency and urgency). There is a 30% reduction in skin collagen. Long-term effects of the menopause include osteoporosis with subsequent pathological fracture (common sites include the distal radius, femoral neck and vertebrae), and an increase in the risk of atherosclerotic cardiovascular disease.

1. A – 17β-Estradiol

Prior to the menopause, 17β-estradiol is the main oestrogen secreted by the ovaries. This is broken down into oestrone, and then oestriol. Gradually, the ovaries become resistant to gonadotropins, so gonadotropin levels become high, which can be measured to confirm the menopause.

2. E – Oestrone

After the menopause, the majority of the body's oestrone is produced in peripheral fat.

3. B – Androstenedione

Oestrone is produced from the androgen androstenedione by the adrenal cortex (70%) and the ovary (30%). Obese women produce more oestrone in the peripheral adipose tissue, which is unopposed by progesterone, and are therefore more at risk of endometrial hyperplasia and endometrial adenocarcinoma.

4. F – Progesterone

During the perimenopausal period, 60% of cycles remain ovulatory. This can be measured by luteal phase progesterone (day 21 of the cycle, or 7 days before menstruation in longer cycles). In the 6 months prior to the menopause, progesterone levels indicative of ovulation occur in 5% of cycles. The estradiol produced by ovarian follicles at this time is insufficient to cause a mid-cycle surge of luteinizing hormone, but is enough to cause some endometrial proliferation.

5. F – Progesterone

The lack of the modifying effect of luteal phase progesterone allows the endometrium to break down, resulting in heavy and irregular bleeding.

Theme 5: Acute pelvic pain

1. L – Torsion of ovarian cyst

Ovarian cysts are fluid-filled sacs that can grow to become as large as a grapefruit. The majority are benign and occur at child-bearing age. Women with ovarian cysts may complain of dull, intermittent, aching pains in the lower abdomen. The woman in this scenario, who has a negative pregnancy test, presents with sudden-onset severe, unilateral, colicky pain with shock. This history indicates torsion of an ovarian cyst. The pain may be intermittent if torsion is incomplete. Vomiting is usual, and tachycardia, hypotension and pyrexia are found on examination. A delay in diagnosis can lead to irreversible ischaemia of the ovary. An urgent laparoscopy is needed and a cystectomy should be performed, although signs of ischaemia or necrosis warrant oophorectomy.

2. J – Pelvic inflammatory disease

Pelvic inflammatory disease describes inflammation of the pelvic organs via sexually transmitted ascending infection from the genital tracts (although some cases occur following descending infections from local organs, such as the appendix). It is most common in 18–25 year olds, with chlamydial infection (50%), gonorrhoea (14%) and bacterial vaginosis being the commonest underlying causes. Risk factors include unprotected sexual intercourse, insertion of intrauterine devices and smoking. Patients present with constant abdominal pain, deep dyspareunia, postcoital or irregular bleeding, menorrhagia or dysmenorrhoea, and a purulent discharge. Women with active infection are systemically unwell with fever, vomiting, anorexia and malaise. On examination, there is lower abdominal tenderness, cervical excitation, tenderness on pelvic examination and pyrexia. A urine sample and high vaginal and endocervical swabs must be taken. Treatment is with appropriate antibiotics (e.g. doxycycline and metronidazole), analgesia, contact tracing and admission to hospital in severe cases. Complications of PID include tubo-ovarian abscess, Fitz-Hugh–Curtis syndrome (perihepatitis leading to perihepatic adhesions), tubal infertility, ectopic pregnancy and chronic pelvic pain.

3. F – Incomplete miscarriage

Miscarriage is the most common complication of pregnancy. It is defined as the loss of pregnancy before 24 weeks. Underlying causes and risk factors of miscarriage include fetal abnormality (50%), infection ('TORCH'), increasing maternal age, maternal illness (diabetes, renal disease), abnormal uterine cavity (intrauterine contraceptive device insertion, congenital septum), antiphospholipid syndrome and intervention (amniocentesis and chorionic villus sampling). Note that exercise, intercourse and emotional trauma *do not* cause miscarriage. Investigation into the underlying cause of miscarriage is performed only if three miscarriages have occurred.

The woman in this scenario has had an *incomplete miscarriage*. This is where some fetal material has been passed, but some products of conception are retained in the uterus (these are visible on ultrasound scanning). The cervical os remains open until all the products have passed (whether that be spontaneous, or with medical or surgical assistance). A *complete miscarriage* is when the mother has experienced bleeding, all the fetal tissue has been passed, there are no products of conception on scanning and the cervical os is closed. In these cases, patients do not required further hospital follow-up. A *threatened miscarriage* is when there is bleeding before 24 weeks, but the fetus is still alive and the cervical os is closed on examination. Only 25% of threatened miscarriages eventually miscarry. An *inevitable miscarriage* describes the scenario where there is bleeding before 24 weeks and the cervical os is dilated. The fetus may still be alive, but miscarriage *will* occur. Finally, a *missed miscarriage* (also known as a delayed or silent miscarriage) is when the fetus dies *in utero* and the cervix stays closed. There may or may not be bleeding in this case.

4. E – Ectopic pregnancy

An ectopic pregnancy is implantation of the embryo outside the uterine cavity, most commonly in the fallopian tube (but it can also happen in the cornua of the uterus, cervix, ovary or abdominal cavity). Ectopics are becoming increasingly common in the UK, with an incidence of 1 in 300 pregnancies. Fifty per cent occur in those with no predisposing risks, but risk factors include pelvic inflammatory disease, previous tubal surgery, previous ectopic pregnancy, assisted reproductive techniques, endometriosis, intrauterine contraceptive device and use of the progesterone-only pill. Presentation is variable and should be suspected in women of child-bearing age with amenorrhoea, abnormal bleeding, and abdominal pain, which can be associated with dizziness, fainting, shoulder pain or collapse. On examination, there is acute abdominal pain with cervical excitation or tender adnexae in a shocked patient. Transvaginal and abdominal ultrasound scans are needed. Management can be medical (methotrexate) or surgical, depending on the scan result, and serial measurements of the human chorionic gonadotropin β-subunit (βhCG) are used to monitor progression. Rhesus D-negative women should be given anti-D antibodies.

Mittelschmerz is a sudden-onset, cramping pelvic pain (midline or unilateral) that occurs at the time of ovulation (day 14). It is more common in teenagers and older women. Persistent mittelschmerz may respond to the combined oral contraceptive pill, as this suppresses ovulation. *Corpus luteum cysts* are usually found in women with irregular cycles or those with amenorrhoea followed by heavy vaginal bleeding. Enlarged or haemorrhagic corpus luteum cysts are the commonest cause of pain in early pregnancy. These are found on ultrasound scan, and are managed conservatively.

Mittelschmerz, from German *mittel* = middle + *schmerz* = pain ('pain that occurs mid-cycle').

Cornua, from Latin *cornu* = horn (as in a musical instrument).

5. A – Acute appendicitis

This patient presents with anorexia, malaise, nausea and abdominal pain that starts centrally and localizes to the right iliac fossa. There is a low-grade pyrexia, tachycardia, localized tenderness and peritonism. This history is strongly suggestive of acute appendicitis. Blood tests would indicate increased white blood cells and inflammatory markers. Urgent general surgical referral for appendicectomy is required. An appendix mass forms when the omentum and bowel surround an inflamed appendix to wall it off. Patients with an appendix mass will have had several days of localized pain and pyrexia with a palpable mass in the right iliac fossa (confirmed with an ultrasound or CT scan). Management is with fluids, analgesia and antibiotics, with consideration of appendicectomy after 6–8 weeks. An appendix abscess is a collection of pus associated with appendicitis. Drainage can be open or ultrasound/CT guided, with antibiotics.

Theme 6: Gametogenesis

1. F – Primordial germ cell

2. K – Spermatozoa

3. I – Spermatid

4. E – Primary spermatocyte

5. C – Polar body

Spermatogenesis occurs when the adult male reaches puberty. It occurs under the influence of testosterone. The whole process of spermatogenesis takes 64 days. Primordial germ cells divide by mitosis and differentiate into spermatogonia, which lie immediately beneath the basement membrane of seminiferous tubules. As spermatogenesis progresses, the germ cells move from the basement membrane into the lumen of the seminiferous tubules. Spermatogonia divide by mitotis and differentiate into primary spermatocytes. Primary spermatocytes contain 46 double-structured chromosomes. These divide by meiosis. The primary spermatocytes initially complete the first meiotic division to give secondary spermatocytes. Secondary spermatocytes therefore contain 23 double-structured chromosomes, which complete the second meiotic division to give spermatids. Spermatids contain 23 single chromosomes. Spermatids undergo spermiogenesis (below) to give spermatozoa.

In summary, every *primary spermatocyte* eventually gives rise to *four spermatid daughter cells*, two with 22 + X chromosomes and two with 22 + Y chromosomes. Spermatozoa are the end-product of spermatogenesis. They have undergone spermiogenesis, which is the process by which spermatids differentiate into the distinctly shaped spermatozoa. Spermatozoa are made up of a head (within which the nucleus lies) capped by the acrosome (containing hydrolytic enzymes), a middle piece that provides power for swimming (generated by large helical mitochondria) and a tail (the propulsion system made up of microtubules).

Oogenesis begins in females during intrauterine life and is a slow process, with many stages of division being arrested for long periods of time. It is more complicated than the male pathway, although the same principles are followed. Primordial germ cells are present in the wall of the yolk sac at the end of the third week of embryological development. They migrate by amoeboid movement to the developing gonads, where they arrive by the beginning of the fifth week. They then divide by mitosis and differentiate into oogonia. Oogonia differentiate into primary oocytes and become surrounded by follicular (epithelial) cells. These are collectively named *primordial follicles*. Primary oocytes contain 46 double-structured chromosomes and enter prophase of meiosis I. Division is arrested at the dictyotene phase of meiosis I, and the first meiotic division is completed only with the pre-ovulatory luteinizing hormone (LH)/follicle-stimulating hormone (FSH) surge to give a secondary oocyte and a polar body. The polar body is merely a useless by-product, which subsequently degenerates.

Secondary oocyte and polar bodies both contain 23 double-structured chromosomes. Meiosis I of the secondary oocyte is completed with the pre-ovulatory LH/FSH surge, but further division of the secondary oocyte occurs only if fertilization occurs. With fertilization, the secondary oocyte divides by meiosis II to give a mature oocyte and a further polar body. The mature oocyte and its polar body both contain 23 single chromosomes. The initial polar body also undergoes meiosis II to give a further two polar bodies, both containing 23 single chromosomes.

Primary oocytes therefore eventually give rise to four daughter cells, all of which contain 22 + X chromosomes. However, only one of these is a mature oocyte, the remaining three daughter cells being polar bodies.

Theme 7: Sexually transmitted infections 2

Remember, if anyone presents with an STI, they are at risk of carrying further infections.

1. C – Chancroid

Chancroid is caused by the Gram-negative bacterium *Haemophilus ducreyi*, and is found mostly in tropical countries. It is an ulcerative condition of the genitalia (single/multiple painful superficial ulcers) and develops within a week of exposure. Inflammation may lead to a phimosis. Enlargement and suppuration of inguinal lymph nodes may occur, leading to a unilocular abscess (bubo) that can rupture to form a sinus. Treatment is with appropriate antibiotics (e.g. erythromycin).

2. D – Chlamydia

Chlamydia is caused by the oculogenital serovars D–K of *Chlamydia trachomatis*. Infection tends to be asymptomatic, although there can be increased vaginal discharge, dysuria and urinary frequency. Ascending infection can cause salpingitis and, if it enters the abdominal cavity, perihepatitis (Fitz-Hugh–Curtis syndrome), which leads to right upper quadrant pain and tenderness. Chlamydial infection is a major cause of infertility and increases the possibility of ectopic pregnancy. In males, symptoms include mucopurulent discharge and dysuria (asymptomatic in 25%). Epididymo-orchitis is a complication. Diagnosis of chlamydia infection is by urine antigen detection or vaginal swab culture. Treatment is with doxycycline.

Chlamydia, from Greek *chlamys* = cloak (as chlamydia is often 'cloaked', i.e. asymptomatic).

Thomas Fitz-Hugh Jr, American physician (1894–1963).

Arthur Curtis, American gynaecologist (1881–1955).

3. A – Bacterial vaginosis

Bacterial vaginosis (BV) is not an STI. It is an infection caused by mixed anaerobic flora (e.g. *Gardnerella* spp. and *Mycoplasma hominis*). It is often asymptomatic, but can cause a creamy-grey discharge with a fishy odour. There is no itching. The risk of preterm delivery and late miscarriage is doubled if BV is present in early pregnancy; however, treatment with antibiotics (metronidazole) does not reduce the perinatal risks, and so should be used only in symptomatic women.

4. Q – Syphilis (specifically secondary syphilis)

This woman has had a painless ulcer followed by systemic symptoms (fever, malaise, headache and skin rash). This history is indicative of secondary syphilis. For more information about syphilis, see 'Sexually transmitted infections 1' (Paper 1 Answers, Theme 4, page 16).

5. P – Scabies

Scabies is caused by the mite *Sarcoptes scabiei*, which burrows into the skin, where the female lays her eggs. Scabies is often an STI, but can be spread throughout households. Patients develop an intense itch, which is worse at night. This is caused by an allergic response to the eggs. The burrows made by the mite tend to be symmetrical and affect finger webs, sides of digits, flexor surfaces of wrists and the penis. Secondary infection of affected areas can occur. Immunocompromised patients can develop a more severe infestation, with thick hyperkeratotic crusting on affected areas. This is known as Norwegian scabies (first described in Norway in 1848 – it was originally thought to be a distant variant of leprosy).

Scabies, from Latin *scabere* = to scratch.

Genital herpes is caused by the DNA-containing herpes simplex virus (HSV) types 1 and 2. The infection remains prevalent due to asymptomatic shedding of the virus. Clinical features of primary infection include dysuria with painful, itchy lesions and occasionally urethral or vaginal discharge. Patients may also complain of constitutional symptoms (fever, headache, malaise and myalgia). Lesions are papular, vesicular or pustular; these crust and heal within 4 weeks. Examination may reveal inguinal lymphadenitis. HSV remains dormant in dorsal root ganglia, and reactivation occurs in 75% of cases. Recurrent attacks tend to be milder, shorter and not associated with systemic features. Diagnosis is by viral swabs. Severe infections can be managed with aciclovir.

Genital warts are most commonly caused by human papillomavirus (HPV) types 6b and 11. Incubation is normally about 3 months, but warts may take up to 2 years to develop. When large warts coalesce, the appearance is known as condylomata acuminata. Genital warts increase in size during pregnancy, and wart-induced obstruction may be an indication for caesarean section. Management options include excision, cautery and caustic agents (podophyllin or imiquimod).

Condylomata acuminata, from Latin *condylomata* = knuckles + *acuminatum* = pointed.

Theme 8: Twins

1. A – Dizygotic dichorionic diamniotic

Dizygotics are the commonest type of twins (60%). They develop due to fertilization of two different ova, from the same or opposite ovaries, by two different sperm, and are therefore not identical. They can be of different sexes and are no more genetically similar than siblings would be. They are *always* dichorionic and diamniotic, which means that each fetus has its own chorion, amnion and placenta. Options B (dizygotic dichorionic monoamniotic) and C (dizygotic monochorionic monoamniotic) are nonsense!

2. F – Monozygotic monochorionic monoamniotic

Monozygotic twins result from the mitotic division of a single fertilized ovum (zygote) into identical twins. They may or may not share the same chorion and amnion, depending on when the mitotic division occurs. Monozygotic monochorionic monoamniotic twins occur rarely when the mitotic division occurs after 8 days. If this occurs prior to the formation of the primitive streak, there will be a single amniotic cavity and chorion. If the division occurs after primitive streak formation, conjoined (Siamese) twins develop.

The term 'Siamese twins' comes from a famous pair of conjoined twins in the nineteenth century, Chang and Eng Bunker, who travelled the world with the circus. They were born in Siam (now Thailand).

3. E – Monozygotic monochorionic diamniotic

Monozygotic monochorionic diamniotic twins result if division occurs between 4 and 7 days (during formation of the inner cell mass). There is a single placenta but, if the amnion has not developed, each fetus will have its own amniotic membrane.

4. A – Dizygotic dichorionic diamniotic

5. D – Monozygotic dichorionic dizygotic

Monozygotic dichorionic dizygotic twins result if the division occurs at less than 3 days after fertilization (at the 'eight-cell' stage). The two embryos implant at separate sites and have a separate chorion, amnion and placenta. They will have the same structural appearance *in utero* as dizygotic twins do, but will be identical.

The incidence of twins is 1 in 100, and of triplets 1 in 1000. Predisposing factors are increasing maternal age and parity, personal or family history, race, and assisted conception (20% of in vitro fertilization (IVF) pregnancies are multiple). Multiple pregnancies need closer monitoring, as fetal and maternal mortality and morbidity is greater. The mother has a greater risk of hyperemesis, miscarriage, hypertension and pre-eclampsia, gestational diabetes, polyhydramnios (especially with monozygotics), anaemia, antepartum and postpartum haemorrhages, and placenta praevia. The fetal risks include increased perinatal mortality, increased congenital abnormality, preterm labour, placental insufficiency or intrauterine growth restriction (especially in monozygotics), malpresentation, twin-to-twin transfusion and vanishing twin syndrome. *Twin-to-twin transfusion* is where, due to anastomosis of vessels in the single placental mass of a monochorionic twin pregnancy, one twin gains at the other's expense. One twin becomes anaemic, hypovolaemic, oligohydramniotic and growth-restricted while the other one develops polycythaemia, hypervolaemia, polyuria and polyhydramnios. Laser ablation of placental vessels can be useful, although there are risks of fetal demise or congenital abnormalities. *Vanishing twin syndrome* is where a fetus in a multiple-gestation pregnancy dies *in utero* and is subsequently reabsorbed by the mother (either partially or completely).

The delivery of twins requires special management. If the first twin is cephalic, a trial of labour is normally attempted regardless of the presentation of the second twin, but there is no definitive evidence comparing vaginal delivery with caesarean section. If the first twin is breech or transverse lie, a caesarean section is indicated. Problems with delivery include cord prolapse, entanglement or knotting, locking, postpartum haemorrhage, thrombosis, fetal distress (especially in the second twin), and inefficient uterine activity after the first twin has been delivered.

Theme 9: Ectopic pregnancy

An ectopic pregnancy is one where the fertilized ovum implants in any tissue other than the uterus. The 'other tissue' is most commonly the fallopian tube, but other sites include the ovary, cervix and abdomen. The incidence of ectopic pregnancy is around 11 per 1000 pregnancies. Patients present with abdominal pain and vaginal bleeding. Initial investigations include a urinary pregnancy test and pelvic ultrasound, followed by a serum βhCG. Management depends upon the clinical state of the patient and her future fertility wishes.

'Ectopic' from Greek *ek* = away from + *topos* = place, i.e. in the wrong place.

All of the following options should be preceded by discussion with a senior doctor.

1. C – Methotrexate injection

This patient has been managed expectantly with 48-hour follow-up because she is clinically stable. The ultrasound scan suggests an ectopic pregnancy in the left ovary, but there is no evidence of rupture, as she is haemodynamically stable and there is no free fluid in the pelvis (free fluid would suggest bleeding). Her serum βhCG has plateaued, which suggests an ectopic pregnancy rather than an intrauterine pregnancy (levels expected to double) or a miscarriage (levels fall).

Medical managment with methotrexate is indicated when:
- The patient is clinically stable with no evidence of active bleeding
- The βhCG is <3000 iu/L (this is the upper limit given by the Royal College of Obstetricians and Gynaecologists, as research has shown higher levels to be associated with more complications and a reduced quality of life due to longer follow-up)
- The ectopic pregnancy is <3 cm diameter on ultrasound or at laparoscopy

Methotrexate is an antimetabolite (a folic acid antagonist) that prevents fetal growth by intefering with DNA synthesis. It is often administered as a single intramuscular injection and the dose is calculated according to body surface area (50 mg/m^2). Serum βhCG is checked on days 4 and 7 post-injection. A 15% drop between these levels is required; otherwise, a second dose is given.

2. A – Laparoscopy ± salpingectomy

There is a purposeful omission of the serum βhCG result in this scenario, as the clinical and radiological findings are sufficient to require a laparoscopy ± proceed to salpingectomy/salpingotomy ('salping-, from Greek *salpinx* = trumpet or tube – describing the shape of the fallopian tube). (This patient's βhCG level was in fact 5131 iu/L.) There is a 20-fold increased risk of ectopic pregnancy in patients who have had one previously. Patients require complete counselling regarding salpingotomy (removal of the ectopic with attempted preservation of the tube) and salpingectomy (removal of tube containing the ectopic). This patient is likely to be a candidate for salpingectomy as her fallopian tube is dilated and therefore damaged. She also may have completed her family. Salpingectomy is found to have a lower postoperative risk of bleeding and fewer incidences of persistent trophoblastic tissue (i.e. unsuccesful removal of ectopic). Salpingotomy is preferable in women who desire future fertility and who have a damaged or absent contralateral tube. It can, however, be a more complicated operation.

Gabriele Fallopio, Italian anatomist (1523–62).

3. G – Urgent laparotomy

This woman requires an emergency laparotomy due to haemodynamic instability and a live, bleeding ectopic pregnancy. Definitive management should, as always, be preceded by ABC. Assess the airway, give oxygen, assess breathing. Insert two large-bore cannulae and take bloods, including a Group & Save blood sample. Start intravenous fluids. Inform your registrar, the on-call anaesthetist and theatre. Experienced surgeons may attempt laparoscopy, but the aim is rapid cessation of bleeding.

4. C – Methotrexate injection

She is still stable with acceptable, but plateaued, βhCG levels. The required 15% fall in βhCG has not been reached (the actual drop here is from 642 to 587 iu/L, or 9%). In these cases (around 15%), a second dose of methotrexate is required. The cramping abdominal pains are likely to be a side-effect of methotrexate (others include conjunctivitis, gastrointestinal upset and stomatitis). Monitoring should continue as described in Case 1 (above), unless there is a clinical indication for intervention. If the second dose of methotrexate is ineffective, she will need surgery. Pregnancy should be avoided for 3 months after methotrexate, and patients should strictly abstain from intercourse until treatment is finished.

5. D – Repeat βhCG in 48 hours

In this case, no mass or free fluid could be seen on ultrasound, and the βhCG results are falling satisfactorily with expectant managment. She can therefore continue with observation by repeating βhCG in 48 hours. Weekly βhCG tests are then taken until levels are <50 iu/L.

Theme 10: Ultrasound scanning in pregnancy

Ultrasonography is an important investigative tool throughout pregnancy that is safe for mother and baby. Abdominal and transvaginal scans are used to assess the uterus and its contents, and the adnexae if necessary to exclude pathology.

1. E – Crown–rump length

An ultrasound scan is the most widely used technique for determination of gestational age. Women are booked for a 'dating' scan before 15 weeks in order to accurately determine gestational age, fetal viability, fetal number and evidence of gross abnormality. This scan is important, as gestation is difficult to calculate accurately beyond 30 weeks. Measurement of the crown–rump length (CRL) is the most accurate measurement of gestational age in the first trimester.

2. D – Biparietal diameter

As the fetus grows, it becomes more flexed in shape. Rather than using CRL, the biparietal diameter (BPD) becomes a more reliable indicator of gestational age from 13 weeks. Nuchal translucency is an effective screening tool for Down's syndrome and is performed at 10–13 weeks. Nuchal translucency measures the lymphatic fluid that has accumulated under the skin at the back of the neck. An increased thickness of this fluid is an indicator of risk of chromosomal abnormality.

3. A – Abdominal circumference

The fetal normality scan (or '20-week scan') is a detailed structural scan performed to detect abnormality. If anomalies are detected, it allows time for parents to make difficult decisions. BPD, head circumference (HC) and femur length (FL) are mandatory measurements. Abdominal circumference (AC) is optional, but is an accurate predictor of intrauterine growth restriction. Ninety per cent of congenital anomalies occur without risk factors, so screening is crucial. The fetal normality scan examines the following:

- head shape and contents: hydrocephalus, anencephaly
- spinal cord: spina bifida
- abdominal shape and contents: exomphalos, gastroschisis
- kidneys and renal pelvis: horseshoe kidney, hydronephrosis
- a four-chamber cardiac view: congenital heart defects
- arms and legs: dwarfism, osteogenesis imperfecta, talipes
- face and lips: cleft lip and palate

4. B – Amniotic fluid volume

Fetal growth scans are undertaken at varying intervals during pregnancy in the third trimester. They may be requested because of suspicion of growth abnormality, such as to detect babies who are small or large for dates, or as monitoring in certain conditions, such as pre-eclampsia or diabetes. Serial scans may be done to monitor growth. Fetal growth scans confirm dates, assess presentation and lie, locate the placental site, and measure biparietal diameter, head circumference, femur length and abdominal circumference. These scans also measure amniotic fluid volume. After 20 weeks, the main source of amniotic fluid is fetal urine (amniotic fluid is cleared by fetal swallowing). Disruption to these mechanisms can alter amniotic fluid volume. Insufficient amniotic fluid (oligohydramnios), if detected after week 12, can be caused by ruptured membranes, fetal kidney abnormalities (polycystic kidneys or renal agenesis) or placental insufficiency. Excess amniotic fluid (polyhydramnios) usually occurs in the third trimester, and is associated with diabetes, macrosomia, problems with fetal swallowing (oesophageal atresia) and multiple pregnancies. The volume is assessed by measuring the deepest pool of liquor that does not contain limbs or cord.

5. C – Biophysical profile

The biophysical profile is an assessment of fetal well-being. It is affected by factors suppressing the fetal central nervous system, such as hypoxia, infection and medication. The assessments look at fetal breathing (which should occur at least once every 30 minutes), fetal movement (at least three should be seen in 30 minutes) and amniotic fluid volume (a 2 cm diameter pool should be seen). A fetal 'non-stress' test is also done, to look for normal accelerations in fetal heart rate in association with movement. This gives reassurance that the fetus is not acidotic or neurologically depressed.

Doppler ultrasound is used to measure the velocity of blood flow during the cardiac cycle in the fetoplacental and uteroplacental circulation. The umbilical artery waveforms are the most reliable in predicting fetal well-being. They give information about vascular resistance in downstream peripheral vessels, such as that which occurs within the placenta. The most useful observation is the absence or reversal of end-diastolic flow, suggesting progressive fetal deterioration.

Theme 1: Abdominal pain

Options

A. Appendicitis
B. Constipation
C. Diabetic ketoacidosis
D. Gastroenteritis
E. Inflammatory bowel disease
F. Intussusception
G. Mesenteric adenitis
H. Mittelschmerz
I. Pancreatitis
J. Pneumonia
K. Urinary tract infection

For each of the following children presenting with abdominal pain, select the most likely diagnosis. Each option may be used once, more than once or not at all.

1. A 4-year-old girl presents to the emergency department with abdominal pain, located in the right loin and flank. She has vomited on two occasions in the last 24 hours, but her mother denies her vomiting up blood. Her temperature is 39.5°C.

2. A 2-year-old boy presents to the emergency department with abdominal pain. For the last 24 hours, he has been screaming and grabbing his abdomen. The episodes last for 15–30 minutes, during which he looks pale and is inconsolable. He then settles for a further 15–30 minutes before the pain starts again.

3. A 5-year-old boy presents to the emergency department with abdominal pain. He has been complaining of central abdominal pain for 24 hours. On examination, he is tender in the right iliac fossa and has a temperature of 37.6°C.

4. A 5-year-old boy presents with abdominal pain. He has had a slight fever and a sore throat for 24 hours and, since this morning, he has complained of central abdominal pain. Examination in the emergency department reveals tenderness throughout the abdomen and pharyngitis. He has a temperature of 39°C.

5. A 5-year-old boy presents with abdominal pain. He has had a slight fever for 24 hours and, since this morning, he has complained of central abdominal pain. His mother reports that he has been more lethargic than usual for the last few weeks. On examination, he has generalized tenderness throughout the abdomen, pharyngitis and laboured breathing.

Theme 2: Apnoea

Options

A. Gastro-oesophageal reflux
B. Hypoglycaemia
C. Intracranial haemorrhage
D. Obstructive sleep apnoea
E. Pertussis
F. Seizure
G. Sepsis

For each of the following scenarios, select the most likely cause of apnoea. Each option may be used once, more than once or not at all.

1. You are called urgently to the postnatal ward. A 24-hour-old infant stopped breathing for a number of minutes. The midwife gave resuscitation breaths, and the baby is now breathing again. The baby was born at term, although the mother's waters broke more than 24 hours prior to delivery. On examination, the baby is cool peripherally and tachycardic.

2. A 6-week-old infant presents to the GP. His mother reports that he is having frequent episodes where he stops breathing for up to 30 seconds. He has occasionally turned blue. He often starts breathing again spontaneously, but sometimes needs a little stimulation. His mother notices that these episodes occur in clusters after feeding.

3. You are called urgently to the postnatal ward. A 24-hour-old infant stopped breathing for a number of minutes. The midwife gave resuscitation breaths, and the baby is now breathing again. He was born at 36 weeks' gestation and weighs 2.4 kg. On examination, he looks jittery, is cool peripherally and is tachycardic.

4. A 6-week-old infant presents to the emergency department. His mother reports that he has had a cough for a few days. The cough occurs in bouts, and a couple of times he has vomited towards the end of the paroxysm. Today, he had a bout of coughing and then stopped breathing and turned blue.

5. A 3-month-old infant presents to the emergency department. He was brought in by ambulance. The paramedic has been performing bag-and-mask ventilation since leaving the family home, as the infant was having a respiratory arrest. On intubating the child, you notice that his frenulum is torn. Once ventilated, examination reveals bruising around the chest wall.

Theme 3: Immunization schedule

Options

A. Diphtheria
B. *Haemophilus influenza* type b
C. Measles
D. Meningococcus C
E. Mumps
F. Pertussis
G. Pneumococcus
H. Polio
I. Rubella
J. Tuberculosis

For each of the following descriptions, select the most likely organism against which protection is given by vaccination. Each option may be used once, more than once or not at all.

1. A live vaccine given intradermally to at-risk babies.

2. An inactivated virus given intramuscularly to all babies at 2, 3 and 4 months, with a preschool booster and a further booster at 13–18 years.

3. An intramuscular vaccine protecting against a bacterial organism given at 3, 4 and 12 months.

4. An intramuscular vaccine protecting against a bacterial organism given at 2, 3 and 4 months, with a preschool booster.

5. An intramuscular vaccine protecting against a bacterial organism given at 2, 3 and 4 months, with a preschool booster followed by a booster at 13–18 years.

Theme 4: Child protection

Options

A. Accidental injury
B. Emotional abuse
C. Fabricated or induced illness
D. Neglect
E. Normal variant
F. Non-accidental poisoning
G. Non-accidental injury (physical abuse)
H. Pathological cause
I. Sexual abuse

For each of the following scenarios, select the most likely description from the above options. Each option may be used once, more than once or not at all.

1. A 2-year-old boy falls out of a first-floor window. His parents say that he was unattended at the time. He sustains a right-sided extradural haematoma resulting in a left hemiplegia.

2. A 3-month-old girl is found to have a fractured humerus. Her father says that she rolled off the changing mat onto a hard wooden floor.

3. A 3-week-old Asian child is referred by the health visitor, who has noticed bruising around the sacrum and buttocks. She suspects that the parents are smacking the baby for crying.

4. A 3-year-old boy is reported to have fallen from his tricycle and has not been using his right arm since. Examination is normal except for a diastolic murmur. X-ray reveals a fractured ulna and radius. The paediatric team perform a skeletal survey, which reveals what look like old skull fractures. The father was on the child protection register when he was a boy, and now the patient is being referred to a named doctor for child protection.

5. A 12-month-old boy presents with a severe cough. On examination, the child is in respiratory distress, and suffers from paroxysms of coughing followed by a whoop. You also notice a widespread nappy rash, which improves rapidly while he is on the ward.

Theme 5: Management of asthma

Options

A. 2–10 puffs of inhaled short-acting β_2-agonist via spacer
B. Increase inhaled steroid to 400 µg/kg/day
C. Inhaled steroid 200–400 µg/kg/day
D. Intravenous aminophylline
E. Intravenous infusion of magnesium sulphate
F. Intravenous salbutamol
G. Intravenous steroid
H. No further management required
I. Nebulized short-acting β_2-agonist
J. Oral leukotriene receptor antagonist
K. Oral steroids
L. Oxygen via facemask, 2–10 puffs of inhaled short-acting β_2-agonist via spacer and oral steroid
M. Oxygen via facemask and 2–10 puffs of inhaled short-acting β_2-agonist via spacer
N. Oxygen via facemask and nebulized short-acting β_2-agonist
O. Oxygen via facemask, nebulized short-acting β_2-agonist and oral or intravenous steroid
P. Regular inhaled short-acting β_2-agonist via a spacer

For each of the following children with asthma, select the next step in the management. Each case option may be used once, more than once or not at all.

1. A 4-year-old boy presents to his GP with a 6-month history of nocturnal cough and intermittent wheeze. On examination, he is small for his age and has mild eczema on his upper limbs.

2. A 3-year-old boy presents with poorly controlled chronic asthma. He is currently being managed with an inhaled short-acting β_2-agonist as required and 400 µg/kg/day of inhaled steroid. His mother wants to know if there is anything else that you can do to help.

3. An 8-year-old girl presents with poorly controlled chronic asthma. She is currently being managed with an inhaled short-acting β_2-agonist as required, 800 µg/kg/day of inhaled steroid, a long-acting β_2-agonist and an oral leukotriene receptor antagonist. Her mother wants to know if there is anything else that you can do to help.

4. A 3-year-old boy presents to his GP with an acute exacerbation of asthma. He has widespread wheeze, is too breathless to talk, and has a heart rate of 140 beats/min and a respiratory rate of 55/min.

5. A 4-year-old boy presents to the emergency department with an acute exacerbation of asthma. He is agitated, with oxygen saturations of 88% in air. He is demonstrating poor respiratory effort, is cyanotic and has a silent chest.

Theme 6: Investigating the febrile child

Options

A. Blood for culture and sensitivity
B. Blood for polymerase chain reaction (PCR)
C. C-reactive protein
D. Chest X-ray
E. Cerebrospinal fluid (CSF) for microscopy, culture and sensitivity
F. CSF for PCR
G. Full blood count
H. Limb X-ray
I. Urine for microscopy, culture and sensitivity

For each of the following children with a fever, select the investigation most likely to lead to a diagnosis. Each option may be used once, more than once or not at all.

1. A 2-year-old girl presents with a 4-day history of fever. The illness started with a cough. Her respiratory rate is 45/min, saturations 94% in air, temperature 38.9°C and capillary refill time 1 s. There are crepitations at the left base on auscultation. Urine is negative on dipstick.

2. A 3-year-old girl presents with a fever for 2 days. She is drowsy and had a seizure causing twitching of the right side of the body for 4 min. Her respiratory rate is 30/min, saturations 98% in air, temperature 38.3°C and capillary refill time 2 s. Urine is negative on dipstick.

3. A 6-month-old boy is admitted with persistent irritability. He is lethargic and is not feeding as well as usual. His respiratory rate is 30/min, saturations 97% in air, temperature 38.0°C and capillary refill time 2 s. Urine reveals leucocytes and nitrites on dipstick.

4. A 3-year-old boy presents with a 1-day history of being unwell. He appears shocked and has a 3-hour-old rash made up of urticaria and purpural spots. His respiratory rate is 30/min, saturations 94% in air, temperature 39.0°C and capillary refill time 5 s. Urine reveals leucocytes on dipstick.

5. A 2½-year-old girl is admitted with a fever for 2 days. She is has stopped walking and cries when changing her clothes. Her respiratory rate is 20/min, saturations 99% in air, temperature 38.7°C and capillary refill time 1 s. Urine is clear on dipstick.

Theme 7: Obesity

Options

A. Acquired hypothyroidism
B. Addison's disease
C. Bulimia nervosa
D. Congenital hypothyroidism
E. Cushing's disease
F. Cushing's syndrome
G. Hyperinsulinaemia secondary to diabetes
H. Lawrence–Moon–Biedl syndrome
I. Obesity secondary to behavioural disorder
J. Polycystic ovarian syndrome
K. Prader–Willi syndrome
L. Primary obesity
M. Tricyclic antidepressant use

For each of the following patients who are clinically obese, select the most likely diagnosis. Each option may be used once, more than once or not at all.

1. An 8-year-old boy is clinically obese. As a baby, he was floppy and difficult to feed. He now has learning difficulties, and is constantly eating despite measures by his parents to hide food out of reach.

2. A 6-year-old boy is clinically obese. His body mass index is above the 95th centile. He has no other medical problems and examination is unremarkable. His mother says that she has tried everything to help him lose weight.

3. A 10-year-old boy is clinically obese and the shortest in his class. He had a renal transplant last year and his mother is worried that he is being bullied.

4. A 17-year-old girl is clinically obese. She has put a lot of weight on over the last year. She says that she is always tired and is becoming more constipated.

5. A 14-year-old girl is clinically obese. She has not started her periods yet and has severe acne. Among her investigations, a high insulin level is found.

121

Theme 8: Heart murmurs

Options

- A. Diastolic – 2nd left intercostal space
- B. Diastolic – 2nd right intercostal space
- C. Diastolic – 5th right intercostal space
- D. Diastolic – apex
- E. Ejection systolic – 2nd left intercostal space
- F. Ejection systolic – 2nd right intercostal space
- G. Pansystolic – 4th right intercostal space
- H. Pansystolic – 5th left intercostal space
- I. Systolic and diastolic – inferior to left clavicle

For each of the following conditions, select the most likely murmur that would be heard on auscultation of the heart (type of murmur – where heard best). Each option may be used once, more than once or not at all.

1. Ventricular septal defect.

2. Mitral stenosis.

3. Aortic stenosis.

4. Patent ductus arteriosus.

5. Pulmonary stenosis.

Theme 9: Diarrhoea

Options

- A. Antibiotics
- B. Cows' milk-free diet
- C. Gluten-free diet
- D. Intravenous rehydration
- E. Laxatives
- F. No management required
- G. Oral rehydration
- H. Pancreatic enzyme supplements
- I. Steroids

For each of the following children presenting with diarrhoea, select the most appropriate first step in the management. Each option may be used once, more than once or not at all.

1. A 5-year-old boy presents with diarrhoea. He has been passing approximately 10 stools per day for the past 2 days. The stools are loose and have at times contained blood. He has had a fever and vomited three times yesterday. He attended a friend's party last

weekend. On examination, he looks unwell. His blood pressure and pulse are normal and his eyes are not sunken. His peripheries are warm, but his lips are slightly dry.

2. An 18-month-old girl presents with diarrhoea. She has been passing 5–10 stools per day for the past 6 months. Her mother reports that the stool is watery, smelly and that there are often food particles visible. The girl is thriving along her centile on the growth chart. On examination, she looks well, her blood pressure and pulse are normal, her eyes are not sunken, her peripheries are warm and her lips are moist.

3. A 16-month-old girl presents with diarrhoea. She has been passing 10–20 stools per day for the past 3 days. The stools are loose and smelly, but no blood is present. Her mother says that she had a fever, is irritable and vomited five times yesterday. She attends a nursery 3 days a week. On examination, she looks unwell, although her blood pressure and pulse are normal. Her eyes are sunken and she is cool around the edges, with a capillary refill time of 3 s. She was recently weighed for an immunization (12 kg), and today she weighs 11.5 kg.

4. A 19-month-old girl presents with diarrhoea. She has been passing 5–10 stools per day for the past few months. Her mother reports that the stool is watery, although occasionally she will pass a large hard stool. The girl is thriving on her growth centiles. On examination, she looks well, her blood pressure and pulse are normal, her eyes are not sunken, her peripheries are warm and her lips are moist.

5. A 4-month-old, breastfed boy presents with diarrhoea. He has been passing 5–10 loose stools per day for the past few months. The stool is watery and at times is flecked with blood. On examination, he looks well, his blood pressure and pulse are normal, his eyes are not sunken, his peripheries are warm and his lips are moist.

Theme 10: Haematology and haematological malignancy

Options

A. Acute lymphoblastic leukaemia
B. Acute myeloid leukaemia
C. α–Thalassaemia
D. β-Thalassaemia
E. Glucose-6-phosphate dehydrogenase deficiency
F. Haemolytic–uraemic syndrome
G. Hodgkin's lymphoma
H. Non-Hodgkin's lymphoma
I. *Plasmodium falciparum* infection
J. Sickle cell disease
K. Spherocytosis
L. Splenic atrophy

For each of the following scenarios, select the most likely diagnosis. Each option may be used once, more than once or not at all.

1. A 2-year-old boy presents with chronic diarrhoea, abdominal distension and failure to thrive. His mother says that he has an itchy, vesicular rash on his upper limbs. A blood film reveals Howell–Jolly bodies and target cells.

2. A 3-year-old boy presents with multiple bruises all over his body. On examination, he has hepatosplenomegaly. Aspiration of bone marrow reveals blast cells containing Auer rods.

3. A 4-year-old boy who has recently emigrated from Africa presents with fever. He is pale and acutely unwell. Blood film reveals signet-ring inclusions.

4. A 6-year-old boy who has recently emigrated from Africa presents with fever. He is pale and acutely unwell. Blood film reveals haemolytic fragments and Heinz bodies.

5. A 15-year-old boy who has recently emigrated from Africa presents with a prolonged history of fever. Examination reveals painless lymphadenopathy in the cervical region. Biopsy of the lymph nodes reveals Reed–Sternberg cells.

Theme 1: Abdominal pain

Abdominal pain is a common problem in children. It is also a highly non-specific symptom, so eliciting a diagnosis can be difficult. Symptoms associated with surgically correctable causes of acute abdominal pain include vomiting of bile, asymmetrical pain, local tenderness and peritonism.

1. K – Urinary tract infection

Urinary tract infections (UTIs) are relatively common in children, with 5% of girls having had a UTI by their second birthday. The most common causative organism is *Escherichia coli*. Other causative pathogens include *Proteus* spp. (more common in boys) and *Pseudomonas* spp. (often associated with structural abnormalities of the urinary tract). Infections located in the lower urinary tract (cystitis) will cause dysuria, urgency, wetting and generalized abdominal pain. This patient has an infection of the upper urinary tract (pyelonephritis), which causes more marked symptoms of high-grade fever and loin pain. NICE guidelines (published in August 2007) have attempted to standardize care of this common problem. Children with atypical or recurrent UTIs should have an ultrasound scan of the abdomen during the acute illness to rule out anatomical anomalies. Investigation for vesicoureteric reflux is no longer required routinely. If the UTI is recurrent or atypical in a child less than 3 years old, they should have renal function investigated with a DMSA scan. (DMSA – dimercaptosuccinic acid – is a radiolabelled compound that becomes fixed in functioning proximal renal tubular cells. DMSA is not taken up by scarred, non-functioning areas of the kidney.) The management of UTI is with oral or systemic antibiotics. Prophylactic antibiotics should not be prescribed routinely following a first UTI.

Mori R, Lakhanpaul M, Verrier-Jones K. Diagnosis and management of urinary tract infection in children: summary of NICE guidance. *BMJ* 2007;**335**:395–7.

2. F – Intussusception

Intussusception is a surgical emergency. It affects children between the ages of 3 months and 3 years (most commonly between 6 and 18 months). Intussusception describes invagination of a proximal portion of bowel (the intussusceptum) into a distal segment (the intussuscipiens), most commonly at the ileocaecal junction. The blood supply to the telescoped bowel is compromised, resulting in tissue ischaemia and eventually necrosis. These children present with recurrent episodes of severe colicky abdominal pain, associated with pallor, screaming and drawing up of the legs. During an episode, the child is pale and draws the legs up. A sausage-shaped mass may be palpable in the right upper quadrant. The passage of blood and mucus per rectum (redcurrant jelly stools) is a late sign. Management is by resuscitation followed by reduction of the intussusception by a rectal air enema. If this is ineffective (25% of cases) then surgical reduction is required. Although intussusception can cause obstruction, these children would be vomiting and have abdominal distension, which is not found in this case.

3. A – Appendicitis

Acute appendicitis is the most common surgical emergency in childhood and adolescence. Inflammation of the appendix occurs secondary to obstruction of the appendiceal opening into the caecum. Obstruction can be by a faecolith (from Latin *faeco* = excrement + Greek *lith* = stone; 'piece of poo'), adhesions or lymphoid hyperplasia. Abdominal pain is initially central, but later shifts to the right iliac fossa due to localized peritonitis. Patients also have anorexia, nausea and vomiting, and a low-grade fever. (Only one-third of cases of appendicitis present with these characteristic findings.) Classically, there is pain over McBurney's point, which is found one-third of the way between the anterior superior iliac spine and the umbilicus. Rovsing's sign, where palpation over the left iliac fossa causes right iliac fossa pain, may also be positive. If the inflamed appendix is adjacent to the bladder or rectum then dysuria or diarrhoea can feature. Management is by appendicectomy.

Charles McBurney, American surgeon (1845–1913).

Niels Thorkild Rovsing, Danish surgeon (1862–1927).

4. G – Mesenteric adenitis

Non-specific abdominal pain is usually vague, central and colicky. Abdominal pain associated with a tachycardia and a flushed appearance often suggests an infective, extra-abdominal cause such as tonsillitis or otitis media. Mesenteric adenitis describes inflammation of the mesenteric lymph nodes that occurs following a viral upper respiratory tract infection. It presents with features similar to acute appendicitis, with the addition of high fever and evidence of viral infection (cervical lymphadenopathy and pharyngitis). Mesenteric adenitis is a self-limiting condition and, if it is suspected, management should initially be conservative to avoid unnecessary laparotomy.

5. C – Diabetic ketoacidosis

A large proportion of children with diabetes present initially with ketoacidosis. Diabetic ketoacidosis is a medical emergency with potentially severe complications. It must be managed carefully with rehydration and correction of the acidosis. Symptoms that suggest a diagnosis of diabetes include polydipsia (excessive thirst), polyuria, lethargy and weight loss. The symptoms of ketoacidosis include abdominal pain, nausea, vomiting and laboured breathing (the body's way of compensating for the acidosis by exhaling excess carbon dioxide). Ketoacidosis is often triggered by an acute infection, such as pharyngitis, which is found in this case.

Theme 2: Apnoea

Although there is no strict definition of apnoea, it can be roughly defined as the cessation of breathing for more than 20 s or for any period where the cessation of breathing is associated with pallor, cyanosis or a bradycardia. The causes of apnoea can be subdivided as follows:

1. Central: defect in neurological drive from respiratory centre
2. Obstructive: temporary blockage of the airway
3. Mixed: combination of central and obstructive.

1. G – Sepsis

With this story, sepsis, congenital pneumonia and meningitis would all be in your differential diagnosis. With a history of prolonged rupture of membranes of greater than 24 hours, sepsis is the most likely cause of apnoea, although it is also a risk factor for congenital pneumonia. You would need to perform a full septic screen, including blood cultures, urine cultures, a lumbar puncture for CSF and a chest X-ray. The commonest organisms causing sepsis in the neonatal period are group B streptococci and coliforms, which are acquired from the birth canal.

2. A – Gastro-oesophageal reflux

Gastro-oesophageal reflux is a common problem in the neonatal period. Most cases in this age group are due to (transient) functional immaturity of the lower oesophageal sphincter and do not require any medical management. Most cases resolve spontaneously by 12 months of age. Complications of reflux include apnoea in infants (this case), failure to thrive, aspiration, oesophagitis (→ pain, bleeding and iron deficiency) and Sandifer's syndrome (dystonic movements of the head and neck).

Gastro-oesophageal reflux can be confirmed by measuring the lower oesophageal pH over a 24-hour period. A pH <4 for over 4 hours is indicative of reflux. Simple measures such as positioning the baby upright after feeding and thickening feeds can help. Medical treatments include drugs that increase gastric motility (erythromycin, metoclopramide or domperidone), antacids (Gaviscon), protein pump inhibitors (omeprazole) and H_2-receptor antagonists (ranitidine). In severe, unresponsive cases, Nissen's fundoplication (where the fundus of the stomach is wrapped around the lower oesophagus to increase the effectiveness of the sphincter) is performed.

Rudolph Nissen, German surgeon (1896–1981).

3. B – Hypoglycaemia

In any emergency, your priority is to assess ABC. Remember always to check a blood sugar (ABC-DEFG: Don't Ever Forget Glucose). In this case, one would list sepsis as a differential, but a blood sugar would confirm the diagnosis rapidly. Hypoglycaemia is defined as blood glucose <2.6 mmol/L. Neonates are commonly asymptomatic when hypoglycaemic, but may present with jitteriness, convulsions, hypotonia, lethargy and apnoea. Infants at risk of hypoglycaemia are babies <37 weeks' gestation, babies <2.5 kg, intrauterine growth restriction and babies born of mothers with diabetes or who were on β-blockers for pre-eclampsia. Prolonged, symptomatic hypoglycaemia can cause permanent neurological disability. Management of hypoglycaemia is by feeding (or intravenous glucose if the infant cannot be fed).

4. E – Pertussis

Respiratory infections associated with apnoea include respiratory syncytial virus (RSV) bronchiolitis and pertussis (whooping cough). Localized airway infections such as tonsillitis, retropharyngeal abscess and epiglottitis can cause obstructive apnoea.

5. C – Intracranial haemorrhage

Physical abuse (non-accidental injury) can present in many ways. This case has many of the classic signs of physical abuse (bruising around the chest wall and torn frenulum). Vigorously shaking babies causes subdural haemorrhage by rupturing the small subdural vessels.

Frenulum, from Latin *frenulum* = little bridle (a bridle being the straps that fit over a horse's head to help control it).

Theme 3: Immunization schedule

The following information is summarized from the NHS website, www.immunisation.nhs.uk.

1. J – Tuberculosis

The BCG (bacille Calmette–Guérin) vaccine protects against tuberculosis. In the UK, BCG is offered to babies who are more likely than the general population to come into contact with someone with TB. The vaccination is usually offered shortly after birth.

2. H – Polio

The live oral polio vaccine has been replaced by IPV (inactivated polio vaccine). This is to remove the risk of vaccine-associated paralytic polio.

3. D – Meningococcus C

Meningococcus (*Neisseria meningitidis*) is a Gram-negative diplococcus that is currently the leading cause of pyogenic meningitis in the UK. There are at least 13 subtypes of meningococcus, which can cause both meningitis and sepsis. This vaccine only protects against meningococcus type C.

4. F – Pertussis

The pertussis vaccine is a suspension of killed organisms. Immunization does not give total protection, and protection is not lifelong. Immunized infants will have a milder illness if they are infected. By having a high level of herd immunity, i.e. immunizing as many children as possible, the most vulnerable group (infants in the first few months of life) are protected.

5. A – Diphtheria (and tetanus)

Diphtheria and tetanus are now rare in developed countries thanks to the protection given by the combined DTaP (diphtheria, tetanus and pertussis) vaccine. This has now been combined with IPV and the *Haemophilus influenzae* type b vaccine (Hib) to make up a pentavalent vaccine.

The current immunization programme (July 2007) is as follows:
- 2 months: DTaP/IPV/Hib, pneumococcal
- 3 months: DTaP/IPV/Hib, meningitis C (MenC)
- 4 months: DTaP/IPV/Hib, pneumococcal, MenC
- 12 months: Hib/MenC
- 13 months: measles, mumps and rubella (MMR), pneumococcal
- preschool: DTaP/IPV, MMR
- 13–18 years: tetanus, diphtheria, IPV

Theme 4: Child protection

Child protection matters are complex and continuously evolving. This is a relatively new field of medical practice, and any healthcare professional working with children needs to be aware of the signs of presentation and the points of referral.

1. D or G – Neglect or non-accidental injury (NAI)

Physical injury can be inflicted deliberately, but can also be caused by a failure to provide a safe environment. The following should initiate a higher level of suspicion:
- discrepancy between injury/presentation and history given
- change in history over time or between different people
- delay in presentation
- unusual reaction to the injury
- repeated injuries
- history of NAI or suspicious injury in a sibling
- other signs of neglect or failure to thrive

2. G – Non-accidental injury

Any fractures in non-mobile children are suspicious. Most fractures in mobile children are accidental. A fall onto a hard surface would not be completely unreasonable, but this question is testing your knowledge of development. Children are able to roll from their front onto their back at 24 weeks and from their back to their front at 28 weeks. It is therefore unlikely that a 3 month old could roll from back to front. The story does not fit with the injury, and therefore you must suspect a non-accidental injury. Remember that developmental milestones are not set in stone and therefore a child protection assessment would include a full assessment of development.

3. E – Normal variant

Alhough you would need to examine this baby to confirm your diagnosis, this sounds like a mongolian blue spot. These are a normal variant that are found more commonly in Asian and Afro-Caribbean children. They usually fade by 1 year of life, but some persist.

4. H – Pathological cause

This child has sustained a serious injury considering the mode of trauma. Child protection should be considered seriously; however, pathological causes should be ruled out. This is a case of osteogenesis imperfecta type I, an autosomal dominant condition. This results in bony fragility, which causes recurrent fractures and deformity. Wormian bones may be seen on skull X-ray (these are irregular, isolated bones found within skull sutures – they are not fractures). The sclerae are blue, and the condition is associated with conductive hearing deafness (50% of cases) and aortic valve regurgitation – hence the diastolic murmur in this case. The 'named doctor' is a consultant (usually paediatric) responsible for giving advice on child protection matters within a hospital.

5. D – Neglect

Neglect can present in many ways: failure to thrive, poor development of emotional attachment, and delayed development, speech and language. In this case, the child has contracted pertussis (whooping cough) because of a failure to attend for immunization. Neglect may also present with inadequate hygiene such as a severe nappy rash, which improves rapidly with adequate care. It is important to note that parents have the right to choose not to have their children immunized; however, in combination with other signs of neglect, it should alert your suspicions to a child who is not being adequately cared for.

Theme 5: Management of asthma

Asthma is the most common chronic respiratory disorder affecting children. The British Thoracic Society guidelines for the management of asthma are the gold standard in the UK (they can be found at www.brit-thoracic.org.uk). All children seen in hospital with an acute exacerbation of asthma should have their long-term management reviewed, their inhaler technique assessed and a clear discharge plan provided along with a follow-up appointment with their GP.

1. P – Regular inhaled short-acting β_2-agonist via a spacer

This boy has a new diagnosis of asthma and should be started on step 1 of the management ladder. He should be reassessed later and, if this has not been effective, then an inhaled steroid should be added. At this age (under 5 years), all inhalers should be given through a spacer device to maximize their effect.

For reference, the management of asthma follows a stepwise approach, summarized as follows:

- Step 1: Short-acting β$_2$-agonist (salbutamol or terbutaline)
- Step 2: Step 1 + low-dose inhaled steroid (budesonide or fluticasone)
- Step 3: Step 2 +
    - ○ <5 years: leukotriene inhibitor (monteleukast)
    - ○ ≥5 years: high-dose inhaled steroid and long-acting β$_2$-agonist
- Step 4: Step 3 + fourth drug (e.g. theophylline or an anticholinergic)
- Step 5: Step 4 + oral steroid (prednisolone)

2. J – Oral leukotriene receptor antagonist

This child is on step 2 of the stepwise approach to managing asthma. He needs escalation to step 3, which at this age involves the use of an oral leukotriene receptor antagonist (e.g. monteleukast). Oral leukotrienes are very useful at this age, as they can be sprinkled into foods such as yoghurt or cereal. Children over 5 years could have the inhaled steroid increased and a trial of a long-acting β$_2$-agonist (e.g. salmeterol or formoterol).

3. K – Oral steroids

This girl is being treated on step 4 unsuccessfully. Step 5 employs an oral steroid (prednisolone). This girl should be referred to a respiratory paediatrician if she is not already being seen by one. She should have her inhaler technique reviewed and compliance checked.

4. L – Oxygen via facemask, 2–10 puffs of inhaled short-acting β$_2$-agonist via spacer and oral steroid

This is a severe exacerbation of asthma. Features of severe asthma are:
- patient is too breathless to talk or feed
- respiration rate ≥50/min
- pulse ≥140/min
- peak flow ≤50% predicted or best

Considering that he is at the GP surgery, he should be managed with the above step (oxygen/inhaled β$_2$-agonist/steroid) and reassessed after 15 minutes. Oxygen should be employed if available. If there is a good response to the bronchodilators and steroid then he could be managed at home with regular β$_2$-agonists and a 3-day course of oral steroid. If the response is poor then he should be referred to a local paediatric unit for assessment and admission.

5. O – Oxygen via facemask, nebulized short-acting β$_2$-agonist and oral or intravenous steroid

This is a life-threatening exacerbation of asthma. Features of life-threatening asthma are:
- fatigue or exhaustion
- decreasing consciousness
- silent chest or poor respiratory effort
- peak flow ≤33% predicted or best

The above measures should be performed (oxygen/nebulized β_2-agonist/ steroid). Frequent use of nebulized short-acting β_2-agonists (salbutamol) is described as 'back-to-back nebs', where each nebulizer is immediately followed by another. This child is very sick, and will probably need admission to a paediatric intensive care unit. He is likely to need intravenous salbutamol and/ or intravenous aminophylline; however, one should reassess response to the initial management prior to commencing these agents. In a child over 5 years, intravenous magnesium sulphate can also be used.

Theme 6: Investigating the febrile child

Infectious diseases remain a major cause of childhood mortality and morbidity in the UK. A fever in a child usually indicates an underlying infection. A full blood count and C-reactive protein (CRP) are very useful in all febrile children without a confirmed focus for infection. However, they will not provide a diagnosis. Neutrophilia suggests a bacterial infection and lymphophilia suggests a viral infection, but these are not hard-and-fast rules. CRP is an acute phase protein produced by the liver. Raised levels are a sign of inflammation, not just infection.

1. D – Chest X-ray

This girl has community-acquired pneumonia. The diagnosis can be made clinically, although radiology can confirm pulmonary consolidation. Tachypnoea is one of the most sensitive signs of pneumonia in children of this age. Attention must be paid to oxygenation, nutrition and hydration. In this case, the patient is not compromised and so can be treated at home with oral antibiotics.

2. F – CSF for PCR

This girl with fever and seizures has viral encephalitis. Warning signs of encephalitis are focal neurological signs, focal seizures and a decreased level of consciousness. The investigation most likely to yield a diagnosis would be CSF for PCR of herpesviruses. She should be treated with intravenous broad-spectrum antibiotics and aciclovir until the results from the CSF are obtained.

3. I – Urine for microscopy, culture and sensitivity

This boy, with fever and a dipstick positive for nitrites and leucocytes, is likely to have a urinary tract infection. Although empirical antibiotics can be commenced, a sample of urine is still required for microscopy, culture and sensitivity, as the child is below 3 years of age (see NICE guidelines). Getting a good-quality urine sample at this age is difficult. Methods include using adhesive bags, clean-catch (sit the child on a sterile pot), catheter insertion or suprapubic aspiration. If the culture is positive in this case then this boy will need investigating for anomalies of the urinary tract.

Richardson M, Lakhanpaul M. Assessment and initial management of feverish illness in children younger than 5 years: summary of NICE guidance. *BMJ* 2007;**334**:1163–4.

4. A – Blood for culture and sensitivity

This boy, who presents with high fever and a purpuric rash, has sepsis caused by the Gram-negative diplococcus *Neisseria meningitidis*. Blood for culture and sensitivity would be the first-line investigation, although PCR can also be employed. Meningococcal disease can present as meningitis, sepsis or both. Evidence shows that children presenting with meningitis alone have a better prognosis.

5. A – Blood for culture and sensitivity

This girl is febrile and is refusing to walk. It is likely, therefore, that she has osteomyelitis or septic arthritis. Radiology will not show any abnormality until later in the disease course. An ultrasound scan of the joints would be more useful. This girl should initially be treated with empirical intravenous antibiotics, but, before this, blood cultures should be sent to look for the offending organism.

Theme 7: Obesity

Body mass index is a standardized measurement used in adults, and can also be used in adolescents and children. A BMI >95th centile in children and >30 kg/m² in adolescents is the definition of obesity. Management options include treating the cause, lifestyle changes, behavioural therapy, physical activity and dietary advice.

1. K – Prader–Willi syndrome

Prader–Willi syndrome can present in the neonatal period with hypotonia and poor feeding. Later in life, children gain excessive weight due to hyperphagia (excessive appetite). Other features include hypogonadism, strabismus, low IQ and characteristic facial features (narrow forehead, olive-shaped eyes, anti-mongoloid slant and carp-shaped mouth).

Laurence–Moon–Biedl syndrome is associated with learning difficulties, but is also characterized by progressive visual impairment (due to retinal changes), digital anomalies (polydactyly and syndactyly), hypogenitalism and nephropathy.

2. L – Primary obesity

Obesity among children is increasing. Primary obesity is the most common cause, and other disorders associated with obesity are rare. Pathological causes account for less than 1% of cases. In most cases, obesity is the result of a positive energy balance that is stored as adipose tissue.

3. F – Cushing's syndrome

Cushing's syndrome describes the clinical features caused by adrenal steroid excess. The most common cause is iatrogenic steroid administration – in this case steroids used in a renal transplant recipient for immunosuppression. Patients present with moon-like faces, plethora, acne, buffalo hump (interscapular fat pad), truncal obesity, growth arrest (i.e. poor height), easy bruising, hypertension, hypogonadism, cataracts and glucose intolerance. The diagnosis of Cushing's syndrome is made by finding a raised 24-hour free urinary cortisol or using the dexamethasone suppression test (not a random cortisol – which is useless, as cortisol has a natural diurnal variation). In the dexamethasone suppression test, there is a high serum cortisol level that is not suppressed by dexamethasone. *Cushing's disease* is excess corticosteroid secretion secondary to a pituitary tumour.

Addison's disease is primary autoimmune-mediated adrenocortical failure. The adrenal cortex can be simplified into secreting three things: glucocorticoids, mineralocorticoids and adrenal androgens. These usually feed back to the anterior pituitary to reduce ACTH (adrenocorticotropic hormone) secretion. Therefore, if the adrenal cortex fails, there are many consequences: reduced glucocorticoids (hypoglycaemia and weight loss), reduced mineralocorticoids (hyperkalaemia, hyponatraemia and hypotension), reduced adrenal androgens (decreased body hair and libido) and ACTH excess (increased pigmentation in sun-exposed areas, pressure areas, palmar creases, buccal mucosa and recent scars). The diagnosis of Addison's disease is by the short Synacthen test. In this investigation, plasma cortisol levels are measured before and half an hour after administration of a single intramuscular dose of ACTH. Normally, the ACTH will result in a rise in cortisol. If there is no rise in cortisol on the second reading, adrenal insufficiency is indicated. Management of Addison's disease is with the replacement of glucocorticoids and mineralocorticoids (with hydrocortisone and fludrocortisone).

Thomas Addison, English physician (1795–1860).

Harvey Cushing, American neurosurgeon and endocrinologist (1869–1939).

4. A – Acquired hypothyroidism

Congenital hypothyroidism presents early in life with coarse facial features, large tongue, hoarse cry, hypotonia, lethargy, umbilical hernia, constipation and prolonged jaundice. Acquired hypothyroidism, which develops later in life, is more common. Iodine deficiency is the commonest cause of acquired hypothyroidism worldwide. Autoimmune disease (Hashimoto's thyroiditis) is the most common cause in childhood and adolescence. Patients present with short stature (due to poor height growth and delayed skeletal growth), intolerance to cold, constipation, lethargy and weight gain. Signs may include goitre, bradycardia and slow relaxation of tendon reflexes. Autoantibodies to thyroid peroxidase (an enzyme required to make thyroxine) may be found. Treatment is with thyroid replacement (thyroxine).

Hashimoto Hakaru, Japanese physician (1881–1934).

5. J – Polycystic ovarian syndrome

The cause of polycystic ovarian syndrome (PCOS) is unknown. Girls with PCOS are classically tall, obese and hirsute. They suffer from amenorrhoea, dysfunctional menstrual bleeding and infertility. Biochemical features include raised testosterone and raised luteinizing hormone. Metabolically, these girls have raised cholesterol levels and insulin resistance, which predisposes them to diabetes. In this case, the raised insulin level is not due to diabetes but to the PCOS. For more information on PCOS, see 'The infertility clinic' (Paper 3 Answers, Theme 10, page 83).

Theme 8: Heart murmurs

Heart murmurs are a relatively common finding in children, and many pathological lesions have distinct patterns of murmurs. Murmurs are caused by turbulent blood flow, usually through valves but also through vessels and heart chambers. Most murmurs are innocent (non-pathological), such as vibratory murmurs and venous hums. The following features suggest an innocent murmur: quiet, asymptomatic, louder during fever/exercise, varying during respiration/posture and systolic.

Heart murmurs are graded according to their intensity:
- Grade I: faint murmur (usually only cardiologists can hear)
- Grade II: quiet murmur
- Grade III: moderate intensity, no thrill
- Grade IV: loud murmur, with a thrill (can be heard by a medical student!)
- Grade V: very loud murmur with a thrill (still requires stethoscope to hear)
- Grade VI: very loud murmur with a thrill (can be heard close to chest wall without a stethoscope)

1. H – Pansystolic – 5th left intercostal space

A ventricular septal defect is the most common congenital cardiac lesion in children. The murmur is pansystolic, which means that it is heard throughout systole. This murmur is caused by shunting of blood from the high-pressure left ventricle to the low-pressure right ventricle.

2. D – Diastolic – apex

Mitral stenosis is almost always caused by rheumatic fever, which in itself is now rare in the UK. The murmur is found at the end of diastole and is heard best in the mitral region (5th intercostal space, left side, midclavicular line – the apex).

3. F – Ejection systolic – 2nd right intercostal space

In mild cases, aortic stenosis will usually cause no symptoms in early life. As the child gets older, the stenosis may become more severe due to calcification of the valve. In critical aortic stenosis, heart failure will ensue rapidly after birth. The murmur is systolic and is heard loudest at the 2nd right intercostal space parasternally (the aortic area). The murmur may be conducted to the carotids and associated with an ejection click.

4. I – Systolic and diastolic – inferior to left clavicle

Patent ductus arteriosus is a common problem in preterm babies. The fetal circulation remains patent, causing heart failure due to blood shunting from the systemic to the pulmonary circulation. The murmur is described as a 'machinery murmur' that is often both systolic and diastolic. It is heard best inferior to the left clavicle.

5. E – Ejection systolic – 2nd left intercostal space

The murmur of pulmonary stenosis is systolic and heard best in the 2nd left intercostal space parasternally (pulmonary area). The degree of pulmonary stenosis varies greatly between patients. Most cases are mild and will not affect the child's health. Critical stenosis will often present rapidly when the ductus arteriosus closes, and will cause early death unless diagnosed early. Management is with dilatation of the stenosis using a balloon or surgical correction.

Theme 9: Diarrhoea

Diarrhoea is defined as stools of increased frequency, volume and fluidity. Acute diarrhoea has a short onset and duration; chronic diarrhoea is present for over 2–3 weeks. Most cases of diarrhoea in children are due to viral infections, and the key is assessing and treating any dehydration.

1. G – Oral rehydration

Using natural routes of hydration/rehydration is always optimal, as there is less risk of electrolyte imbalance. This child has gastroenteritis, likely to be bacterial in origin. Although he is unwell, he has not yet become dehydrated. At this point, no treatment would be required except advice to his parents about good hydration and handwashing. Antibiotics and adsorbent or stool-bulking drugs (e.g. loperamide) should be avoided in gastroenteritis. Organisms that cause bacterial gastroenteritis include *Campylobacter*, *Salmonella* and *Shigella* spp., and *Escherichia coli*. The most serious complication of bacterial gastroenteritis (other than profound dehydration) is haemolytic–uraemic syndrome, which can cause acute-onset renal failure and anaemia.

2. F – No management required

This is a case of 'toddler's diarrhoea'. Most cases of toddler's diarrhoea can be diagnosed clinically, often with the description of food in the diarrhoea ('carrots and peas' diarrhoea) in the otherwise-well child. However, it is important not to miss more sinister diagnoses. Many centres will send stool for blood, ova and parasites, pH, bacterial cultures and reducing substances (sugars suggestive of carbohydrate malabsorption). No management is required except reassurance that the child is normal. Most cases resolve with age.

3. G – Oral rehydration

This girl has gastroenteritis, most likely caused by a virus. Many children receive intravenous rehydration too early. With patience and perseverance, most cases of gastroenteritis can be managed with oral rehydration/hydration. If the child is under 2 years of age and refusing oral fluids then a nasogastric tube can be sited, thus allowing the gut to be used for fluid intake. This girl is dehydrated, as she has sunken eyes and dry mucous membranes. Weights are very useful in children, and in this case we can see that she is less than 5% dehydrated (mild dehydration). If she had severe dehydration (>10% weight loss) then one would consider intravenous rehydration slowly over 24–48 hours. The most common cause of viral gastroenteritis is rotavirus, which, along with RSV bronchiolitis, keeps paediatric wards and GP surgeries busy during the winter months. There is hope of a rotavirus immunization in the near future.

4. E – Laxatives

This is a case of overflow diarrhoea secondary to constipation. Constipation is a vicious cycle in this age group: children learn that it is painful to pass large hard stools, and so retain the stool, which gradually becomes harder, thus making the child more constipated. Eventually, these children lose sphincter tone, and proximal soft stools bypass the impacted stool. Treatment is complex and reassurance is very important. Laxatives such as Movicol (polyethylene glycol) and lactulose work by holding water in the stool (osmotic laxatives). These agents require a good fluid intake to work. It is important to inform the parents that the overflow diarrhoea may get a little worse before the constipation improves. Treatment can take months to years to complete.

5. B – Cows'-milk-free diet

Proteins found in cows' milk, and occasionally soy-based milk, can cause an enterocolitis in the first few months of life. Stool should be sent for culture and *Clostridium difficile* toxin. Management is with a trial of casein- or whey-based formula, or by eliminating cows' milk from the diet of a breastfeeding mother. There are other, more sinister, causes of rectal bleeding in infants that should be considered. These include haemorrhagic disease of the newborn, anal fissures, volvulus, intussusception, polyps, Meckel's diverticulum and infection.

Theme 10: Haematology and haematological malignancy

1. L – Splenic atrophy

Howell–Jolly bodies are basophilic nuclear remnants in the cytoplasm and are a sign of asplenism (as the spleen normally removes such fragments). Causes of splenic atrophy and asplenism include surgical removal of the spleen, sickle cell disease and coeliac disease (this case). The rash on the upper limb is dermatitis herpetiformis (which confusingly has nothing to do with herpes) and is associated with coeliac disease. Target cells are red blood cells, which demonstrate increased staining in the middle of an area of pallor. They are found in obstructive liver disease, sickle cell disease, asplenism, thalassaemia and iron-deficiency anaemia.

2. B – Acute myeloid leukaemia

Leukaemia is caused by the proliferation of a single bone marrow stem cell following malignant transformation. Acute myeloid leukaemia (AML) is caused by the proliferation of myeloid precursor cells. The presentation of AML is variable. Many sufferers are completely asymptomatic and are diagnosed incidentally, whereas others become very unwell, very quickly. Marrow failure caused by blast infiltration results in anaemia, thrombocytopenia and neutropenia (resulting in the clinical features of easy bleeding, bruising and multiple infections). Investigation usually shows a significantly raised white blood cell count. Cellular inclusions called Auer rods that are seen on microscopy are pathognomonic of AML. The management of AML involves blood and platelet transfusion, treatment of secondary infections and chemotherapy. Stem cell transplantation may be considered. The prognosis of AML is worse than that of acute lymphoblastic leukaemia (ALL). This condition is generally seen in adulthood and is rapidly fatal if untreated. Patients with Down's syndrome are at increased risk of both ALL and AML, with the risk of AML being highest in the first 3 years of life.

Acute lymphoblastic leukaemia is the most common leukaemia in children, and is caused by the clonal proliferation of lymphoid precursor (blast) cells that have been arrested at an early stage of development. The blast cells infiltrate the marrow and lymphoid tissue, causing pancytopenia and lymphadenopathy respectively. The central nervous system (CNS) can also be affected, causing headache, vomiting, meningism, cranial nerve palsy and seizures. Treatment is with supportive measures such as transfusion and antibiotics, and with chemotherapy. Chemotherapy is traditionally delivered in three main stages: remission induction, consolidation and maintenance, which can be for a number of years. Since patients with ALL are at high risk of developing neurological disease, they are often given CNS prophylaxis in the form of intrathecal methotrexate and radiotherapy. The prognosis of ALL is good with appropriate treatment.

3. I – *Plasmodium falciparum* infection

This boy has malaria. Malaria is caused by *Plasmodium* parasites, which are transmitted through the bite of the female *Anopheles* mosquito. The incubation period is 3 weeks. Patients present with abrupt-onset fever and rigors. The fever peaks every 3 or 4 days. Other features are abdominal pain, diarrhoea, headache and flu-like symptoms. Malaria is diagnosed on thick and thin blood films. Thick films allow detection of parasites; thin films reveal the species responsible and the determination of parasitaemia (measured as the percentage of erythrocytes infected). Complications of malaria include haemoglobinuria ('black water fever' – from severe haemolysis), acute renal failure and cerebral malaria (fits and coma). Cerebral malaria is the main cause of death. Treatment is with oral or intravenous quinine, as there is such a high rate of choloroquine resistance in *P. falciparum*. Side-effects of quinine include tinnitus, deafness and nausea. (Quinine overdose results in heart block.) Exchange transfusion may be required if the parasitaemia exceeds 10%.

4. E – Glucose-6-phosphate dehydrogenase deficiency

Glucose-6-phosphate dehydrogenase (G6PD) is an enzyme that reduces oxidative stress by reducing glutathione levels within red cells. G6PD deficiency is an X-linked disorder common in West Africa, southern Europe, the Middle East and south-east Asia. Patients are usually asymptomatic until oxidative stress causes haemolytic anaemia. Common triggers include fava broad beans (broad bean-induced haemolysis is termed *favism*), drugs (including antimalarials and sulphonamide antibiotics) and infections. Treatment is supportive, although transfusions may be required for acute haemolytic crises. Heinz bodies are denatured haemoglobin aggregates that are found in the cytoplasm of red blood cells. They result from oxidant stress (e.g. G6PD deficiency) or haemolysis. Recessive carriers of the G6PD mutation are protected against malaria.

5. G – Hodgkin's lymphoma

Lymphomas are diseases caused by malignant proliferation of the lymphoid system. Hodgkin's lymphoma classically presents with asymmetrical painless lymphadenopathy, usually in the form of a single rubbery lymph node in the cervical, axillary or inguinal region, which may become painful after alcohol ingestion. Disease spread to the mediastinal nodes may occur and cause dyspnoea and superior vena cava obstruction. Approximately 20% of patients suffer systemic symptoms such as weight loss, sweating, fever, pruritis and general lethargy (these are known as 'B' symptoms). Diagnosis is usually based on lymph node biopsy showing pathognomonic Reed–Sternberg cells. CT scanning can help confirm the diagnosis, and is often used for staging. Early-stage disease is managed with radiotherapy alone. In advanced and bulky disease, the combination of radiotherapy and chemotherapy is often employed. The prognosis of Hodgkin's lymphoma is good, with a 70% chance of cure even in later stages of disease. Increasing age and the presence of systemic symptoms indicate a poorer prognosis.

Thomas Hodgkin, British physician (1798–1866).

Other haematological terms

- Anisocytosis: red cells are of varying sizes (haemoglobinopathies and anaemias)
- Basophilic stippling: RNA inclusion bodies in the cytoplasm
- Burr cells: crimpled cell membrane
- Helmet cells: red cell fragments indicating microangiopathic haemolysis (HUS)
- Poikilocytosis: red cells are of varying shapes
- Schistocytes: fragmented cells
- Spherocytes: small, spherical, densely stained cells

Poikilocyte, from Greek *poikilos* = irregular.

Aniocytosis, from Greek *anisos* = unequal.

Schistocyte, from Greek *schistos* = split.

Theme 1: Vomiting

Options

- A. Appendicitis
- B. Duodenal atresia
- C. Exomphalos
- D. Gastroenteritis
- E. Gastro-oesophageal reflux disease
- F. Gastroschisis
- G. Incarcerated inguinal hernia
- H. Intussusception
- I. Malrotation with volvulus
- J. Meckel's diverticulum
- K. Overfeeding
- L. Pyloric stenosis
- M. Sepsis
- N. Testicular torsion
- O. Urinary tract infection

For each of the following infants presenting with vomiting, select the most likely diagnosis. Each option may be used once, more than once or not at all.

1. A 2-month-old boy presents with vomiting. He has been vomiting milk up to five times a day for the last 2 days. The vomiting is associated with loose stools and he has been having up to 10 motions a day for 3 days. His temperature is 37.1°C. On examination, his blood pressure and pulse are normal, his eyes and fontanelle are not sunken, his peripheries are warm and his lips are moist.

2. A 2-month-old boy presents with vomiting. He has had bilious vomiting for the past 24 hours. On examination, he looks very unwell, his blood pressure is normal, he is tachycardic, his eyes and fontanelle are sunken, and his capillary refill time is 5 s. He has a firm mass in his groin.

3. A 2-month-old boy presents with vomiting. He vomits small amounts of milk into his mouth, which he then swallows. This has been a problem since the first few weeks of life. He is often very irritable after feeds. On examination, his blood pressure and pulse are normal, his eyes and fontanelle are not sunken, his peripheries are warm and his lips are moist.

4. A 2-month-old boy presents with vomiting. He is described as a 'greedy baby'. He vomits large amounts of milk after feeds. This has

been a problem since the first few weeks of life. On examination, his blood pressure and pulse are normal, his eyes and fontanelle are not sunken, his peripheries are warm and his lips are moist.

5. A 2-month-old boy presents with vomiting. This has steadily been getting worse over the last 2 weeks. He is now eager for feeds, and shortly after taking milk will forcefully vomit. On examination, his blood pressure is normal, he is tachycardic, his eyes and fontanelle are not sunken, his peripheries are warm and his lips are moist. However, he has lost weight since he was last weighed at 6 weeks of age.

Theme 2: The child with a limp

Options

    A. Developmental dysplasia of the hip
    B. Fracture
    C. Genu varus
    D. Ligament strain
    E. Osgood–Schlatter disease
    F. Osteomyelitis
    G. Perthes' disease
    H. Septic arthritis
    I.   Slipped upper femoral epiphysis
    J. Spontaneous haemarthrosis
    K. Talipes equinovarus
    L. Transient synovitis

For each of the following children presenting with a limp, select the most likely diagnosis. Each option may be used once, more than once or not at all.

1. A 14-year-old boy presents with a limp and left knee pain of 24 hours' duration. He is systemically well and is afebrile. On examination, he appears overweight. His left leg is externally rotated and shorter than the right.

2. A 6-year-old boy presents with groin pain and a limp. The groin pain is exacerbated with exercise. On examination, you notice a leg-length discrepancy. He is systemically well and afebrile. There is no history of medical problems.

3. A 12-year-old boy presents with hip pain and a limp of acute onset. He denies pain at rest. He has been unwell for the few days prior to admission with a low-grade fever and a coryzal illness. He is reluctant for you to move the affected leg, which has a decreased range of movement.

4. An 18-month-old boy presents with a limp. Since waking this morning, he has not been using his left leg. He has a temperature of 39.5°C and looks systemically unwell. You attempt to examine the range of movement of the affected limb, but this elicits severe pain. The left knee is red, hot and swollen.

5. A 16-month-old boy presents with a limp. His mother has noticed that, since he started walking 2 months ago, he has had a limp, although it does not appear to cause him any discomfort. He is systemically well and is afebrile.

Theme 3: Cough

A. Aspiration of vomit
B. Asthma
C. Bronchiolitis
D. Croup
E. Cystic fibrosis
F. Foreign-body inhalation
G. Pertussis
H. Pneumonia

For each of the following children presenting with a cough, select the most likely diagnosis. Each option may be used once, more than once or not at all.

1. An 18-month-old girl presents with a recurrent cough, which is occasionally productive. She is small for her age. Her mother reports episodes of wheeze.

2. A 2-year-old boy presents with a cough. The cough has been present for the last 3 days. He was previously well. On examination, he has a temperature of 38.9°C and a respiratory rate of 55/min. There is no wheeze.

3. A 4-year-old boy presents with a recurrent cough, which is worse at night. He is small for his age. The cough has been present for the last 12 months and interrupts his sleep.

4. A 6-month-old presents with a cough. The illness began 4 days ago with a runny nose and a mild fever. Over the last 24 hours, he has developed a high-pitched cough associated with a wheeze. On examination, crepitations are heard throughout the lung fields.

5. A 2-year-old boy presents with a cough, which started suddenly yesterday afternoon. He is otherwise well and has a temperature of 36.5°C. On examination, there are reduced breath sounds on the right side.

Theme 4: Chromosomal disorders

Options

    A. 45XO
    B. 47XXX
    C. 47XXY
    D. 47XY (13)
    E. 47XY (18)
    F. 47XY (21)
    G. 69XXY
    H. Fragile X syndrome

For each of the following scenarios, select the most likely karyotype. Each option may be used once, more than once or not at all.

1. You are performing the postnatal check on a 3-day-old girl. She has swollen hands and feet, and you find it difficult to palpate her femoral pulses.

2. You are asked to see a 1-hour-old baby. He is dysmorphic, with a small chin and low-set ears. He also has a small head and rocker-bottom feet.

3. A 15-year-old boy presents to the general paediatrics clinic. He and his family are concerned as he has not entered puberty yet. He is tall for his age and has small, firm testes. He is a shy boy and has had some behavioural problems at school.

4. You are asked to see a 1-hour-old baby. He is dysmorphic with a round face. On examination you notice that he is very floppy.

5. A 5-year-old boy presents to the outpatient clinic. He has learning difficulties, a large head and large testicles. He has quite a characteristic facial appearance, with a prominent forehead and large ears.

Theme 5: Arthritis

Options

A. Acute rheumatic fever
B. Enteropathic arthritis
C. Haemarthrosis
D. Hand–foot syndrome
E. Leukaemia
F. Monoarticular juvenile idiopathic arthritis
G. Pauciarticular juvenile idiopathic arthritis
H. Polyarticular juvenile idiopathic arthritis
I. Psoriatic arthropathy
J. Reactive arthritis
K. Septic arthritis
L. Still's disease
M. Systemic lupus erythematosus
N. Transient synovitis

For each of the following children presenting with painful joints, select the most likely diagnosis. Each option may be used once, more than once or not at all.

1. A 12-year-old boy presents with painful joints. He recently had a bout of gastroenteritis, which he blames on a 'dodgy doner kebab'. His stools were loose and contained blood. On examination, both his knee joints are tender and hot.

2. A 12-year-old boy presents with painful joints. He is known to have sickle cell disease and was out sledging today in the freshly fallen snow. The joints of his fingers on both hands are now red, hot and swollen.

3. A 12-year-old boy presents with painful joints. For 2 months, he has complained of having painful wrist joints. Both wrists are affected, and on examination they appear red, hot and swollen. He is otherwise systemically well and has had no recent illness.

4. A 12-year-old boy presents with painful joints. He recently had a sore throat, which was confirmed as a streptococcal infection on throat swab. He has an unusual rash over his trunk and upper limbs associated with a fever. The rash is made up of pink rings and is not itchy.

5. A 12-year-old boy presents with painful joints. He recently had a bout of gastroenteritis, which he blames on a 'dodgy doner kebab'. His stools were loose and contained blood. He says that his stools had contained blood for at least a month prior to the bout of gastroenteritis. On examination, both knee joints are tender and hot.

Theme 6: Jaundice in the newborn

Options

- A. Abdominal X-ray
- B. Abdominal ultrasound
- C. Blood cultures
- D. C-reactive protein
- E. Conjugated bilirubin level
- F. Full blood count
- G. Group and Coombs' testing
- H. Metabolic screen
- I. No further investigation required
- J. Sweat test
- K. Thyroid-stimulating hormone (Guthrie card)
- L. TORCH screen
- M. Unconjugated bilirubin level
- N. Urea and electrolytes

For each of the following neonates/infants presenting with jaundice, select the most likely investigation that will reveal the underlying cause. Each option may be used once, more than once or not at all.

1. You are asked to see an 18-hour-old baby urgently on the delivery suite. He stopped breathing for a few seconds and needed stimulation to terminate the apnoea. He is jaundiced, irritable and not feeding well. His mother's waters broke over 24 hours before he was born.

2. You perform a baby check on a 12-hour-old baby. He is clinically well but significantly jaundiced. His mother is from India and had two children before moving to the UK.

3. A GP refers a 5-week-old infant who is jaundiced. His mother reports that his stools are white like chalk. On examination, the infant is clinically well but markedly jaundiced.

4. A health visitor refers a 10-day-old infant who is clinically well but jaundiced. The jaundice was first noticeable after 3 days when a bilirubin level was sent and found to be below the treatment level. He was initially breastfed, but his mother has just given up and started bottle feeding as he was not gaining weight.

5. You are asked to see a 24-hour-old newborn baby. He is small for dates and was born at 37 weeks' gestation. On examination, you notice that he has a small head and is jaundiced. Palpation reveals a large liver. While you are present, the baby has a seizure.

Theme 7: Seizures

Options

A. Anaesthesia and intubation
B. Intravenous dextrose
C. Intravenous lorazepam
D. Intravenous phenytoin
E. No treatment required
F. Oral antipyretics
G. Oral antibiotics
H. Oral diazepam
I. Rectal diazepam
J. Rectal paraldehyde

For each of the following children, select the most appropriate next step in management once airway, breathing and circulation have been assessed and facial oxygen has been applied. Each option may be used once, more than once or not at all.

1. A 3-year-old boy presents with fitting. There is no history of epilepsy and he is on no medication. The seizure started 5 minutes ago and has now stopped. He is very hot to touch and on examination you notice an inflamed left ear drum. His mother says that he has been pulling at his ear all day. His blood sugar is 5.0 mmol/L.

2. A 3-year-old boy presents with fitting. There is no history of epilepsy and he is on no medication. He started fitting 40 minutes ago. The seizure is still continuing despite attempts at medical termination. His blood sugar is 4.7 mmol/L.

3. A 3-year-old boy presents with fitting. There is no history of epilepsy and he is on no medication. He started fitting 15 minutes ago. The ambulance crew has given a single dose of rectal diazepam en route. On your arrival, the emergency department registrar has had two attempts at inserting a cannula, but has been unsuccessful. His blood sugar is 5.6 mmol/L.

4. A 3-year-old boy presents with fitting. There is no history of epilepsy and he is on no medication. He started fitting 20 minutes ago. He had an intravenous cannula sited on arrival and his blood sugar is 4.5 mmol/L. He has had two doses of intravenous lorazepam, but continues to fit.

5. A 3-year-old boy presents with fitting. There is no history of epilepsy and he is on no medication. His mother says that he has been having these fits for a few months. They always occur when he has hurt himself. Today, he bumped his head and started crying. He then stopped breathing and turned blue. On falling to the floor, there was a brief period where he was twitching his legs. He has now fully recovered. His blood sugar is 3.5 mmol/L.

Theme 8: Fever and a rash

Options

A. Fifth disease
B. Hand, foot and mouth disease
C. Henoch–Schönlein purpura
D. Kawasaki's disease
E. Measles
F. Meningococcal sepsis
G. Mumps
H. Roseola
I. Rubella
J. Scarlet fever
K. Varicella

For each of the following descriptions, select the most likely diagnosis. Each option may be used once, more than once or not at all.

1. A 2½-year-old boy presents with a fever and a rash. The rash is found mostly on his trunk, and is made up of papules, vesicles and pustules. There are lots of scratch marks over his torso. The onset of fever coincided with the rash.

2. A 2½-year-old boy presents with a fever and a rash. Five days ago, he was in contact with a girl at nursery who has chickenpox. His mother says that, after this contact, he became miserable and had a runny nose; a few days later, he developed a pink rash moving from his face down to his trunk. On examination, he has some white spots in his mouth.

3. A 2½-year-old boy presents with a fever and a rash. On the day prior to his admission, he had been a little irritable and had a high fever. He had vomited once. The following morning, he was not rousable and had a red rash over his lower limbs. On examination, he is cold and tachycardic and has a capillary refill time of 5 s.

4. A 2½-year-old boy presents with a fever and a rash. He had been a little hot this morning, but his mother sent him to nursery after giving him some paracetamol. She has now brought him to the emergency department because she is concerned that he has been slapped around the face at nursery.

5. A 2½-year-old boy presents with a fever and a rash. His mother is concerned that he is having an allergic reaction, as he has been hot all day, has a red rash that feels like goose-pimples, and now his tongue is red and swollen. You examine his throat, which reveals an inflamed pharynx.

Theme 9: Failure to thrive

Options

A. Antiretrovirals
B. Cardiac catheter laboratory – plugging
C. Cardiothoracic surgery
D. Change in milk formula
E. Creon with feeds
F. Fundoplication
G. Gluten-free diet
H. No treatment required
I. Oral metoclopramide
J. Oral metronidazole
K. Oral nystatin
L. Oral omeprazole
M. Oral rifampicin, isoniazid and pyrazinamide
N. Psychological intervention
O. Total parenteral nutrition

For each of the following children presenting with failure to thrive, select the next step in management. Each option may be used once, more than once or not at all.

1. A 4-month-old boy is failing to thrive. He has gastro-oesophageal reflux, shown on pH studies, and is being treated with feed thickeners, antacids, a proton pump inhibitor and a hypermotility drug. He continues to cry and arch his back after feeds. He has also occasionally stopped breathing and becomes cyanosed after feeds.

2. A 6-month-old girl is failing to thrive. On examination, she is small and breathless. Examination of the chest reveals a murmur heard throughout systole and diastole.

3. A premature infant develops necrotizing enterocolitis. A laparotomy is performed and the majority of the small and large bowel is resected.

4. A 2-year-old girl is failing to thrive. She has chronic diarrhoea and bloating. She is originally from India and arrived in the UK 12 months ago. An upper gastrointestinal endoscopy is performed and a duodenal biopsy is taken, which reveals partial villous atrophy with motile trophozoites.

5. A 2-year-old girl is failing to thrive. She has chronic diarrhoea and bloating. She is originally from India and arrived in the UK 12 months ago. An upper gastrointestinal endoscopy is performed and a duodenal biopsy is taken, which reveals total villous atrophy and no organisms.

Theme 10: Haematuria

Options

A. Benign familial haematuria
B. Drug ingestion
C. Food ingestion
D. Glomerulonephritis
E. Haemolysis
F. Haemorrhagic cystitis
G. Henoch–Schönlein purpura
H. Hypercalciuria
I. Nephrotic syndrome
J. Polycystic kidney disease
K. Porphyria
L. Renal/bladder tumour
M. Rhabdomyolysis
N. Stress haematuria

For each of the following scenarios, select the most appropriate diagnosis. Each option may be used once, more than once or not at all.

1. A 12-year-old boy presents to the clinic having recently started treatment for tuberculosis. He has developed painful purple lesions on his lower limbs and reports that he has started 'weeing blood'. The urine dipstick is negative for blood, protein, leucocytes and nitrites.

2. A 15-year-old boy reports that his urine has turned red. He has not changed his diet and is otherwise clinically well. He is a regular cross-country runner and took part in a road race the day before presentation. A urine dipstick is positive for blood and negative for protein, leucocytes and nitrites. He is followed up, and two repeat urine samples have no blood in them.

3. A 16-year-old girl has recently been started on the oral contraceptive pill. She presents shortly after with abdominal pain and vomiting. She reports that her urine has turned red. A dipstick is negative for blood, protein, leucocytes and nitrites.

4. A 3-year-old boy presents with red urine. He is clinically well, although he did have a perioral rash with yellow crusting 2 weeks prior to admission. He is systemically well and has no other symptoms. On examination, you find no signs other than a raised blood pressure. Urine is positive for blood and protein, but negative for leucocytes and nitrites. A full blood count is normal, with a normal blood film.

5. A 4-year-old boy returns to the ward after surgery to remove a brain tumour. The nursing staff notice that his urine is red. A urine sample is taken, and is positive for blood but negative for protein, leucocytes and nitrites.

Theme 1: Vomiting

1. D – Gastroenteritis

This history (vomiting and diarrhoea in an afebrile baby) is suggestive of gastroenteritis. A malrotation of the gut would usually present with bilious vomiting. Infective causes such as meningitis and a urinary tract infection should be in your differential diagnosis, but the lack of pyrexia in this case makes these less likely. Gastroenteritis is unusual in this age group, although it is more common in bottle-fed infants. The most important step is assessing and treating any degree of dehydration and ruling out more sinister infective causes. Educating parents how to sterilize bottles is important in preventing gastroenteritis.

2. G – Incarcerated inguinal hernia

This child is unwell. Bilious vomiting in this age group is a sign of bowel obstruction and should be taken very seriously. In this case, the infant has an incarcerated inguinal hernia, as revealed by the firm mass in the groin. (Testicular torsion can present with a firm mass in the scrotum with vomiting, but this is unlikely to be bilious.) As the bowel becomes obstructed, huge volumes of fluid shift into the bowel, which becomes oedematous and inflamed. The first step in managing this child is treating the severe dehydration, followed by reduction of the hernia and possible resection of necrotic bowel. There has been more than one cardiorespiratory arrest due to incarcerated inguinal hernias – so take them seriously!

3. E – Gastro-oesophageal reflux disease

True vomiting is the forceful ejection of stomach contents. Gastro-oesophageal reflux disease (GORD) is technically not vomiting but rather regurgitation, where stomach contents are ejected effortlessly. In infants, the lower oesophageal sphincter is not competent, so the passive reflux of acidic gastric contents into the oesophagus and oral cavity can cause significant symptoms. Aspiration can occur with GORD, causing chronic cough, wheeze and recurrent pneumonia in childhood. The first steps in management are conservative, e.g. propping the child up in a baby chair after feeding, nursing in a prone position and adding feed thickeners. Later steps include antacids (Gaviscon), prokinetics (erythromycin), H_2-receptor antagonists (ranitidine) and proton pump inhibitors (omeprazole). Cases resistant to medical management can be treated with surgery (Nissen's fundoplication).

4. K – Overfeeding

Overfeeding with milk is rare in breastfed babies. In bottle-fed babies, taking excessive volumes of milk causes distension of the stomach, which then ejects (vomits) the milk. A good feeding history is essential in any baby presenting with vomiting. Infants should take 150 180 mL/kg/day of milk.

5. L – Pyloric stenosis

The presentation of non-bile-stained projectile vomiting soon after feeds in a hungry baby is indicative of pyloric stenosis. Pyloric stenosis is hypertrophy of the circular muscle of the pylorus causing gastric outflow obstruction. It characteristically presents between 2 and 7 weeks of age and it most commonly affects firstborn males (4M:1F). Apart from projectile vomiting, affected babies may be constipated and lose weight. Often, these children are not clinically dehydrated, as the body compensates for the chronic fluid loss. A characteristic hypochloraemic, hypokalaemic, metabolic alkalosis results from vomiting stomach acid. Pyloric stenosis is diagnosed by giving the baby a 'test feed': when the baby is given milk, visible gastric peristalsis may be seen over the epigastrium, and the pylorus is felt as an olive-shaped mass in the upper abdomen. If the diagnosis is in doubt, an ultrasound scan can be performed. After initial rehydration, management is by Ramstedt's pyloromyotomy (where the muscle of the pylorus is cut longitudinally down to the mucosa). The baby can tolerate milk feeds a few hours after the operation.

Duodenal atresia is the congenital absence or closure of a portion of the duodenum. Around one-third of babies with duodenal atresia have trisomy 21 (Down's syndrome). Affected babies present at birth with bile-stained vomiting and abdominal distension. Diagnosis is confirmed by the presence of a double-bubble sign on the abdominal X-ray. This represents the presence of air in the stomach and proximal duodenum only, and not in the distal intestines. Treatment is by duodeno-duodenostomy.

Gastroschisis (Greek *gastro* = belly + *schisis* = cleft; 'split belly') is a defect in the anterior abdominal wall adjacent to the umbilicus. Abdominal contents, such as the liver and intestines, can herniate through this defect, but there is no sac covering the contents. Management of gastroschisis is by immediately covering the exposed viscera with Clingfilm, followed by surgical repair. Gastroschisis is rarely associated with other congenital malformations.

Exomphalos is the herniation of abdominal contents through the umbilicus. The herniated viscera are surrounded by a sac (the amnion), and this structure is known as an omphalocele. Surgical closure of the defect is required. Fifty per cent of cases of exomphalos are associated with other congenital malformations, such as trisomies and cardiac defects.

Meckel's diverticulum is a congenital diverticulum that contains gastric-type mucosa. It is an example of a true diverticulum (Latin *diverticulum* = by-road). A true diverticulum incorporates all the layers of the wall from which it arises. Conversely, a false diverticulum is made up of only the inner layer of the normal bowel wall, an example being colonic diverticula. There is a rule of 2's surrounding Meckel's diverticulum: it is found 2 feet proximal to the ileocaecal junction, it is 2 inches in length and it occurs in 2% of the population. Most Meckel's diverticula are incidental findings, but the commonest presentation is painless rectal bleeding. Some may present with acute inflammation, similar to acute appendicitis. Because Meckel's diverticula contain gastric mucosa, they are susceptible to peptic ulceration. Diagnosis is confirmed by a technetium-

99m (^{99m}Tc) scan. The radiolabelled technetium is taken up only by gastric-type mucosa, so the scan will highlight the stomach as well as a diverticulum in the right iliac fossa. Treatment is by resection if required.

Johann Friedrich Meckel, German anatomist (1781–1833).

Theme 2: The child with a limp

1. I – Slipped upper femoral epiphysis

Slipped upper femoral epiphysis describes posterolateral displacement of the femoral head. Slippage occurs though the femoral head growth plate. It occurs most commonly in boys aged 10–15 years during their adolescent growth spurt, and is associated with obesity, microgenitalia, hypothyroidism and a tall stature. Twenty per cent of cases are bilateral. Slipped upper femoral epiphysis presents with a limp and hip pain referred to the knee. It may follow minor trauma. There may be restriction in abduction and internal rotation of the hip. The diagnosis is confirmed on a lateral view X-ray of the affected hip. Management is by surgical pinning of the epiphysis. Complications of a slipped upper femoral epiphysis include premature epiphyseal fusion and avascular necrosis.

2. G – Perthes' disease

Perthes' disease (or Legg–Calvé–Perthes disease) is a degenerative disease of the hip. There is ischaemia of the femoral head involving the epiphysis and adjacent metaphysis (resulting in avascular necrosis). This is followed by revascularization and reossification over 2–3 years. Perthes' disease is five times more common in boys and usually occurs between 2 and 10 years of age. It presents with insidious-onset hip pain (which may be referred to the knee) and a limp. It is bilateral in 10% of cases. Diagnosis is by lateral X-ray of the affected hip, which shows an increased density and reduced size of the femoral head. The femoral head later becomes fragmented and irregular.

Management in mild disease is by bed rest and traction. In more severe cases, the femoral head needs to be 'covered' by the acetabulum so that it can act as a mould for the reossifying epiphysis. This is achieved by maintaining the hip in abduction or by surgical femoral osteotomy. The prognosis of Perthes' disease is usually good. However, if the child is under 6 years, or if more than half of the epiphysis is involved, there is an increased risk of deformity of the femoral head, with subsequent degenerative osteoarthritis in adult life.

Georg Clemens Perthes, German surgeon (1869–1927).

3. L – Transient synovitis

Transient synovitis (irritable hip) is the most common cause of acute hip pain in prepubescent children (between 3 and 8 years), and often follows a viral infection. It is often a diagnosis of exclusion. Features include sudden-onset hip pain that radiates to the knee, mild fever, a slight limp and a reduced range of movement, especially external rotation. There is no pain at rest and minimal systemic symptoms. Investigations, such as full blood count, acute phase proteins, joint X-ray and blood cultures, are negative. Ultrasound investigation may demonstrate a small effusion. Management is with analgesia, bed rest and skin traction. Irritable hip usually resolves in 7–10 days.

4. H – Septic arthritis

Septic arthritis is a medical emergency. It often affects a single joint and should always be considered with the presentation of a hot, swollen, tender joint with a restricted range of movement in the unwell patient. Septic arthritis is an infection within the synovial joint, most often caused by *Staphylococcus aureus* infection. It is most common in the hip and knee. Risk factors for developing septic arthritis include being very old or very young, intravenous drug use, diabetes and having pre-existing joint complaints. X-ray is normal in the early stages, but an ultrasound scan should be performed and joint aspiration done to culture organisms. Management of septic arthritis is with surgical washout of the joint and intravenous antibiotics (e.g. flucloxacillin and benzylpenicillin) until the patient is clinically well, followed by a few weeks of oral antibiotics. Complications of septic arthritis include joint destruction (leading to arthritis), spread of infection to the bone (osteomyelitis) and ankylosis (bony fusion across the joint).

5. A – Developmental dysplasia of the hip

Developmental dysplasia of the hip (DDH, or congenital dislocation of the hip) is a spectrum of disorders ranging from partial subluxation to frank dislocation of the hip. It is thought that high concentrations of the maternal hormone relaxin contribute to the laxity of the hip joint. DDH is found in 1 in 1000 births, and it is six times more common in females. The left hip is more likely to be dislocated than the right. Risk factors for DDH include a positive family history, breech delivery, spinal/neuromuscular abnormalities (e.g. spina bifida and talipes equinovarus) and oligohydramnios.

Neonatal screening for DDH is by two methods: Barlow's test (the hip can easily be displaced posteriorly out of the acetabulum on adduction of the leg with posterior pressure) and Ortolani's manoeuvre (the femoral head can be reduced back into the acetabulum on abduction of the leg with anterior pressure). These tests are routinely done at birth and 6 weeks of age. These manoeuvres have a good positive predictive value (i.e. if the examination is positive, the patient has DDH) but a very poor negative predictive value (i.e. many patients with a normal examination are later found to have DDH). DDH may present with asymmetrical skinfolds, limited abduction, shortening of the affected limb and limp. If spotted early, DDH responds to conservative treatment. The hips can be placed in abduction (using a Craig's splint) or the child can be put in a restraining device (Pavlik harness) for several months. Progress should be monitored by ultrasound or X-ray. If conservative measures fail, open reduction and femoral osteotomy may be required. Necrosis of the femoral head is a potential complication of DDH.

Sir Thomas Barlow, English physician and paediatrician (1845–1945).

Marino Ortolani, Italian paediatrician (1904–83).

In *talipes equinovarus* ('clubfoot'), the foot is inverted and plantarflexed. Talipes is the commonest congenital abnormality, occurring in around 1 in 500 births. Half of cases are bilateral. Clubfoot may be secondary to intrauterine compression (from oligohydramnios) or a neuromuscular disorder (such as spina bifida). This condition must be managed, otherwise the deformity will persist. Options include passive stretching and strapping. If deformity is severe then corrective surgery is required.

Osgood–Schlatter disease is a condition characterized by transient inflammation of the growth plate (i.e. osteochondritis) of the tibial tuberosity where the patellar tendon attaches. It is most common in active boys in their early teens. Features include pain and swelling around the tuberosity that is worse on activity, especially leg extension. Treatment is with rest and analgesia.

Spontaneous haemarthrosis describes recurrent acute swellings in joints of children due to underlying haemophilia. Trivial trauma may result in bleeding into the joint, most commonly the knee, and this is known as haemarthrosis. Haemophilia is an X-linked recessive deficiency of factor VIII or IX. Recurrent haemarthroses result in pain, stiffness and early osteoarthritis.

Genu varus (or bowlegs) is a deformity characterized by medial angulation of the lower leg at the knee (the term 'valgus' describes the opposite deformity). The most common cause of genu varus is rickets, which is a deficiency of vitamin D resulting in a lack of calcium absorption with subsequent skeletal and dental deformities. Another cause of genu varus in children is *Blount's disease*, where asymmetrical growth of the tibial physis results in a progressive varus deformity at the knee (i.e. the lateral part of the tibia grows quicker than the medial side). Blount's disease is more common in Scandinavian and Afro-Caribbean children.

The original Latin words *varus* and *valgus* had the opposite meaning to their modern use in medicine. *Varus* meant 'knock-kneed' and *valgus* meant 'bowlegged', because the Latin words actually described the position of the leg at the hip joint rather than at the knee joint. (Latin *genu* = knee.)

Talipes equinovarus, from Latin *talus* = ankle + *pes* = foot + *equinus* = horse-like + *varus* = inward (inward turning of the ankle and foot, like a horse).

Walter Putnam Blount, American orthopaedic surgeon (1900–92).

Robert Bayley Osgood, American orthopaedic surgeon (1873–1956).

Carl Schlatter, Swiss physician (1864–1934).

Theme 3: Cough

1. E – Cystic fibrosis

Cystic fibrosis (CF) is the commonest autosomal recessive condition in Caucasian populations in the UK, affecting 1 in 2500 live births. CF is caused by an abnormal gene coding for the cystic fibrosis transmembrane regulator protein (CFTR), located on chromosome 7. CFTR is a cyclic adenosine monophosphate (cAMP)-dependent chloride channel blocker. The most common mutation in CF is the ΔF508 mutation. The poor transport of chloride ions and water across epithelial cells of the respiratory and pancreas exocrine glands in CF results in an increased viscosity of secretions. The range of presentations is varied, including recurrent chest infections, failure to thrive from malabsorption and liver disease. In the neonatal period, infants may present with prolonged neonatal jaundice, bowel obstruction (meconium ileus) or rectal prolapse.

The gold standard investigation for CF is the sweat test. The abnormal function of sweat glands results in an excess concentration of sodium chloride (NaCl) in sweat. Sweat is stimulated by pilocarpine iontophoresis, collected on filter paper and analysed.

Normal sweat NaCl concentration   10–14 mmol/L
Sweat NaCl concentration in CF   80–125 mmol/L

At least two sweat tests should be performed, as diagnostic errors and false positives are common.

Management options in CF include physiotherapy (for respiratory secretions), antibiotics (for prophylaxis and treatment of lung infections) and pancreatic enzyme supplements (to prevent malabsorption). Complications include diabetes mellitus, hepatic cirrhosis, infertility in males, severe pulmonary hypertension and cor pulmonale, and chronic lung infections (*Pseudomonas* spp. and *Burkholderia cepacia*). Many cases of CF are now being picked up early since the introduction of a national screening programme assessing immunoreactive trypsin (IRT) levels on the Guthrie card at day 8 of life. IRT is a pancreatic enzyme with levels that are raised in CF.

2. H – Pneumonia

Fever and a respiratory rate >50/min in a child under 3 years is strongly suggestive of pneumonia. Lower respiratory tract infections (pneumonias and chest infections) can be caused by both viruses and bacteria. Although aspiration can cause similar findings, there are no risk factors in this case that suggest aspiration (e.g. neurological pathology). Chest signs such as crepitations are less reliable in children, and often will not be heard at all. It is paramount that you check respiratory rate, as most children with pneumonia will be tachypnoeic. Upper respiratory tract infections (URTIs) can cause very similar findings, but the child is less likely to be tachypnoeic. Evidence of lower respiratory tract infections may be seen on chest X-ray. Treatment of bacterial infections is with appropriate antibiotics (and oxygen if required).

3. B – Asthma

This boy has asthma. Asthma can present in a number of ways, including cough (often worse at night), wheeze, shortness of breath and failure to thrive. Sleep is interrupted, which can affect school performance. Note that gastro-oesophageal reflux can also cause a night cough and should be considered as a differential.

Asthma is the commonest chronic illness in childhood, affecting up to 15% of all children. The underlying pathophysiology is chronic inflammation of the bronchial mucosa, with airway hyperreactivity. Trigger factors (e.g. exercise, viral infections, allergens, cold air and severe emotions) cause bronchoconstriction, mucosal oedema and excess mucus production. This leads to airway narrowing and the typical features of asthma. Asthma is associated with atopy, a condition where individuals produce substantial amounts of immunoglobulin (IgE) antibodies following trivial exposure to everyday antigens. It tends to run in families. Other atopic conditions include allergic rhinitis (obstruction of nostrils causing sniffing, sneezing and a runny nose), eczema, allergic conjunctivitis, urticaria/angioedema and food/drug allergies. When allergic rhinitis occurs only in summer due to high pollen counts, it is known as 'hay fever'. If it occurs throughout the year, it is called 'perennial rhinitis'.

A diagnosis of asthma can be confirmed by demonstrating reversible airflow obstruction using a peak flow meter (this can only be done above the age of 5 years). If peak flow significantly improves following administration of a bronchodilator then asthma is suggested. The management of asthma follows a stepwise approach, summarized as follows:

- Step 1: Short-acting β_2-agonist (salbutamol or terbutaline)
- Step 2: Step 1 + low-dose inhaled steroid (budesonide or fluticasone)
- Step 3: Step 2 +
  - o <5 years: leukotriene inhibitor (monteleukast)
  - o ≥5 years: high-dose inhaled steroid and long-acting β_2-agonist
- Step 4: Step 3 + fourth drug (e.g. theophylline or an anticholinergic)
- Step 5: Step 4 + oral steroid (prednisolone)

Acute exacerbations of asthma may require admission to hospital. Immediate treatment of acute asthma is with high-flow oxygen (via a facemask), bronchodilating nebulizers (β_2-agonists and anticholinergics) and steroids. Features of severe asthma are being too breathless to talk or feed, respiration rate ≥50/min, pulse ≥140/min and peak flow ≤50% predicted or best. Features of life-threatening asthma are fatigue/exhaustion, decreasing consciousness, a silent chest, poor respiratory effort and a peak flow ≤33% predicted or best.

4. C – Bronchiolitis

Bronchiolitis is very common. It keeps paediatric wards busy during the winter months and can be life threatening, especially to at-risk groups (premature babies, heart disease, etc.). Bronchiolitis is caused by viruses, most commonly respiratory syncytial virus (RSV). Respiratory distress (intercostal recession, head bobbing and nasal flaring) and wheezing are caused by obstruction of the small airways. Auscultation may reveal fine inspiratory crepitations. Bronchiolitis can be confirmed by taking swabs of nasopharyngeal secretions. Most infants do not require admission, although some may need support for hydration and oxygenation. Antibiotics, steroids and bronchodilators are not effective.

5. F – Foreign body

Foreign-body inhalation is most common in toddlers, as they are prone to putting objects in their mouths. The most common offenders are small toys and peanuts. Most foreign bodies present immediately. However, some may be delayed by weeks to months before symptoms develop. At the time of swallowing, the child has sudden-onset cough, wheeze or breathlessness. If the object is stuck in the larynx, it causes a croupy cough and stridor. If the object becomes stuck in the bronchus, there may initially be no symptoms until an infection develops several days later. Inhaled foreign bodies may be diagnosed by radiography, but rigid bronchoscopy will confirm the diagnosis and remove the offending object.

For information on the diagnosis and investigation of respiratory problems, in children and adults, put your textbooks away and use the excellent British Thoracic Society (BTS) guidelines, which can be found online at www.brit-thoracic.org.uk (cited September 2007).

Theme 4: Chromosomal disorders

1. A – 45XO (Turner's syndrome)

Most cases of Turner's syndrome result in early miscarriage (approximately 95%). Despite this, the incidence remains approximately 1 in 2500 liveborn females. The features of Turner's syndrome are lymphoedema of the hands and feet in the neonatal period, webbed neck (*in utero* oedema causes the webbing), short stature, wide carrying angle, widely spaced nipples, coarctation of the aorta and infertility. Girls with Turner's syndrome will have normal to low-normal intelligence.

Henry Turner, American endocrinologist (1892–1970).

2. E – 47XX (18) (Edwards' syndrome)

Most children with Edwards' syndrome die early in infancy, with fewer than 10% surviving beyond 1 year of age. The clinical features of Edwards' syndrome are low-set ears, small chin, microcephaly, overlapping fingers, rocker-bottom feet, cardiac defects (especially ventricular septal defects), renal anomalies and learning disability.

Patau's syndrome, or 47XX (13), is characterized by structural defects of the brain, small eyes, polydactyly and cardiac/renal malformations. Most babies with Patau's syndrome do not survive beyond 1 year of age.

John Hilton Edwards, British geneticist (1928–2007).

Klaus Patau, German geneticist (1908–75).

3. C – 47XXY (Klinefelter's syndrome)

Klinefelter's syndrome is the most common cause of male hypogonadism, occurring in 1–2 per 1000 male births. These patients have small, firm testes, are tall, and have behavioural problems, delayed speech and gynaecomastia. Testosterone therapy is sometimes used to improve the development of secondary sexual characteristics.

47XXX (*triple X syndrome*) is the presence of an extra X chromosome in females. Although some patients have mild learning disabilities, most do not have any

The diagnosis of rheumatic fever is made using the modified Duckett Jones criteria, requiring either two major criteria *or* one major and two minor criteria *plus* evidence of streptococcal infection (e.g. anti-streptolysin-O titres).

Modified Duckett Jones criteria

Major:
- pancarditis
- polyarthritis
- Sydenham's chorea (St Vitus' dance)
- erythema marginatum
- subcutaneous nodules

Minor:
- fever
- arthralgia
- high erythrocyte sedimentation rate (ESR) or white cell count (WCC)
- heart block

In this case, the boy has erythema marginatum, arthralgia and a fever.

Pancarditis can present with murmurs, including mitral regurgitation, aortic regurgitation (in 50%) and the Carey Coombs murmur (a soft mid-diastolic murmur that occurs due to nodule development on mitral valve leaflets). Sydenham's chorea includes choreiform movements, emotional lability and explosive speech. The polyarthritis is often fleeting, affects the large joints and is characteristically responsive to aspirin. Subcutaneous nodules are small, firm and painless, and are best felt over the tendons or bones.

The treatment of rheumatic fever requires antibiotics (usually penicillin), analgesia, NSAIDs and bed rest. Steroids are sometimes indicated in severe cases. Following the acute phase, patients require prophylactic antibiotics prior to invasive procedures such as tooth extraction in order to protect against bacteraemia and subsequent bacterial endocarditis.

Chorea, from Latin *chorea* = dance.

Saint Vitus' dance (*chorea sancti viti* in Latin) was a festival of the Middle Ages celebrating Vitus the patron saint of dancers, actors and comedians.

Carey Franklin Coombs, English cardiologist (1879–1932).

T Duckett Jones, American physician (1899–1954).

Thomas Sydenham, English physician (1624–89).

5. B – Enteropathic arthritis

Enteropathic arthritis is an asymmetrical oligoarthritis predominantly affecting the larger joints of the lower limb. It occurs with underlying inflammatory bowel disease. It is difficult to distinguish between ulcerative colitis (UC) and Crohn's disease from the history, although UC is more commonly associated with bloody stools. Other extraintestinal features of inflammatory bowel disease include clubbing, erythema nodosum (painful lesions on the lower legs), anterior uveitis (inflammation of the anterior eye causing acute pain, photophobia and blurring), ankylosing spondylitis, hepatobiliary disease (primary biliary cirrhosis), pyoderma gangrenosum (deep, necrotic ulcers with a dark-red border usually occurring on the leg) and perianal disease (skin tags, fissures and fistulae).

Theme 6: Jaundice in the newborn

As many as 50% of newborn babies will be clinically jaundiced in the first week of life. Bilirubin is produced by the breakdown of fetal haemoglobin (HbF), which is replaced with adult haemoglobin (HbA). Most infants will not need any intervention or any investigation as long as they do not break any of the following rules:

- Jaundice is not apparent in the first 24 hours of life.
- The infant is clinically well, and remains clinically well.
- The serum bilirubin is below treatment level.
- The jaundice has resolved by 14 days.

High levels of unconjugated bilirubin can cross the blood–brain barrier and cause permanent neuronal damage (kernicterus). Jaundice can be treated with phototherapy, which converts unconjugated bilirubin into non-toxic isomers that are excreted. In reality, one would rarely perform a single blood test in an infant with jaundice, instead ordering a battery of them together as a 'jaundice screen'. In this question, the examiner is looking to see if you can assess the diagnosis and the investigation that comes with it. Always remember to take a serum bilirubin level, as this will determine if phototherapy is required.

1. C – Blood cultures

This infant is likely to have a bacterial sepsis associated with prolonged rupture of membranes. Common organisms include group B streptococci, *Escherichia coli*, *Listeria* spp., *Staphylococcus aureus* and other streptococci. A full blood count and C-reactive protein may be helpful, but will not provide a diagnosis. A blood culture is needed. Intravenous empirical antibiotics should be started immediately. Use of the polymerase chain reaction (PCR) is starting to play more of a role in identifying organisms causing sepsis, but is currently not available in all centres.

2. G – Group and Coombs' testing

This is likely to be a case of rhesus disease of the newborn. The mother's blood group should be taken, along with a group and Coombs' test performed on the baby's blood. The blood group will tell you if they have the same blood group and rhesus status; the Coombs' test will tell you if there is a reaction occurring between the two. Rhesus disease is now uncommon in the UK due to the use of anti-D immunoglobulins in rhesus D-negative mothers to prevent the production of antibodies. All pregnant women have their blood group taken early in pregnancy, and then infants of rhesus-negative mothers will have blood taken from the umbilical cord immediately after birth. (Some slip through the net.)

3. B – Abdominal ultrasound

The most important diagnosis to rule out is biliary atresia. Any baby jaundiced beyond 14 days of life should have conjugated bilirubin levels measured. If there is a high conjugated fraction (>18% and >20 μmol/L) then biliary atresia is likely. This, however, does not confirm the diagnosis, as there are other causes of a conjugated jaundice. Biliary atresia can be seen on liver ultrasound or on a non-excreting hydroxyiminodiacetic acid (HIDA) scan. If biliary atresia is diagnosed early enough (before 6–8 weeks), surgery can be performed and will result in a relatively good outcome.

4. I – No further investigation required

This is most likely to be a case of breastfeeding jaundice. There are many hypotheses regarding why breastfeeding can cause jaundice, but all are still yet to be proven. The key here is that the infant is well, that the jaundice was not present in the first 24 hours after birth and that it is below treatment level. If the jaundice is still present after 14 days, he will need to have conjugated bilirubin levels.

5. L – TORCH screen

All the congenital infections cause jaundice. The mnemonic TORCH is used:
- **T** Toxoplasmosis
- **O** Other (e.g. syphilis)
- **R** Rubella
- **C** Cytomegalovirus (CMV)
- **H** Herpes simplex

The most common of these is CMV, which may be associated with hepatomegaly. Features common to all TORCH infections are low birth weight, prematurity, jaundice, microcephaly, seizures, anaemia, failure to thrive and encephalitis.

Theme 7: Seizures

In any seizure, the priority is first to assess and rule out any compromise of airway, breathing and circulation. Check for and treat any hypoglycaemia (ABC-DEFG: Don't Ever Forget Glucose). The Advance Life Support Group has drawn up algorithms for managing both paediatric and adult seizures. Make sure that you are familiar with these. For more information on the management of seizures, see the SIGN (Scottish Intercollegiate Guidelines Network) guidelines (www.sign.ac.uk).

1. F – Oral antipyretics

This boy has most likely had a febrile convulsion. For a seizure to be defined as febrile, the child must be developmentally normal and between the ages of 6 months and 5 years. There is often a family history of febrile seizures. Evidence suggests that antipyretics such as paracetamol and ibuprofen do not reduce the risk of febrile convulsions (so if you marked '*no treatment required*', give yourself the mark). However, if a child is in pain (earache in this case) or has a fever then symptomatic relief is appropriate. Acute otitis media does not routinely need antibiotic management.

2. A – Anaesthesia and intubation

This boy is in status epilepticus. Status epilepticus is defined as generalized convulsions lasting 30 minutes or longer, or successive convulsions lasting over 30 minutes without recovery between seizures. When a child has been fitting for a period of longer than 20 minutes, an anaesthetist should be contacted, as there is a good chance that the child will need rapid anaesthesia (by rapid sequence induction) for intubation and ventilation.

3. I – Rectal diazepam

Benzodiazepines are the mainstay of early seizure treatment. They can be given intravenously (lorazepam), rectally (diazepam) or buccally (midazolam). Getting intravenous access is important, but if this is not possible then there are other routes of administering antiepileptic medications. The jury is still out on whether rectal diazepam or buccal midazolam is superior. Either is appropriate. One must be very aware that benzodiazepines, by any route, can cause respiratory depression. When a child is fitting, you should continually reassess ABC and keep an appropriately sized bag and mask to hand.

4. J – Rectal paraldehyde

This child is not yet in status epilepticus, but is still having a significant seizure that requires terminating. He has had two doses of benzodiazepine, and so the next step is a rectal dose of paraldehyde. If this is not successful then a phenytoin infusion should be administered. Failing this, the next step is intubation and ventilation.

5. E – No treatment required

This child is having breath-holding attacks. These usually commence in the first few years of life. They are often preceded by physical or emotional trauma. After a brief period of crying, the child will hold their breath and will become cyanotic. They will then become hypotonic and potentially lose consciousness. Some children subsequently display seizure-like activity (tonus or clonus). No investigation or treatment is required. Behavioural steps may help, and some families find that blowing on the face or splashing the face with water may terminate the event.

Theme 8: Fever and a rash

1. K – Varicella

Chickenpox is caused by the varicella zoster virus, which is spread via the respiratory route with an incubation period of 14–21 days. Clinical features include fever and an itchy rash found predominantly on the trunk and scalp. The rash is made up of pustules and vesicles, which eventually crust over. The onset of fever coincides with the pustular phase of the rash. Complications of chickenpox include secondary bacterial infection (staphylococcal or streptococcal), pneumonitis and conjunctival lesions. Encephalitis is a rare complication that presents with ataxia several weeks after infection. Purpura fulminans (widespread vasculitis of the skin and subcutaneous tissues) and stroke are very rare complications.

In immunocompromised patients, primary varicella infection can result in disseminated haemorrhagic infection with a 20% mortality rate. If a pregnant woman develops chickenpox in the first trimester, there is a 2% risk that the baby will develop fetal varicella syndrome (characterized by limb hypoplasia, microcephaly, cataracts, growth retardation and skin scarring). Treatment of chickenpox is generally supportive, although the antiviral aciclovir should be given to adolescents and immunocompromised individuals. Human varicella zoster immunoglobulins are administered prophylactically to immunocompromised patients who are at high risk of infection.

2. E – Measles

Measles (morbilli) is caused by an RNA virus that is transmitted by droplet infection. There is an incubation period of 10–12 days. The incidence has decreased since introduction of the vaccine. Children with measles tend to be miserable, with fever, coryza, cough, conjunctivitis, and a maculopapular rash that starts at the face and spreads downwards onto the trunk. The fever and coryza precede the rash by around 4 days. Koplik's spots (white pinhead spots on the buccal mucosa) are pathognomonic for measles. Complications of measles include otitis media, pneumonitis, myocarditis and encephalitis. Encephalitis, which occurs in 1 in 5000 cases a few weeks after initial infection, is characterized by headache, lethargy, convulsions and coma. Long-term sequelae of measles encephalitis include epilepsy, deafness, hemiplegia and learning difficulties. Subacute sclerosing panencephalitis (SSPE) is a very rare complication that begins 7 years after initial infection. Features include gradual loss in neurological function, progressing to dementia and death. Management of measles is symptomatic and children should be isolated. Measles is a notifiable disease.

Henry Koplik, American physician (1858–1927).

3. F – Meningococcal sepsis

Meningococcal disease is caused by the Gram-negative diplococcus *Neisseria meningitidis*. Meningococcal disease can present with meningitis alone (15%), septicaemia alone (25%), or both meningitis and septicaemia (60%). The incubation period is 2–10 days. Affected children often present with non-specific symptoms: headache, poor feeding, lethargy and photophobia. This is followed by shock, fever and a non-blanching purpuric rash. Examination signs include Kernig's sign (when the hip is flexed with the knee bent, pain is felt on attempting to straighten the leg) and Brudzinski's sign (flexion of the neck causes the leg to be drawn up due to meningeal irritation). A bulging fontanelle, neck stiffness and opisthotonus (lying with an arched back) are late signs. The offending organism can be cultured (from pharyngeal swabs, blood cultures, aspirates of skin lesions or cerebrospinal fluid), although diagnosis is increasingly relying on PCR. Treatment is with resuscitation and immediate intravenous antibiotics, e.g. cefotaxime. Complications include brain damage, deafness, blindness, loss of digits or limbs, adrenal haemorrhage (Waterhouse–Friderichsen syndrome), and death.

Josef Brudzinski, Polish paediatrician (1874–1917).

Carl Friderichsen, Danish paediatrician (1886–1979).

Vladimir Mikhailovich Kernig, German neurologist (1840–1917).

Rupert Waterhouse, English physician (1873–1958).

4. A – Fifth disease

Fifth disease (also known as erythema infectiosum or slapped-cheek syndrome) is caused by droplet-borne parvovirus B19 infection (now called erythrovirus). It has an incubation period of 6–14 days. Affected children present with an appearance of slapped cheeks followed by a maculopapular rash on the limbs, malaise and fever. Complications include arthralgia and aplastic anaemia. All children with fifth disease should have a full blood count to exclude pancytopenia from aplastic anaemia.

Fifth disease is so called because it is the fifth of the six classic childhood skin rashes (the others being measles, chickenpox, rubella, scarlet fever and roseola infantum).

5. J – Scarlet fever

Scarlet fever is caused by the group A β-haemolytic streptococcus (*Streptococcus pyogenes*), which has an incubation period of 7 days. Children present with tonsillitis, an erythematosus rash predominantly on the trunk and a sore coated tongue (strawberry tongue). Desquamation (peeling) of the skin of the palms and soles may occur towards the end of the illness. Diagnosis is made by finding raised anti-streptolysin O (ASO) titres or by culturing group A streptococci from throat swabs. Complications include otitis media, acute nephritis and rheumatic fever.

Roseola infantum (exanthema subitum) is caused by human herpesviruses (HHV) 6 and 7, and presents with high fever and malaise followed by a generalized macular rash. Diagnosis is confirmed by finding evidence of the virus in serum.

Hand, foot and mouth disease is caused by enteroviruses (e.g. coxsackievirus). It results in a painful papulovesicular eruption on the palms, soles, mucous membranes and occasionally the buttocks.

Theme 9: Failure to thrive

1. F – Fundoplication

This child has severe gastro-oesophageal reflux disease, which is being managed medically. Feed thickeners make milk more viscid and reduce reflux into the oesophagus. Antacids and proton pump inhibitors (e.g. omeprazole) do not prevent reflux, but rather reduce the acidity of the stomach contents and therefore reduce irritation within the gullet. Hypermotility drugs (e.g. metoclopramide) reduce the tone in the pylorus and aid emptying of the stomach to reduce reflux. All of these steps have failed in this child, and he is symptomatic with failure to thrive and apnoeas after feeds. The next step in management is surgical correction – fundoplication – which involves wrapping the fundus of the stomach around the lower part of the oesophagus.

2. B – Cardiac catheter laboratory – plugging

This child has a patent ductus arteriosus causing heart failure. Heart failure commonly causes failure to thrive for two reasons: first, the workload of the heart is raised due to increased right atrial filling pressures; and second, these children are often too breathless to feed effectively. The heart failure should initially be treated with diuretics, such as furosemide and spironolactone. The patent ductus should then be plugged via a catheter inserted into the femoral artery. Only if this fails should open cardiothoracic surgery be performed.

3. O – Total parenteral nutrition

Necrotizing enterocolitis (NEC) is a life-threatening condition occurring in the neonatal period. It occurs primarily in premature infants who are milk-fed. The exact cause is not yet known. There is ischaemia of the bowel and infection by bowel organisms. Babies present with bile-stained vomiting, bloody diarrhoea and abdominal distension. This is rapidly followed by shock. Abdominal X-ray shows dilated bowel loops and thickening of the bowel wall with intramural air. Management is initially medical with broad-spectrum antibiotics to cover both aerobes and anaerobes, but often the affected bowel needs to be resected. If only small lengths of bowel remain then nutrition is not possible through the gut. Nutrition therefore needs to be provided parenterally (intravenously) – usually through a central line. Calories, fat, protein, vitamins and minerals all need to be administered. These children often have a stormy course, as they get frequent central line infections.

4. J – Oral metronidazole

This girl has giardiasis (also known as beaver fever). The motile trophozoites and the villous atrophy are diagnostic. *Giardia lamblia* is a flagellate protozoal parasite, passed via the faeco-oral route, which attaches itself to the intestinal wall but does not invade it. Chronic infection causes malabsorption, particularly of carbohydrates and fat. The malabsorption of fat can result in deficiency of fat-soluble vitamins (vitamins A, D, E and K). A duodenal biopsy identifying trophozoites suggests giardiasis. Stool cultures can be taken to look for cysts. Treatment is with oral metronidazole.

5. G – Gluten-free diet

Causes of villous atrophy include coeliac disease, temporary gluten intolerance secondary to gastroenteritis, cows'/soya milk intolerance, giardiasis, severe combined immunodeficiency, post-chemotherapy, kwashiorkor and tropical sprue. The most common cause would be coeliac disease, especially with a history of chronic diarrhoea, abdominal distension and failure to thrive.

Coeliac disease ('coeliac', from Greek *koiliakos* = abdominal), which affects 1 in 1000 in the UK, is caused by an adverse immunological response to the gliadin fraction of gluten. Children normally present with failure to thrive following the introduction of the gluten cereals barley, wheat and rye. Symptoms include general irritability, diarrhoea, abdominal distension, buttock wasting, iron-deficiency anaemia and growth failure. Diagnosis is by jejunal biopsy, which demonstrates villous atrophy and crypt hyperplasia, although screening for autoantibodies is often performed in the first instance (anti-gliadin and anti-endomyseal antibodies). Treatment is with a lifelong gluten-free diet, and results in rapid resolution of symptoms. Conditions that are associated with coeliac disease include small-bowel lymphoma, dermatitis herpetiformis (an intensely itchy vesicular rash found on the extensor surfaces) and other autoimmune diseases (e.g. thyroid disease, pernicious anaemia and vitiligo).

Theme 10: Haematuria

Haematuria can be described as either microscopic (>5 red cells per high-power field) or macroscopic (visible to the naked eye). Remember that red urine is not always blood; other causes include drug ingestion (below), porphyrinuria, methaemoglobinaemia and food ingestion (beetroots and blackberries). All patients with significant haematuria should have the following investigations performed: blood pressure, full blood count, serum creatinine and C3 levels, urine for culture, 24-hour urine collection for creatinine, protein and calcium, and an ultrasound scan of the urinary tract.

1. B – Drug ingestion

This boy is being treated for tuberculosis. The antituberculous drug rifampicin commonly causes red urine and purple tears as side-effects. Other anti-tuberculous drugs (and their side-effects) are isoniazid (hepatitis and peripheral neuropathy), pyrazinamide (hepatitis, photosensitivity and gout), streptomycin (nephrotoxicity and ototoxicity) and ethambutol (optic neuritis). The painful purple lesions on the legs are erythema nodosum (Henoch–Schönlein purpura could be a differential, but the dipstick is negative for blood). Causes of erythema nodosum include sarcoidosis, leprosy, inflammatory bowel disease, streptococcal throat infections, tuberculosis and certain drugs (sulphonamide antibiotics and the oral contraceptive pill). Trauma is *not* a cause.

Theme 1: Constipation

Options

- A. Anal dilatation
- B. Behavioural therapy
- C. Bowel resection
- D. EDTA chelation
- E. Gastrograffin enema
- F. Laxatives
- G. Manual evacuation
- H. Oral enzyme supplements
- I. Thyroid-stimulating hormone
- J. Thyroxine

For each of the following children with constipation, select the next most appropriate step in management. Each option may be used once, more than once or not at all.

1. A 12-year-old boy is constipated. He opens his bowels on average once each week. He describes this as being incredibly painful, 'like a tearing pain'. On wiping, he has noticed blood on the toilet paper. Examination is very painful, and a skin tag is present at the anal verge.

2. A 6-year-old boy is constipated. He is a challenging child who has some behavioural problems and has recently started eating dirt from the garden. He presents to the emergency department with acute-onset abdominal pain, vomiting and headache. On examination, he is unable to walk properly. You perform a full blood count, which reveals a haemoglobin of 8.4 g/dL with a mean cell volume of 72 fL.

3. A newborn presents having failed to open his bowels by 48 hours of life. On performing a rectal examination, you note a normal-sized rectum. When you withdraw the examining finger, there is an explosion of meconium from the rectum.

4. A 6-month-old boy presents with constipation. He recently moved from China. He has coarse facial features and a large tongue. He is behind on his developmental milestones. Examination is un-remarkable except for an umbilical hernia.

5. A newborn presents having failed to open his bowels by 48 hours of life. Apart from this, he is clinically well. He has an older sibling with cystic fibrosis.

Theme 2: Anaemia

Options

A. Haemoglobin electrophoresis
B. No investigation at this point
C. Plasma viscosity
D. Schilling test
E. Serum ferritin levels
F. Serum folate levels
G. Serum iron levels
H. Serum lead levels
I. Serum urea and creatinine

For each of the following cases presenting with anaemia, select the investigation most likely to give a diagnosis at this point. Each option may be used once, more than once or not at all.

1. A 4-year-old girl presents with acute-onset pain in the fingers of her left hand. She had been playing in the snow with her brothers earlier that day. She is normally fit and well, but was feeling under the weather a week ago, with a high temperature and flushed cheeks. A full blood count reveals a haemoglobin of 5 g/dL.

2. A 4-year-old girl presents with a fever and productive cough, and is found to have a lower respiratory tract infection. A routine full blood count reveals microcytic hypochromic anaemia. She is described as a fussy eater by her mother, although she has a tendency to eat inappropriate items such as soil and paper. There is no history of medical problems.

3. A 15-year-old girl is found to be anaemic on her annual assessment. On examination, you notice that she is mildly jaundiced. Her haemoglobin is 9.2 g/dL, with a mean cell volume of 102 fL. She has been treated for Graves' disease in the past.

4. A 4-month-old boy presents with failure to thrive. You find hepatosplenomegaly on examination. A full blood count reveals haemoglobin 10.0 g/dL and mean cell volume 72 fL. A blood film confirms hypochromia.

5. A 6-year-old girl who was previously well presents to the paediatrics clinic with long-standing abdominal pain. Her parents have noticed her eating inappropriate substances such as paper and paint. A social history elicits that her performance at school has deteriorated recently. Routine investigations reveal hypochromic microcytic anaemia.

Theme 3: Stridor

Options

A. Inhaled salbutamol
B. Intramuscular adrenaline
C. Intramuscular and nebulized adrenaline
D. Intravenous broad-spectrum antibiotics
E. Intravenous steroids
F. Intubation and ventilation
G. Intubation, ventilation and intravenous broad-spectrum antibiotics
H. Nebulized steroids
I. No management required
J. Oral antihistamine
K. Oral antihistamine and intravenous steroids
L. Oral antihistamine and nebulized steroids
M. Oral antihistamine and adrenaline
N. Oral antihistamine, intravenous steroids and adrenaline
O. Oral antihistamine, nebulized steroids and adrenaline
P. Rigid bronchoscopy

For each of the following children presenting with stridor, select the management steps that you would take after applying oxygen. Each option may be used once, more than once or not at all.

1. An 18-month-old girl presents with a cough and stridor. The cough is described as 'barking' in nature. She has a temperature of 38°C and is restless. She does not appear systemically unwell and is not cyanotic, but there is moderate stridor on exertion.

2. A 3-year-old girl presents with stridor of a few hours' duration. She has been well for the last few days. She has a temperature of 39.5°C. She is sat on her mother's knee with her head leaning forward, is very quiet and is drooling. On examination, she is systemically unwell and has a quiet stridor and reduced air entry bilaterally.

3. A 16-month-old girl presents with stridor. She was with her family this afternoon at a picnic in the park. Since having lunch an hour ago, she developed swelling of her face and lips. She has a red rash over her trunk and limbs. On examination, she is pale, tachycardic and oedematous. She has a quiet stridor with reduced air entry bilaterally.

4. A 4-year-old girl presents with stridor of a few hours' duration. She has been unwell for a few days, complaining of a sore throat. She has a temperature of 39.5°C. She is sat on her mother's knee, is very irritable, with her head tilted to one side, and is drooling. On examination, she appears systemically unwell and has a quiet stridor but good air entry bilaterally.

5. A 21-month-old girl presents with a cough and stridor. This developed while she was having lunch with her family at home an hour ago. On examination, she is systemically well and has a quiet bilateral stridor with reduced air entry on the right.

Theme 4: Developmental assessment

Options

    A. Newborn baby
    B. 1 month
    C. 6 weeks
    D. 3 months
    E. 6 months
    F. 9 months
    G. 12 months
    H. 15 months
    I. 18 months
    J. 2 years
    K. 2 ½ years
    L. 3 years
    M. 4 years
    N. 5 years

For each of the following stages, select the age at which you would expect to see this stage in development. Each option may be used once, more than once or not at all.

1. Can draw a triangle.

2. Can walk alone, feet apart, arms assisting balance.

3. Is able to babble loudly with repetitive syllables e.g. 'dad-dad', 'adaba', 'agaga'.

4. Can hop on one foot.

5. Is able to fix and follow an object through 180° in the horizontal plane.

Theme 5: Oedema

Options

A. Anaemia
B. Angioedema
C. Glomerulonephritis
D. Heart failure
E. Henoch–Schönlein purpura
F. Kwashiorkor
G. Liver failure
H. Marasmus
I. Nephrotic syndrome
J. Protein-losing enteropathy
K. Renal failure
L. Thyrotoxicosis
M. Turner's syndrome

For each of the following cases, select the most likely diagnosis. Each option may be used once, more than once or not at all.

1. An 18-month-old boy presents with oedema. He has chronic diarrhoea and is listless and irritable. He had been breastfed until recently. On examination, despite being of African origin, he has hair with a red tinge. His skin is tight and cracked in places. A urine dipstick is negative for protein.

2. A 4-year-old boy presents with oedema. He is clinically unwell with severe abdominal pain, fever and guarding. Urine is positive for protein and his serum albumin level is low.

3. A 9-year-old boy presents with oedema, just a day after being diagnosed with tonsillitis by his GP. The oedema is most marked around his lips and face. He is clinically unwell with an urticarial rash and wheeze. A urine dipstick is negative for protein.

4. A 5-year-old girl presents with oedema. This is most marked over her lower lip, where she was hit by her brother. The oedema is not itchy and there is no inflammation. She has no wheeze audible. A urine dipstick is negative for protein.

5. A 6-month-old girl presents with oedema. She is failing to gain weight and appears very short of breath. Examination is normal except for peripheral oedema. A urine dipstick is negative for protein.

Theme 6: Diagnosis of electrolyte imbalance

Options

A. Central diabetes insipidus
B. Diabetes mellitus
C. Glucocorticoid deficiency
D. Hypervolaemic hypernatraemia
E. Hypervolaemic hyponatraemia
F. Hypovolaemic hypernatraemia
G. Hypovolaemic hyponatraemia
H. Nephrogenic diabetes insipidus
I. Psychogenic polydipsia
J. Pyloric stenosis
K. Syndrome of inappropriate antidiuretic hormone secretion

For each of the following cases, select the most likely diagnosis. Each option may be used once, more than once or not at all.

1. A mother brings her 12-year-old son to the emergency department as she is concerned that he is drinking excessively. He drinks 4 litres of water a day and passes a similar volume of urine. On examination, he looks clinically well and is not dehydrated. Blood tests reveal Na$^+$ 152 mmol/L (range 135–145 mmol/L). On restricting his fluid intake, his urinary specific gravity remains low. On administration of desmopressin, concentration of the urine occurs.

2. A 5-year-old girl is admitted with gastroenteritis. She is passing 5–10 loose stools a day and is not passing urine as frequently as normal. Her observations are pulse 100 beats/min and capillary refill time <2 s. Her mucous membranes are dry and she reports feeling thirsty. The emergency department SHO takes bloods, which reveal a sodium concentration of 148 mmol/L.

3. A 6-year-old girl is admitted feeling acutely unwell. She has a temperature of 38.2°C and is breathing quickly. Clinically, she appears well hydrated. A cannula is sited to commence intravenous antibiotics. Blood is sent for analysis, which reveals a serum sodium concentration of 128 mmol/L. Urea and creatinine are normal. A urine dipstick reveals a high specific gravity.

4. A mother brings her 14-year-old son to the emergency department as she is concerned that he is drinking excessively. He drinks 4 litres of water a day and passes a similar volume of urine. On examination, he looks clinically well and is not dehydrated. You admit him for investigation. Blood tests reveal Na$^+$ 129 mmol/L (range 135–145 mmol/L). On restricting his fluid intake, his urinary specific gravity increases.

5. A 3-week-old male infant presents with severe vomiting. On examination, he is shocked and hypotensive. You insert a cannula and send bloods for electrolytes, which reveal a normal pH, K$^+$ 5.9 mmol/L (range 3.5–4.5 mmol/L), Na$^+$ 118 mmol/L and glucose 5.8 mmol/L.

Theme 7: Management of electrolyte imbalance

A. Fluid restriction
B. Hydrocortisone
C. Intravenous furosemide
D. Intravenous hypertonic saline
E. Low-sodium diet
F. Nasal desmopressin administration
G. Oral rehydration
H. Oral sodium supplementation
I. Pyloromyotomy
J. Stool-forming agent
K. Subcutaneous insulin

For each of the following cases, which are the same as in the previous question, select the next most appropriate management option. Each option may be used once, more than once or not at all.

1. A mother brings her 12-year-old son to the emergency department as she is concerned that he is drinking excessively. He drinks 4 litres of water a day and passes a similar volume of urine. On examination, he looks clinically well and is not dehydrated. Blood tests reveal Na$^+$ 152 mmol/L (range 135–145 mmol/L). On restricting his fluid intake, his urinary specific gravity remains low. On administration of desmopressin, concentration of the urine occurs.

2. A 5-year-old girl is admitted with gastroenteritis. She is passing 5–10 loose stools a day and is not passing urine as frequently as normal. Her observations are pulse 100 beats/min and capillary refill time <2 s. Her mucous membranes are dry and she reports feeling thirsty. The emergency department SHO takes bloods, which reveal a sodium concentration of 148 mmol/L.

3. A 6-year-old girl is admitted feeling acutely unwell. She has a temperature of 38.2°C and is breathing quickly. Clinically, she appears well hydrated. A cannula is sited to commence intravenous antibiotics. Blood is sent for analysis, which reveals a serum sodium concentration of 128 mmol/L. Urea and creatinine are normal. A urine dipstick reveals a high specific gravity.

4. A mother brings her 14-year-old son to the emergency department as she is concerned that he is drinking excessively. He drinks 4 litres of water a day and passes a similar volume of urine. On examination, he looks clinically well and is not dehydrated. You admit him for investigation. Blood tests reveal Na$^+$ 129 mmol/L (range 135–145 mmol/L). On restricting his fluid intake, his urinary specific gravity increases.

5. A 3-week-old male infant presents with severe vomiting. On examination, he is shocked and hypotensive. You insert a cannula and send bloods for electrolytes, which reveal a normal pH, K$^+$ 5.9 mmol/L (range 3.5–4.5 mmol/L), Na$^+$ 118 mmol/L and glucose 5.8 mmol/L.

Theme 8: Congenital heart disease

Options

A. Atrial septal defect
B. Atrioventricular septal defect
C. Coarctation of the aorta
D. Critical aortic stenosis
E. Patent ductus arteriosus
F. Pulmonary atresia
G. Tetralogy of Fallot
H. Transposition of the great vessels
I. Truncus arteriosus
J. Ventricular septal defect

For each of the following scenarios, select the most likely congenital heart defect. Each option may be used once, more than once or not at all.

1. A 4-month-old girl presents with breathlessness. Her health visitor is concerned, as she is failing to thrive. Over the last 2 months, there have been intermittent episodes of her turning blue, especially when she is upset. These episodes resolve spontaneously. A chest X-ray reveals a boot-shaped heart.

2. You are asked to see a 2-day-old baby girl. She is tachycardic and cool to the touch. There is no murmur and no cyanosis. The femoral pulses are difficult to palpate.

3. A 4-month-old girl presents with breathlessness. Her health visitor is concerned, as she is failing to thrive. The parents deny any episodes of cyanosis. On examination, there is a moderate pansystolic murmur at the lower left sternal edge associated with a parasternal thrill. A chest X-ray reveals cardiomegaly.

4. You are asked to see a 2-day-old baby girl. She is tachycardic and cool to the touch. There is no murmur, but she looks blue. The femoral pulses are palpable.

5. A 4-month-old girl presents with breathlessness. Her health visitor is concerned, as she is failing to thrive. The parents deny any episodes of cyanosis. On examination, she has a loud murmur present throughout systole and diastole, heard best just inferior to the left clavicle. A chest X-ray reveals moderate cardiomegaly.

Theme 9: Organisms associated with paediatric pathology

A. *Campylobacter jejuni*
B. *Clostridium difficile*
C. *Mycobacterium tuberculosis*
D. *Mycoplasma pneumoniae*
E. *Neisseria meningitides*
F. *Pneumocystis jiroveci*
G. *Salmonella typhi*
H. *Streptococcus pneumoniae*
I. *Treponema pallidum*

For each of the following descriptions, select the most appropriate organisms. Each option may be used once, more than once or not at all.

1. A Gram-positive bacillus causing gastroenteritis.

2. A spiral-shaped bacterium causing syphilis.

3. A Gram-positive coccus causing respiratory infection.

4. A Gram-negative comma-shaped bacterium causing gastroenteritis.

5. A cell-wall-deficient bacterium causing respiratory infection.

Theme 10: The crying baby

Options

A. Constipation
B. Gastro-oesophageal reflux
C. Incarcerated inguinal hernia
D. Infantile colic
E. Intussusception
F. Maternal drug use
G. Non-accidental injury (shaken baby)
H. Sepsis
I. Teething
J. Urinary tract infection

For each of the following babies presenting with intractable crying, select the most likely diagnosis. Each option may be used once, more than once or not at all.

1. A 4-month-old baby presents with intractable crying. His mother describes him as a very 'sicky baby' who has chronic hiccups. Examination is unremarkable.

2. A 4-week-old baby presents with intractable crying for the last 2 weeks. He has episodes, usually after feeds, where he is inconsolable and pulls his legs up to his chest. There is no vomiting and his stools are normal. Examination is unremarkable.

3. A 6 month old presents with intractable crying for the last month. His mother says that he is also drooling excessively. The crying may occur at any time during the day. The baby is happy only when he has something in his mouth.

4. A newborn baby is admitted to the neonatal unit as he is small for gestation. After a number of days, he becomes very irritable. He has a high-pitched cry and has diarrhoea. He is difficult to settle to sleep, yet is persistently yawning. The observations are stable, with a temperature of 36.7°C.

5. A newborn baby is admitted to the neonatal unit from the maternity unit. His mother's waters broke more than 24 hours before delivery. Eighteen hours after delivery, he becomes very irritable, with a high-pitched cry. His temperature is 38.3°C.

Theme 1: Constipation

1. F – Laxatives

This patient has an anal fissure. An anal fissure is a longitudinal tear at the anal margin that occurs after passing a constipated stool. Tears usually occur at the posterior margin, and multiple fissures may occur with Crohn's disease. Patients present with a stinging pain on defecation that can last up to 2 hours. This may be associated with small amounts of fresh bleeding and pruritus. On examination, the anal sphincter is in spasm and there may be a sentinel pile protruding from the anus (this represents a torn tag of the anal epithelium). Anal fissures cause a vicious cycle in constipation, because the child learns that it will be very painful to pass the hard constipated stools. This exacerbates the constipation as more fluid is withdrawn from the already hard stool. As the constipation worsens, the hard stool reopens the fissure when it is passed. Small anal fissures heal spontaneously. Management options include treating the underlying constipation with laxatives. If this does not work, topical preparations that relax the anal sphincter can be used, such as glyceryl trinitrate (GTN) or diltiazem pastes. Chronic recurring fissures may need excision.

2. D – EDTA chelation

This boy presents with features of encephalopathy, which are likely to be due to underlying lead poisoning given the history of pica (eating non-nutritive substances). Pica can be both a sign and a cause of lead poisoning. Lead poisoning affects the nervous, gastrointestinal and haematological systems. Affected children present with encephalopathic signs or behavioural problems. The diagnosis of lead poisoning can be confirmed definitively by measuring blood lead levels. Other blood tests will reveal hypochromic microcytic anaemia, and a blood film demonstrates basophilic stippling (the presence of granules within the cytoplasm of red blood cells). Treatment is with chelation of the lead using ethylenediamine tetraacetic acid (EDTA).

3. C – Bowel resection

This patient has Hirschprung's disease. Hirschprung's disease is a congenital absence of ganglion cells from the parasympathetic myenteric plexus of the large bowel, resulting in a narrowed, contracted segment. Without innervations, the bowel is spastic and has no peristalsis. This abnormally innervated bowel extends proximally from the rectum for a variable distance. Hirschprung's disease often presents in neonates with abdominal distension, bile-stained vomiting or failure of passage of meconium. Rectal examination shows a narrowed segment, and removal of the examining finger is often followed by a gush of stools and flatus. Occasionally, Hirschprung's disease can present later in childhood with chronic constipation and abdominal distension without soiling. Diagnosis is by rectal biopsy, which demonstrates the absence of ganglion cells in the affected mucosa. Definitive management is by excision of the abnormal bowel with re-anastomosis to the anus (end-to-rectum anastomosis). Before surgery, temporary decompression of the colon can be brought about by rectal bowel washouts using physiological or 0.9% saline.

Harald Hirschprung, Danish paediatrician (1830–1916).

4. J – Thyroxine

This child has congenital hypothyroidism (formerly known as cretinism). Congenital hypothyroidism has a number of causes, including embryological maldescent of the thyroid, maternal iodine deficiency and dyshormonogenesis (an autosomal recessive inborn error of thyroid hormone synthesis). Congenital hypothyroidism is now routinely screened for in neonates with the Guthrie test (along with phenylketonuria). Children with congenital hypothyroidism present with hypotonia, coarse facial features, delayed closure of the anterior fontanelle, a hoarse cry, dry skin, hypothermia, prolonged jaundice, umbilical hernia, short stature, developmental delay, constipation and learning difficulties. If thyroxine treatment is started early enough (usually the first weeks of life) then learning difficulties can be minimized and sometimes entirely prevented. Bone age is used to monitor thyroxine therapy to ensure that there is no under- or overtreatment.

Robert Guthrie, American microbiologist (1916–95).

5. E – Gastrograffin enema

Around 10% of infants with cystic fibrosis (CF) will present with meconium ileus, where a thick meconium plug causes intestinal obstruction. Affected babies will present with bile-stained vomiting and abdominal distension, and there will be no record of passage of meconium. Initial management is with a gastrograffin enema, which is both diagnostic and therapeutic. If the child is peritonitic, a gastrograffin enema is contraindicated and a laparotomy and bowel resection should be performed. In all cases, these children should be immediately started on prophylactic flucloxacillin to protect lung function, and a sweat test performed at 6 weeks of life to confirm the diagnosis of CF.

The following is a good review on chronic constipation:

Rubin G, Dale A. Clinical review: Chronic constipation in children. *BMJ* 2006;**333**:1051–5.

Theme 2: Anaemia

1. A – Haemoglobin electrophoresis

This is a case of sickle cell anaemia with dactylitis induced by low temperatures. The infection the week before may have been secondary to erythrovirus (formally known as parvovirus), which can cause an aplastic crisis (a reduction or total absence of haematopoietic cell lines of the marrow leading to pancytopenia).

Sickle cell disease is a homozygous inheritance of faulty β-globin genes that is commonest in African, Mediterranean and Middle Eastern countries. A single amino acid substitution (glutamine → valine) results in an abnormal haemoglobin (HbS) that becomes insoluble in its deoxygenated state and causes sickling (crescentic shaping) of red blood cells. Sickled cells can become trapped in the microcirculation, leading to thrombosis and ischaemia. Such vaso-occlusive crises include dactylitis (swelling and pain in the digits) and priapism (prolonged erection). Management of acute painful crises is by analgesia, warmth and rehydration. Diagnosis of sickle cell disease can be made by several methods: blood film appearance, haemoglobin electrophoresis or using screening methods where the blood is deoxygenated to induce sickling. Electrophoresis has two general applications. The first is the diagnosis of haemaglobinopathies, including sickle cell disease, by separating the abnormal haemoglobins at an alkaline pH. The second is in the investigation of myeloma to detect monoclonal immunoglobulins characteristic of the disease.

2. B – No investigation at this point

Investigation of iron-deficiency anaemia will reveal a hypochromic microcytic anaemia. However, this will not *confirm* the diagnosis, as there are other causes of hypochromic microcytic anaemia (e.g. thalassaemias and anaemia of chronic disease). Ferritin is a plasma protein that carries iron, and levels are reflective of total body iron stores. A low serum ferritin (in association with hypochromic microcytic anaemia) is the most useful test in confirming iron-deficiency anaemia. However, ferritin is an acute-phase protein and concentrations are raised in chronic inflammation or acute infection, such as here.

The question asks about which investigation you would perform at this point. This child is clinically unwell with pneumonia, and therefore the ferritin will most likely be high or normal. One should wait until the child has improved clinically before measuring the serum ferritin level. Oral iron is given to correct iron deficiency, and should produce a haemoglobin rise of 1 g/dL per week of therapy. Iron should be continued for a further 3–6 months after normal haemoglobin levels are attained to ensure that iron stores are replenished.

The girl in this question eats inappropriate foods. The compulsion to eat non-nutritive substances, such as paint, paper and soil, is called *pica* and is strongly associated with iron-deficiency anaemia.

Pica, from Latin *pica* = magpie. A bird that is reported to eat almost anything!

3. D – Schilling test

This patient has anaemia with macrocytosis (a high mean cell volume – the normal range being 80–90 fL). Considering her previous history of autoimmune disease, the likely cause of her features is pernicious anaemia. Pernicious anaemia is an autoimmune disease of the gastric parietal cells, which normally produce intrinsic factor (IF). IF is required for the absorption of vitamin B_{12} in the terminal ileum. In pernicious anaemia, because no IF is made, the serum vitamin B_{12} level is very low. Around 90% of patients demonstrate anti-parietal antibodies (but some normal people also have these), and 60% are found to have anti-IF antibody (which is a more specific marker). Although most patents with pernicious anaemia complain of lethargy and general malaise, specific features of vitamin B_{12} deficiency include peripheral neuropathy, smooth tongue, angular stomatitis, depression, dementia and subacute degeneration of the spinal cord. The blood film is likely to show macrocytic (increased mean cell volume) megaloblastic anaemia with hypersegmented neutrophil nuclei (>6 lobes). In addition, serum vitamin B_{12} levels are low and ferritin levels are normal, reflecting normal iron stores. Serum vitamin B_{12} levels can be measured directly, but this option is not provided.

The two-part Schilling test can be used to diagnose vitamin B_{12} deficiency. It can also help define whether this is due to pernicious anaemia or problems of the terminal ileum. Patients are initially given intramuscular vitamin B_{12}. This occupies all the vitamin B_{12}-binding sites in the plasma, so any further absorbed vitamin B_{12} is immediately excreted via the kidneys. Oral vitamin B_{12} labelled with radioactive cobalt is then administered. If the patient starts excreting radiolabelled vitamin B_{12} in the urine, then they do not have a problem with vitamin B_{12} absorption. In those who do not excrete vitamin B_{12}, the second part of the test is performed. This time, oral radiolabelled vitamin B_{12} *and* IF are given. If the patient now starts excreting radiolabelled vitamin B_{12}, pernicious anaemia is confirmed. If there is still no excretion, an underlying bowel-related problem is the cause of poor vitamin B_{12} absorption. Pernicious anaemia is rare in this age group, and usually occurs in the female population aged over 50 years. There is an increased risk associated with autoimmune diseases such as vitiligo, thyroid disease and Addison's disease. Jaundice occurs due to haemolysis of the ineffective products of erythropoiesis by the spleen. Treatment of pernicious anaemia is with 3-monthly intramuscular injections of hydroxocobalamin, a vitamin B_{12} analogue.

Viktor Theodor Schilling, German haematologist (1883–1960).

fL = femtolitres. The prefix *femto* denotes 10^{-15} (a quadrillionth).

Femto, from Danish and Norwegian *femten* = 15.

4. A – Haemoglobin electrophoresis

This child has thalassaemia. β-thalassaemia major is an autosomal recessive disorder in which there is a complete lack of production of the haemoglobin β-globin chain. It occurs mainly in Mediterranean and Middle Eastern families and is due to a point mutation on chromosome 11. Because patients with β-thalassaemia major have mutations on both alleles and cannot synthesize any β-globin, they cannot produce functioning adult haemoglobin (HbA – $\alpha_2\beta_2$). This condition typically presents within the first year of life when the production of fetal haemoglobin (HbF – $\alpha_2\gamma_2$) begins to fall. Affected children become generally unwell and fail to thrive secondary to severe microcytic anaemia. Ferritin levels are normal, since there is no iron deficiency. A compensatory increase in the synthesis of HbF and haemoglobin A_2 (HbA$_2$ – $\alpha_2\delta_2$) occurs, which can be detected on serum electrophoresis.

Clinical features include failure to thrive, lethargy, pallor and jaundice. On examination, there is often hepatosplenomegaly (secondary to extramedullary haematopoiesis), with bossing of the skull and long-bone deformity (due to excessive intramedullary haematopoiesis). The treatment of β-thalassaemia major is with regular blood transfusions, aiming to maintain the haemoglobin concentration above 10 g/dL, or with allogenic bone marrow transplantation. Regular iron-chelation therapy (with desferrioxamine) is required to prevent iron overload and deposition in vital organs such as the heart, liver and endocrine glands. If untreated, death is inevitable in the first years of life.

β-thalassaemia minor describes people heterozygous for the β-chain chromosomal mutation. Affected persons have only a mild anaemia and are usually asymptomatic.

α-thalassaemia is commonest in Asian populations. There are four α-globin genes. The presence of defects in all four genes results in Hb Barts (tetramers of γ chains), which does not carry oxygen effectively, and results in death *in utero*. The presence of defects in three of the four genes results in HbH (tetramers of β chains), which causes chronic moderate haemolysis. Defects in only one or two of the four α-chain genes result in subclinical hypochromic microcytic anaemia. Treatment options are as for β-thalassaemia.

Leukaemia can also present with hepatosplenomegaly and anaemia. It would therefore be prudent to perform a blood film to identify blast cells.

Thalassaemia, from Greek *thalassa* = sea + *haima* = blood. It is so called as the disease is especially prevalent in 'countries by the sea' (i.e. the Mediterranean).

5. H – Serum lead levels

This girl has pica (the compulsive eating of non-nutritive substances). Of these, she is known to eat paint, which contains lead. Lead poisoning affects the brain, gut and blood. Children can present with a varied spectrum of symptoms ranging from abdominal pain to encephalopathy and behavioural problems. Examination may reveal a bluish line along the gums. Lead poisoning is not as common as it used to be, as household plumbing no longer uses lead pipes. A blood film may reveal basophilic stippling (multiple scattered granules throughout the cytoplasm of erythrocytes); however, this may also be seen in thalassaemia and other forms of anaemia. Diagnosis is made by measurement of serum lead levels. However, early lead poisoning can also be demonstrated by finding reduced concentrations of haem precursors (e.g. free protoporphyrin). Treatment is with chelating (binding) agents such as EDTA that speed up the excretion of lead.

Chelation, from Greek *chele* = claw.

Theme 3: Stridor

Stridor is a respiratory noise made on inspiration. Stridor implies extrathoracic airway obstruction. The intensity (volume) of the stridor is not a good clinical indicator of the degree of obstruction; indeed, a quiet stridor with reduced air entry is a very worrying sign. Any child with a stridor should never have their oropharynx examined unless there is a consultant anaesthetist and ENT surgeon present to manage the airway (even if you think that it is croup). This is because examination can stimulate total obstruction of an already compromised airway in acute epiglottitis.

1. H – Nebulized steroid

Croup (laryngotracheobronchitis) typically follows a viral upper respiratory tract infection and accounts for 95% of laryngeotracheal infections in children. The main causative pathogen is the parainfluenza virus. It commonly affects children under the age of 2 years and can be very distressing for parents. These children often have a barking cough, harsh stridor and a low-grade fever (compared with the high-grade fever in epiglottitis). Various croup scores have been devised to assess the degree of stridor, cyanosis, respiratory distress, air entry and consciousness. Management options include humidified air and steroids (nebulized or oral) to relieve the inflammation. In severe cases, the airway compromise can be significant enough to require adrenaline. Antibiotics are of no use.

2. G – Intubation, ventilation and intravenous broad-spectrum antibiotics

This is a case of acute epiglottitis, a bacterial infection caused by *Haemophilus influenzae* type b. Differentiating epiglottitis from a retropharyngeal abscess or bacterial tracheitis can be difficult clinically. In epiglottitis, the patient inevitably needs intubation to protect the airway. Antibiotics are required to treat this bacterial infection.

3. N – Oral antihistamine, intravenous steroids and adrenaline

This girl is having a severe anaphylactic reaction. The treatment is not dependent on the cause (bee sting, food reaction, etc.). Anaphylaxis is an immunoglobulin E (IgE)-mediated immunological reaction that is precipitated by allergen exposure (type I hypersensitivity). Release of inflammatory mediators, such as histamine and prostaglandins, results in vasodilatation and smooth muscle contraction, with symptoms ranging from mild irritation to anaphylactic shock and death. Such reactions are potentially life-threatening and should be treated aggressively. Oxygen is required to prevent hypoxia, along with systemic administration of antihistamines, steroids and adrenaline. This girl may well need intubating and ventilating if the above steps are not rapidly successful.

4. D – Intravenous broad-spectrum antibiotics

The child has a retropharyngeal abscess that presents with fever, drooling, dysphagia and stridor. (The relatively long history makes acute epiglottitis unlikely.) Occasionally, the head may be tilted to one side and the neck may be stiff. A lateral X-ray of the neck shows an increase in the 'soft tissue' shadow between the vertebral column and the air in the pharynx. Invariably, the abscess will need incising with antibiotic cover.

5. P – Rigid bronchoscopy

This girl has inhaled a foreign body, with typical presenting symptoms (cough, stridor and *unilateral* reduced air entry). A chest X-ray may locate the foreign object, but it will need to be removed by rigid bronchoscopy under anaesthesia. Foreign bodies that have been swallowed can also be removed by endoscopy, although those that have already passed through the lower oesophageal sphincter are managed conservatively with serial X-rays to ensure that they are moving along the gastrointestinal tract.

Theme 4: Developmental assessment

The assessment of development falls into four key areas:
- gross motor (including posture)
- fine motor and vision
- language
- social behaviour and play

The following has been taken from Sheridan's description of child development (Sheridan MD, Frost M, Sharma A. *From Birth to Five Years, Children's Developmental Progress*, 4th edn. London: Routledge, 1997). This is a comprehensive description of child development in an easy format. The only way to learn how to assess development is to practise by seeing lots of normal children.

1. N – 5 years

At 5 years of age, one would expect a child to be able to walk on a narrow line and to stand on one foot with arms folded, to be able to build elaborate models when shown (e.g. three steps with six cubes), and to be able to colour pictures neatly and to draw squares and triangles. Their speech is fluent, and they will enjoy reading or being told stories that they act out later. They are able to give their full name, age and often their birthday.

2. H – 15 months

The stages one would expect a child to take to fully mobilizing are:

6 months   take their own weight when held to stand
9 months   able to pull to stand, holding on to support for a few moments
12 months crawling on hand and knees, shuffles on buttocks or 'bear-walks', cruising
15 months walks alone, feet apart, arms assisting balance
18 months walks well, carrying toy

3. F – 9 months

The language milestones at various ages are:

6 months   vocalizes, e.g. a-a, muh, goo
9 months   babbles with repetitive syllables (da-da), understands no and bye-bye
12 months babbles loudly and incessantly in conversational cadences; vocalization contains most vowels and many consonants; waves goodbye, understands simple instructions (e.g. 'come to mummy)
18 months uses 6–20 recognizable words; understands many more

4. M – 4 years

Hopping on one foot is a gross motor skill. Other gross motor skills expected by 4 years are climbing ladders and trees, the ability to stand, walk and run on tiptoe, sitting with knees crossed and showing increasing skill in ball games (throwing, catching, bouncing, kicking, etc.).

5. D – 3 months

At 6 weeks, the child can fix and follow 90° through the horizontal plane. This is increased to 180° by 3 months.

Theme 5: Oedema

Oedema is the accumulation of excess interstitial fluid. Its causes can be subdivided into those due to increased interstitial pressure and those due to low plasma protein concentrations. Low plasma protein levels can be caused by increased losses, decreased production or impaired lymphatic flow.

1. F – Kwashiorkor

Kwashiorkor is a clinical diagnosis. It is caused by severe protein deficiency due to poor nutrition – specifically protein–calorie malnutrition. There is often adequate calorie intake but inadequate protein in the diet. Kwashiorkor is therefore more common in developing countries where carbohydrates are the staple diet. Oedema often masks the poor weight gain. Clinical features are chronic diarrhoea, irritability, listlessness, apathy and anorexia. Classically, these children have sparse discoloured hair, are oedematous, have tight skin and have abdominal distension. Marasmus is caused by total calorie malnutrition and does not cause oedema. Children with marasmus look emaciated and do not demonstrate abdominal distension.

Kwashiorkor, from Ghanaian = displaced child – so-called as it affects children who have newly been displaced from breastfeeding.

Marasmus, from Greek *marasmos* = waste away, decay.

2. I – Nephrotic syndrome

Nephrotic syndrome is diagnosed if a patient has the triad of peripheral oedema, hypoalbuminaemia and proteinuria. About 85% of cases are caused by minimal-change glomerulonephritis. Loss of immunoglobulins in the urine puts these patients at high risk of pneumococcal and *Haemophilus* infections. In this case, the child is acutely unwell with abdominal pain associated with fever and guarding, which may be due to peritonitis. Treatment of nephrotic syndrome is with salt restriction and replacement of fluids with human albumin solution. Oral fluids often need to be restricted. Steroids are used to induce remission. Prophylactic penicillin should be started in all cases of nephrotic syndrome because of the risk of sepsis and peritonitis.

3. B – Angioedema

This boy is having an anaphylactic reaction, possibly from recently prescribed antibiotics. The swelling is caused by histamine release in response to a specific allergen. Management is with antihistamines (chlorphenamine), steroids and adrenaline, depending on the severity of the anaphylactic reaction.

4. B – Angioedema

Hereditary angioedema is a rare and potentially fatal autosomal dominant deficiency of the C1-esterase inhibitor. The C1-esterase inhibitor acts as a mediator of complement proteins of the immune system, and a lack of this protein allows the complement system to go unchecked, with an accumulation of vascoactive inflammatory mediators. This can result in intermittent itchy swelling of the face, lips, pharynx and limbs, along with abdominal pain, vomiting and diarrhoea. Attacks of hereditary angioedema can be mistaken for anaphylaxis, and repeated doses of antihistamine and adrenaline are given with no effect. There is often no identifiable trigger for attacks of hereditary angioedema, although recognized precipitators include minor trauma and strenuous exercise. Acute attacks last 2 or 3 days, but can be treated with intravenous C1-esterase inhibitor concentrate. Long-term management with anabolic steroids (e.g. danazol) helps promote synthesis of C1-esterase inhibitor. Laryngeal oedema is the most concerning complication, and can be fatal.

5. D – Heart failure

This child has peripheral oedema, shortness of breath and failure to thrive. Differentials would include Turner's syndrome, anaemia and heart failure. Turner's syndrome is a chromosomal disorder (45 XO), and these girls often present as neonates with oedema. It is the *in utero* oedema that causes the webbed neck classically seen. Anaemia has to be very severe to cause oedema, and is unlikely to cause such drastic symptoms. This child's oedema is thus most likely to be due to congenital heart disease. The most common congenital heart condition is a ventricular septal defect (VSD). If the VSD is large, it can cause heart failure, presenting with shortness of breath, which is worse on feeding, and failure to thrive. VSDs are usually associated with a pansystolic murmur, although large VSDs have an exceptionally quiet murmur or no murmur at all. This is because very little turbulent flow is created by such a large defect. Treatment of heart failure is complex, but diuretics are the first-line agents.

Theme 6: Diagnosis of electrolyte imbalance

1. A – Central diabetes insipidus

This is a case of central diabetes insipidus (CDI). Diabetes insipidus presents with polyuria, polydipsia, frequency, nocturia and nocturnal enuresis. Differentials include nephrogenic diabetes insipidus (NDI), psychogenic polydipsia and diabetes mellitus. CDI is caused by a deficiency of antidiuretic hormone (ADH – also known as arginine vasopressin, AVP) secretion from the posterior pituitary. NDI is caused by insensitivity to ADH in the collecting ducts of the kidney. Causes of CDI include idiopathic, hypothalamic disease, head injury and meningoencephalitis.

The diagnosis of DI is confirmed using the water deprivation test. The patient is deprived of water, and the urine and plasma osmolalities are measured every 2 hours. If there is a raised plasma osmolality (>300 mmol/kg) in the presence of urine that is not maximally concentrated (i.e. <660 mmol/kg) then the patient has DI. At this point in the test, the patient is given an intramuscular dose of desmopressin (a synthetic analogue of ADH). If the patient now starts concentrating their urine then they have cranial DI. If the urine osmolality remains <660 mmol/kg then NDI is confirmed. Dipstick analysis of specific gravity allows for a bedside test for urinary osmolality. A low specific gravity indicates dilute urine and a high specific gravity indicates concentrated urine. The treatment of cranial DI is with desmopressin, although in mild cases hydration may be maintained orally. NDI is improved by thiazide diuretics.

2. F – Hypovolaemic hypernatraemia

This girl has gastroenteritis causing diarrhoea; however, she is not vomiting. She has become mildly dehydrated due to the loss of fluids in the loose stool. This loss of fluids has caused a hypovolaemic hypernatraemia. The clinical examination reveals a mild case of dehydration, and, as the child is not vomiting, a trial of oral rehydration therapy is indicated. If this fails then intravenous fluids could be used. Oral fluids are encouraged in such cases like this, as the electrolyte disturbance will be corrected naturally.

3. K – Syndrome of inappropriate antidiuretic hormone secretion

Syndrome of inappropriate antidiuretic hormone secretion (SIADH) is the inappropriate secretion of excess ADH. This causes retention of fluid in the kidneys, which results in hyponatraemia by diluting the serum (there is no absolute sodium loss). In children, the aetiology includes intracranial disease (head injury, meningitis, space-occupying lesions and haematomas), pulmonary disease and drugs. The diagnosis is one of exclusion, and should be made only if the child is not dehydrated or oedematous and there is no renal, adrenal, pituitary or thyroid dysfunction. Many cases require no management, but treatment of more marked cases is by restricting oral intake of fluids. Management should be monitored with daily weights and serial serum and urine osmolality and electrolyte analysis. In severe cases, if there are complications such as seizures, then more aggressive management may be required with hypertonic saline and concurrent furosemide. However, this should be done with extreme caution, as rapid correction of low sodium can result in central pontine myelinolysis (damage to the nerve sheath of the brainstem, resulting in paralysis, dysphagia, dysarthria or locked-in syndrome).

4. I – Psychogenic polydipsia

Psychogenic polydipsia is a relatively rare problem. It involves drinking excessive volumes of fluid without the physiological stimulus to do so. In children, it may be a sign of emotional difficulties – but it may well be an isolated problem in children who simply enjoy drinking a lot. Diagnosis is made using the water deprivation test, which assesses urinary concentration on restricting fluid intake. In psychogenic polydipsia, the previously dilute urine becomes concentrated. If the urine remains dilute then diabetes insipidus is more likely. Treatment is with restriction of daily fluid intake.

5. C – Glucocorticoid deficiency

This baby has congenital adrenal hyperplasia (CAH) causing glucocorticoid (cortisol) and mineralocorticoid (aldosterone) deficiency. CAH is an autosomal recessive deficiency in the enzyme 21-hydroxylase. This enzyme is required to synthesize mineralocorticoids and glucocorticoids (but not adrenal androgens) from the hormone precursor 17-hydroxyprogesterone. Because there is a lack of mineralocorticoids and glucocorticoids, there is no negative feedback on the anterior pituitary, resulting in increased secretion of adrenocorticotropic hormone (ACTH). The high ACTH then causes an increased secretion of adrenal androgens, since this does not require the deficient hormone. The androgens result in the physical features of CAH, namely ambiguous genitalia (in girls), precocious puberty (in girls), accelerated growth in childhood and virilization. Patients who are steroid-deficient can present with a salt-losing crisis. This presents with hypotension, features of dehydration, vomiting, shock and collapse. The aldosterone deficiency will result in a high serum potassium and low sodium. Infants with CAH may present with genital hypertrophy and hypoglycaemia.

The diagnosis of CAH is suggested by finding a raised concentration of the hormone precursor 17-hydroxyprogesterone. The priority here is resuscitation with intravenous fluids swiftly followed by intravenous hydrocortisone. Long-term treatment is with hydrocortisone and fludrocortisone to replace the deficient steroids.

Theme 7: Management of electrolye imbalance

For explanations, see Theme 6: 'Diagnosis of electrolyte imbalance'.

1. F – Nasal desmopressin administration

2. G – Oral rehydration

3. A – Fluid restriction

4. A – Fluid restriction

5. B – Hydrocortisone

Theme 8: Congenital heart disease

Approximately 1% of newborn babies will have some form of congenital heart disease. Ventricular septal defect (VSD) is the most common, accounting for 25–30% of lesions. Cardiac disease is commonly associated with chromosomal and genetic conditions.

Circulatory changes at birth. In the fetus, left atrial pressure is low, as little blood returns from the lungs. The pressure in the right atrium is much higher, as it receives all the systemic venous blood and placental blood. Blood therefore passes from the right atrium to the left atrium via the flap valve of the foramen ovale. The ductus arteriosus connects the pulmonary artery to the aorta, so blood entering the pulmonary artery enters the aorta directly. Both the foramen ovale and ductus arteriosus help blood bypass the lungs. After birth, when the baby starts to breathe, resistance to pulmonary blood flow falls and the volume of blood passing through the lungs rises massively (leading to a high left atrial pressure). Conversely, the right atrial pressure falls, as there is no blood returning to the heart from the placental circulation. The immediate pressure differences that occur after birth between the right and left atria cause the flap valve of the foramen ovale to close (and become the fossa ovalis). The ductus arteriosus closes within a few hours of birth via a prostaglandin-mediated mechanism (becoming the ligamentum arteriosus). Some babies with congenital heart lesions rely upon the ductus arteriosus to maintain circulation. These babies deteriorate rapidly when the duct closes.

Foramen, from Latin *foramen* = hole or window.

1. G – Tetralogy of Fallot

Tetralogy of Fallot is the most common congenital cyanotic heart disease, the other being transposition of the great vessels (see below). The tetralogy comprises:
- large VSD
- pulmonary stenosis
- aorta that overrides the VSD
- right ventricular hypertrophy

Patients with tetralogy have hypercyanotic spells, characterized by cyanosis, breathlessness and pallor. These can lead to myocardial ischaemia and death. Examination may reveal clubbing and a loud, long ejection systolic murmur heard best in the 3rd intercostal space with a single heart sound. Chest X-ray may reveal a 'boot-shaped' heart, where the normally convex-shaped pulmonary artery on the left heart border becomes a concavity. Congenital cyanotic heart conditions can result in clubbing.

Etienne-Louis Fallot, French physician (1850–1911).

2. C – Coarctation of the aorta

In coarctation of the aorta, the degree of stenosis of the aorta will affect the presentation. Severe stenosis will present soon after birth (when the ductus arteriosus closes). The femoral pulses are weak on examination due to reduced blood flow in the aorta distal to the stenosis. In addition, the blood pressures are higher in the arm than in the leg. Heart failure and a murmur (over the back) may or may not be present. Milder stenosis may not present until adulthood with heart failure, a murmur and hypertension. Chest X-ray in coarctation may demonstrate 'rib notching' due to the development of large intercostal collateral arteries running under the ribs posteriorly in an attempt to bypass the stenosis. Management is with surgical ligation or balloon dilatation of the stenosis. *Critical aortic stenosis* can also present with a shocked neonate with femoral pulses that are difficult to palpate. The difference clinically is that in critical aortic stenosis the radial/brachial pulses would also be difficult to palpate.

3. J – Ventricular septal defect

VSDs may be perimembranous (adjacent to the tricuspid valve: 80%) or muscular (completely surrounded by muscle: 20%). Small VSDs are usually asymptomatic. Large VSDs are almost always membranous. They present with heart failure (breathlessness, difficulty feeding, excessive sweating, recurrent upper and lower respiratory tract infections, and failure to thrive) due to left-to-right shunting of blood. Examination may reveal either an ejection systolic murmur (small defect) or a loud pansystolic murmur (larger defect). If uncorrected, irreversible pulmonary hypertension ensues, with eventual reversal of the shunt (becoming right to left) known as Eisenmenger's syndrome. Surgical correction of the VSD should be performed prior to the development of Eisenmenger's syndrome. VSDs are often missed on examination soon after birth, as the pressure gradient across the ventricles required for shunting takes time to develop.

There are two types of atrial septal defect (ASD): ostium primum (deficiency of the atrioventricular septum) and ostium secundum (deficiency of the foramen ovale and the surrounding atrial septum). Examination features include a fixed, widely split second heart sound (due to the right ventricular stroke volume being equal in both inspiration and expiration) and an ejection systolic murmur heard best in the 3rd left intercostal space (due to increased right ventricular outflow secondary to the left-to-right shunt). Increased flow across the tricuspid valve leads to a rumbling mid-diastolic murmur.

Victor Eisenmenger, Austrian physician (1864–1932).

4. H – Transposition of the great arteries

With these symptoms, sepsis is the most likely diagnosis, and so this child should be commenced on intravenous antibiotics until an echocardiogram can be performed to confirm transposition of the great arteries (TGA). This is a more difficult question, as pulmonary atresia could present in a similar fashion. However, this question tests your knowledge of incidences. Pulmonary atresia is less common, therefore TGA is the *most* likely diagnosis. In TGA, the great vessels are reversed (transposed), with the aorta coming off the right ventricle and the pulmonary artery off the left ventricle. Affected children are therefore dependent on the ductus arteriosus (duct-dependent) to supply oxygenated blood to the systemic circulation. As the duct closes after birth, the baby will become profoundly cyanotic and acidotic. Chest X-ray shows a characteristic narrow mediastinum with an 'egg-on-side' appearance of the heart shadow. The 'switch operation' (surgical swapping of the pulmonary artery and aorta) is required as definitive management.

5. E – Patent ductus arteriosus

Normally, the ductus arteriosus will close in the first few days of life. This is caused by constriction of the vessel as the blood passing through it changes from deoxygenated to oxygenated. The vessel later fibroses. Patent ductus arteriosus (PDA) is more common in premature infants, but does occur in term babies. Features of PDA include a continuous machinery-sounding murmur inferior to the left clavicle. If the PDA is significant, massive left-to-right shunting of blood causes heart failure. Management is with indometacin (a prostaglandin synthetase inhibitor that closes the defect) or surgical ligation.

Theme 9: Organisms associated with paediatric pathology

1. B– *Clostridium difficile*

2. I – *Treponema pallidum*

3. H – *Streptococcus pneumoniae*

4. A – *Campylobacter jejuni*

5. D – *Mycoplasma pneumoniae*

Medically important bacteria can be classified depending on their morphology and staining reactions. In clinical life, a microbiologist will be at hand to type organisms; however, organism classification comes up in exams. There is no easy way to overcome this – you just have to learn them. For more information, see Elliott T, Hastings M, Desselberger U. *Lecture Notes on Medical Microbiology*, 3rd edn. Oxford: Blackwell Science, 1997.

Gram-positive cocci

Staphylococcus:	S. aureus, S. epidermis
Streptococcus:	S. pneumoniae, S. pyogenes

Gram-positive bacilli

Bacillus:	B. anthracis, B. cereus
Clostridium:	C. difficile, C. tetani, C. perfringens
Corynebacterium:	C. diphtheriae
Listeria:	L. monocytogenes

Gram-negative diplococci

Neisseria:	N. meningitides, N. gonorrhoeae

Gram-negative bacilli

Escherichia:	E. coli
Klebsiella:	K. pneumoniae
Proteus:	P. mirabilis
Salmonella:	S. typhi
Shigella:	S. sonnei
Yersinia:	Y. enterocolitica, Y. pestis
Pseudomonas:	P. aeruginosa
Bordatella:	B. pertussis
Haemophilus:	H. influenzae
Legionella:	L. pneumophila

Gram-negative comma-shaped/curved bacteria

Vibrio: V. cholerae
Campylobacter: C. jejuni
Helicobacter: H. pylori

Spiral-shaped bacteria

Treponema: T. pallidum
Borrelia: B. burgdorferi

Acid-fast bacteria

Mycobacterium: M. tuberculosis

Cell-wall-deficient bacteria

Mycoplasma: M. pneumoniae

Pneumocystis jiroveci (formerly *P. carinii*) is a yeast-like fungal infection and not a bacterium. *Pneumocystis* is responsible for infections (mainly pneumonia) in immunocompromised hosts.

Theme 10: The crying baby

Eliciting the cause of intractable crying in young infants poses a diagnostic challenge. It is thought that as many as 60% of afebrile children presenting with prolonged crying will have an underlying diagnosis.

1. B – Gastro-oesophageal reflux

Gastro-oesophageal reflux disease (GORD) is a common problem. Gastric contents reflux into the oesophagus and often into the mouth itself. It is caused by transient relaxation of the lower oesophageal sphincter and occurs most commonly after feeds when the stomach is full. Typical symptoms include regurgitation, vomiting, failure to thrive, irritability during and after feeds, arching, food refusal, excessive hiccups, iron-deficiency anaemia and aspiration pneumonia. Children can, however, present with more unusual symptoms such as wheeze, cough, apnoea, cyanotic episodes and sleep disturbance.

2. D – Infantile colic

The cause of colic in infants is unknown. It presents in the first few weeks of life and occurs in as many as 20% of babies. The child is irritable and inconsolable during episodes of screaming, and often pulls the legs up to the chest. Stools are normal and there is no vomiting. Examination is also normal. Treatment is supportive, and colic usually resolves by the fourth month of life.

3. I – Teething

Some babies are born with teeth (neonatal teeth). These are a third set of teeth, separate from milk teeth and adult teeth. Neonatal teeth are often removed, as there is a risk of aspiration and they can also cause problems with breast-feeding. The primary set of teeth (milk teeth) usually erupts at approximately 6 months, but this is variable. There is often an increase in salivation, and relief with chewing on various objects. The erupting teeth may be visualized on examination.

4. F – Maternal drug use

This is a case of opioid withdrawal in the infant of a heroin user. Maternal use of illicit drugs (e.g. cocaine, opiates and marijuana) is associated with infantile irritability. The key features of this scenario that make drug withdrawal more likely than meningitis or sepsis are the lack of fever, being small for gestation and frequent yawning.

5. H – Sepsis

Most cases of neonatal sepsis present in the first 48 hours of life (peak at 18 hours). Prolonged rupture of membranes (PROM) increases the risk of early sepsis. Prophylactic antibiotics should be commenced if PROM is associated with any other risk factors for sepsis, such as prematurity (<37 weeks), low birth weight (<2.5 kg), maternal fever, foul-smelling amniotic fluid or maternal colonization with group B streptococci. Differentiating clinically between neonatal sepsis and neonatal meningitis is difficult, although both are treated with the same antibiotics. Sepsis is 10 times more common than meningitis in newborns.

Theme 1: Scrotal pain and swelling

Options

   A. Epididymo-orchitis
   B. Hydrocele
   C. Incarcerated inguinal hernia
   D. Non-strangulated inguinal hernia
   E. Orchitis
   F. Spermatocele
   G. Strangulated inguinal hernia
   H. Testicular torsion
   I. Testicular trauma
   J. Testicular tumour
   K. Torsion of the hydatid of Morgagni
   L. Varicocele

For each of the following scenarios, select the most likely diagnosis. Each option may be used once, more than once or not at all.

1. A mother brings her 15-month-old boy to the emergency department. She is concerned about a swelling in his scrotum. On examination, there is a smooth left-sided mass. You can feel above the mass, but are unable to feel the testicle behind it. The swelling transilluminates with a pen torch.

2. A 15-year-old boy presents to the clinic. He complains of a chronic ache in his scrotum. On examining the scrotum, you notice a large, soft, left-sided mass. You can get above the mass and it does not transilluminate with a pen torch. It does not exhibit a cough impulse.

3. A 16-year-old boy presents with a 10-hour history of scrotal pain and malaise. The pain is severe and radiates into the abdomen. On examination, the left testicle is tender and swollen. Lifting the left testicle results in relief of the pain.

4. A 12-year-old boy presents with sudden-onset scrotal pain. It first started when a football hit him in the groin at school. This started in the last 4 hours. The pain is severe and radiates into the abdomen. On examination, the left testicle is tender and swollen. The cremasteric reflex of the left testicle is absent.

5. A 14-year-old boy presents with a 24-hour history of scrotal pain. His mother reports that he was ill 5 days ago with a temperature, when 'his glands were up'. On examination, his left testicle is tender and swollen.

Theme 2: Acid–base disturbances

Options

  A. Diabetic ketoacidosis
  B. Hypoxia
  C. Metabolic acidosis with respiratory compensation
  D. Metabolic acidosis without respiratory compensation
  E. Metabolic alkalosis with respiratory compensation
  F. Metabolic alkalosis without respiratory compensation
  G. Normal blood gas
  H. Pyloric stenosis
  I. Respiratory acidosis with metabolic compensation
  J. Respiratory acidosis without metabolic compensation
  K. Respiratory alkalosis with metabolic compensation
  L. Respiratory alkalosis without metabolic compensation

For each of the following scenarios, select the most appropriate description of blood gas. Each option may be used once, more than once or not at all.

Reference ranges (*arterial*): Po_2 > 11.0 kPa, Pco_2 4.6–6.0 kPa, bicarbonate 22–28 mmol/L, pH 7.35–7.45.

1. You see a 6-week-old baby with vomiting. The blood gas analyser has broken, so you cannot get a blood gas. You send some blood instead to biochemistry for electrolytes. The results are phoned through as Na$^+$ 138 mmol/L, K$^+$ 2.9 mmol/L, chloride 75 mmol/L, bicarbonate 34 mmol/L, creatinine 60 µmol/L and urea 5.9 mmol/L.

2. You are called to see a child with diabetes who has diarrhoea and vomiting. Her mother reports that she is drowsy and that her 'sugars' have been high. You take a venous blood gas. The results show pH 7.38, Pco_2 4.9 kPa, Po_2 3.9 kPa, bicarbonate 22 mmol/L and base excess –0.9.

3. You are called to see a child with diabetes who has diarrhoea and vomiting. Her mother reports that she is drowsy and that her 'sugars' have been high. Results of a venous blood gas are pH 7.24, Pco_2 3.2 kPa, Po_2 3.9 kPa, bicarbonate 14 mmol/L and base excess –8.5.

4. You are called to see a 5-year-old boy in the emergency department. You are told by the attending SHO that he has a fever of 39.8°C associated with a petechial, purpuric rash. His capillary refill time is 5 s. An arterial blood gas shows pH 7.3, Pco_2 4.9 kPa, Po_2 22.4 kPa, bicarbonate 16 mmol/L and base excess –4.5.

5. A 13-year-old girl attends the emergency department for treatment of a self-harm injury. The attending doctor notices pitting of the teeth. A venous blood gas shows pH 7.47, Pco_2 7.2 kPa, Po_2 4.6 kPa, bicarbonate 31 mmol/L and base excess +3.6.

Theme 3: Sore throat

Options

A. Acute epiglottitis
B. Candidal infection
C. Diphtheria
D. Gastro-oesophageal reflux
E. Infectious mononucleosis
F. Quinsy
G. Retropharyngeal abscess
H. Streptococcal tonsillitis
I. Viral pharyngitis

For each of the following patients with a sore throat, select the most likely diagnosis. Each option may be used once, more than once or not at all.

1. A 7-year-old boy from India presents to the emergency department. He has been generally lethargic for a few days, with a mild sore throat. Over the last few hours, his sore throat has suddenly become much worse and he has a temperature of 39.6°C. There is no stridor, and examination of his throat shows a grey membrane covering his tonsils. He has a past medical history of asthma and has never been immunized.

2. A 7-year-old boy from India presents to the emergency department. He was lethargic and had a fever for 2 days before developing a sore throat. His GP diagnosed tonsillitis this morning, and so commenced oral antibiotics. He has now developed a widespread maculopapular rash. He has a past medical history of asthma and has never been immunized.

3. A 7-year-old boy from India presents to the emergency department. His mother describes that he has become very unwell very quickly. It started with a high fever and a sore throat. He is now very quiet and is drooling while sitting upright on the edge of the bed. You briefly examine him, and he appears shocked and tachypnoeic and has a very faint stridor. He has a past medical history of asthma and has never been immunized.

4. A 7-year-old boy from India presents to the emergency department. He has had a sore throat for 24 hours. He is drooling, as it is painful to swallow. On examination, he is systemically well and he is not shocked. There is no stridor, and examination of his throat demonstrates inflamed tonsils with a bulge from the right soft palate. His uvula is deviated to the left and his breath smells very bad. He has a past medical history of asthma and has never been immunized.

5. A 7-year-old boy from India presents to the emergency department. He complains of having a sore throat for the last 2 weeks. On examination, he is systemically well and he is not shocked. There is no stridor, and examination of his throat shows non-inflamed tonsils with white exudates. He has a past medical history of asthma and has never been immunized.

Theme 4: Illnesses protected against by immunization

Options

A. Diphtheria
B. *Haemophilus* epiglottitis
C. *Haemophilus* meningitis
D. Measles
E. Mumps
F. Pertussis
G. Polio
H. Pneumococcal pneumonia
I. Rubella
J. Tetanus
K. Tuberculosis

For each of the following cases, select the most likely diagnosis. Each option may be used once, more than once or not at all.

1. A 5-year-old boy from Uganda presents to the GP with a sore throat. He has been generally unwell for the previous 3 days with a fever and a mild sore throat. Today, he has deteriorated. He is restless and febrile and his sore throat is severe. There is currently no stridor, and examination of the throat reveals a white membrane covering a red pharynx.

2. A 6-year-old boy from a travelling family presents to the emergency department having had what appeared to be a fit. He is very rigid, arching his body and hyperextending his neck. He is unable to speak, as his face is locked into a permanent smile. You notice a small wound on his leg, which his mother says has been there for a few days.

3. An 18-month-old boy, whose mother is a nurse, is admitted to the paediatric ward. He presents with a headache, mild fever and lethargy. A blood culture is taken and a lumbar puncture performed. The CSF has a very high lymphocyte count, high protein and low glucose. Antibiotics are commenced but stopped when all the cultures come back negative. Despite treatment the patient continues to deteriorate.

4. A 7-year-old boy from China presents with a history of headache, muscle pain and neck stiffness. Three days after the onset of these symptoms his left leg becomes weak. On examination, he has a flaccid paralysis and loss of reflexes of the left leg. Sensation is normal in the limb.

5. A 5-year-old unimmunised boy presents to the GP with a chronic cough. His mother reports that he has had this cough for 3 months. It started with a normal 'cold and cough', but he has not managed to shake it off. For the first 4 weeks, the cough would occur in bursts and he would get very distressed, occasionally going blue and vomiting.

Theme 5: The febrile child

Options

A. Bacterial endocarditis
B. Cat-scratch fever
C. Kawasaki's disease
D. Malaria
E. Malignancy
F. Meningitis
G. Pneumonia
H. Rheumatic fever
I. Osteomyelitis
J. Scarlet fever
K. Tuberculosis
L. Urinary tract infection

For each of the following children presenting with a fever, select the most likely diagnosis. Each option may be used once, more than once or not at all.

1. An 11-year-old-girl who has just returned from Africa presents with a 6-week history of fever, which is worse at night. There are no other features, except that you notice that the girl has a painful purple rash on the lower limbs.

2. An 11-year-old girl from the UK presents with a fever for the last 6 days. She complains that her eyes have been itchy and red, and that her lips are sore. On examination, you note bilateral cervical lymphadenopathy and a widespread rash, and that the skin on her hands is peeling.

3. An 11-year-old girl who has just returned from Africa presents with a 6-week history of fever, which is worse at night. She reports being more tired than usual. There are no other features and there are no dermatological findings on examination.

4. An 11-year-old girl from the UK presents with a fever of 8 days' duration. On examination, she has a temperature of 38.7°C and has painful, hot lymph nodes in the left axilla. There is a small wound on the back of her left hand.

5. An 11-year-old girl who has just returned from Africa presents with a 6-week history of fever. She reports being more tired than usual. On examination, she has widespread cervical and supraclavicular lymphadenopathy, which is not painful on palpation.

Theme 6: Modes of inheritance

Options

A. An acquired condition rather than an inherited one
B. Autosomal dominant
C. Autosomal recessive
D. Mitochondrial
E. Uniparental disomy
F. X-linked dominant
G. X-linked recessive
H. Y-linked inheritance

For each of the following conditions, select the mode of inheritance. Each option may be used once, more than once or not at all.

1. Sickle cell disease.

2. Prader–Willi syndrome.

3. Marfan's syndrome.

4. Duchenne muscular dystrophy.

5. Williams' syndrome.

Theme 7: Headaches

Options

  A. Acute sinusitis
  B. Alcohol intoxication
  C. Febrile illness
  D. Head injury
  E. Idiopathic intracranial hypertension
  F. Intracranial mass
  G. Meningitis alone
  H. Meningitis and septicaemia
  I. Migraine
  J. Stress headache
  K. Subarachnoid or intracerebral haemorrhage

For each of the following children with a headache, select the most likely diagnosis. Each option may be used once, more than once or not at all.

1. A 3-year-old girl presents with a 3-day history of a runny nose. For the last 24 hours, she has had a high fever and a severe frontal headache with toothache.

2. A 5-year-old girl presents with a 2-week history of moderately severe headache. The pain is present most mornings and is located on the crown of the head. Her mother has noticed that she has a fine tremor of the right hand on using cutlery. For the last month, the girl has become more clingy and withdrawn than usual.

3. A 6-year-old girl presents with acute-onset headache. She has been febrile since waking 3 hours ago. She is now resisting movement of her neck. On examination, she is cool peripherally and has a dark-red rash on her legs that does not disappear with pressure.

4. A 13-year-old girl is brought to the emergency department by her mother. She has had a severe headache since waking 3 hours ago. She has also been vomiting. Yesterday afternoon, when she returned from her friend's house, her mother noticed that she was behaving oddly before sloping off to bed early. On examination, her temperature is 37.2°C. She has no focal neurological signs and there is no neck stiffness or photophobia.

5. A 4-year-old girl presents to the emergency department with acute-onset headache. She avoids bright lights and has been vomiting since her arrival. She is unable to move the right side of her body and is unable to speak. On examination, her temperature is 36.8°C and there is no neck stiffness. She makes a full recovery within 48 hours.

Theme 8: Dysuria

Options

A. Intravenous cephalosporin
B. Intravenous amoxicillin
C. Intravenous gentamicin
D. No treatment required
E. Oral cephalosporin
F. Oral ciprofloxacillin
G. Oral erythromycin
H. Oral metronidazole
I. Oral oestrogen
J. Oral nystatin
K. Oral tetracycline
L. Surgical correction
M. Topical nystatin
N. Topical oestrogen

For each of the following cases, select the most appropriate first step in management. Each option may be used once, more than once or not at all.

1. A 15-year-old girl complains of pain on urinating and back pain. She has a temperature of 39.5°C and is tender in the right flank on examination. She is not vomiting. A urine dipstick is positive for leucocytes, blood and nitrites.

2. A 5-year-old girl complains of pain on urinating. On examination of the genitalia, the labia have the appearance of not being fully formed, with surrounding mild inflammation. A urine dipstick reveals no blood, nitrites or leucocytes.

3. A 5-year-old girl complains of pain on urinating, suprapubic abdominal pain and having to pass urine more frequently. She has a temperature of 37.8°C. She is otherwise systemically well and examination of the genitalia is normal. A urine dipstick reveals leucocytes and nitrites.

4. A 15-year-old girl complains of pain on urinating. Her temperature is 37.0°C and she is otherwise systemically well. She is pregnant at 12 weeks' gestation. Cell culture reveals an intracellular organism.

5. A 2½-year-old boy complains of infrequent penile pain on passing urine. His mother is concerned as his foreskin is non-retractile. There is no local inflammation or scar tissue and the microscopy, culture and sensitivity of urine are negative.

Theme 9: Short stature

Options

- A. Chronic illness
- B. Congenital hypothyroidism
- C. Constitutional delay
- D. Cushing's syndrome
- E. Familial short stature
- F. Growth hormone deficiency
- G. Malnutrition
- H. Prader–Willi syndrome
- I. Trisomy 21
- J. Turner's syndrome

For each of the following children who present with short stature, select the most likely diagnosis. Each option may be used once, more than once or not at all.

1. A 14-year-old boy who is overweight repeatedly attends hospital with severe exacerbations of his asthma. On examination, you notice that he is particularly short for his age.

2. A 16-year-old boy is concerned as he is the smallest in his class. He has not yet entered puberty. His father tries to be reassuring, mentioning that he was also late beginning puberty.

3. A 15-year-old girl is concerned as she is the smallest in her class. She has not yet entered puberty. There is no family history of delayed puberty. On examination, you hear a systolic murmur that radiates to the back.

4. An 18-month-old boy with a cleft palate presents with short stature. He had frequent episodes of hypoglycaemia as a neonate.

5. A 9-month-old is admitted to the ward for investigation of his failure to thrive. On examination, he has a large tongue and an umbilical hernia.

Theme 10: Petechiae and purpura

Options

A. Aplastic crisis
B. Disseminated intravascular coagulation
C. Drugs
D. Henoch–Schönlein purpura
E. Idiopathic thrombocytopenic purpura
F. Increased superior vena cava pressure
G. Malignancy
H. Meningococcal septicaemia
I. Non-accidental injury
J. Thrombotic thrombocytopenic purpura
K. Wiskott–Aldrich syndrome

For each of the following children presenting with a non-blanching rash, select the most likely diagnosis. Each option may be used once, more than once or not at all.

1. A 2-year-old boy presents acutely unwell. He has a temperature of 39.5°C and is shocked. Examination of the lower limbs and trunk reveals widespread purpura. Broad-spectrum antibiotics are commenced, and blood cultures reveal Gram-positive cocci.

2. You are asked to see a 3-year-old boy in the emergency department. The referring doctor is worried about physical abuse, as this boy has presented three times in the last 2 months with 'viral-sounding illnesses' and on two occasions bruising was noticed. Today, he presented with a fever and coryzal symptoms. His mother also reports that he 'just hasn't been himself' recently, as he is lethargic during the daytime. On examination, there is widespread bruising over his upper and lower limbs and there is a ring of petechiae around this wrist where his mother says 'his brother grabbed him this morning'. His full blood count shows a platelet count of 30×10^9/L (range 200–400 $\times 10^9$/L) and a white cell count of 54×10^9/L (range 4–11 $\times 10^9$/L).

3. A 4-year-old boy presents with a long history of coughing. Over the last 2 days, he has been having paroxysms of coughing followed by an inspiratory 'whoop' with occasional vomiting. His mother is worried that he has developed meningitis. On examination, he is afebrile and has petechiae on his upper chest and face.

4. You are asked to see a 3-year-old boy who has a ring of petechiae around his wrist where his mother says 'his brother grabbed him this morning'. He had a viral illness 5 days ago, but has now recovered. Blood tests are performed that reveal normal haemoglobin and renal function. The platelet count is 30×10^9/L and the white cell count is 9×10^9/L.

5. A 4-year-old boy is unable to weight bear on his right leg. He has a temperature of 38.7°C, and examination of the lower limbs demonstrates an urticarial rash that in places is becoming purpuric.

Theme 1: Scrotal pain and swelling

1. B – Hydrocele

Hernias and hydroceles are the most common causes of inguinal masses in boys. To differentiate between a hydrocele and an inguinal hernia:

- A hernia will transmit a cough impulse; hydroceles will not.
- You cannot 'get above' a hernia, but you can with a hydrocele.
- The testis can be palpated separately with a hernia; it cannot with a hydrocele.
- A hernia does not transilluminate with a pen torch; a hydrocele will.

A hydrocele is a collection of serous fluid in the tunica vaginalis, a membrane that covers the testis. Hydroceles can be primary or secondary to an underlying cause. Primary hydroceles (as in this case) are tense, painless, fluctuant swellings that transilluminate. Because the fluid surrounds the testicle, the underlying testis is not palpable; however, the epididymis above can be felt as a separate structure. Primary hydroceles are benign, but can be surgically excised if desired. (Simple aspiration of the cyst will result in re-accumulation of fluid.) A secondary hydrocele can occur when the membranous sac around the testis becomes filled with exudates secondary to tumours or inflammation of the underlying testis or epididymis. Secondary hydroceles are usually small and lax. An ultrasound scan should be performed in all adults presenting with a hydrocele to exclude an underlying tumour. Secondary hydroceles require treatment of the underlying condition.

2. L – Varicocele

The differential diagnoses here would be a varicocele or a testicular tumour. An inguinal hernia is ruled out as you can get above the lesion, and hydrocele and spermatocele are ruled out as the mass does not transilluminate. Testicular tumours are usually painless, and this boy is relatively young for such a diagnosis.

The term varicocele describes varicosities in the pampiniform venous plexus, the network of veins that drains the testicle. It usually occurs on the left side and is present in 10% of males. Patients present with a scrotal swelling on standing that feels like a 'bag of worms', and they may experience a heavy, dragging sensation. Varicoceles are usually harmless, but have been associated with defective spermatogenesis, rendering some patients subfertile (although this is a contentious issue). Varicoceles can be diagnosed by ultrasound, which shows venous dilatation greater than 2 mm. Management is by reassurance and wearing supportive underwear. If a patient desires treatment then radiological embolization of the left testicular vein, or ligation and division of the testicular veins, can be performed.

3. A – Epididymo-orchitis

In the final three cases, including with semi-acute-onset scrotal pain, your first action should be to provide adequate analgesia and organize an urgent testicular ultrasound. Epididymo-orchitis (inflammation of the epididymis and testis) presents with a painful swelling of the epididymis with constitutional symptoms, such as pyrexia and malaise. Patients may also exhibit a secondary hydrocele. Because epididymo-orchitis is usually a consequence of ascending infection (e.g. from a urinary tract infection or sexually transmitted urethritis), there may also be a history of dysuria or urethral discharge. Prehn's sign (relief of pain on elevation of the testes) can help clinically diagnose epididymo-orchitis. However, when someone presents with a painful, swollen testicle, it is important to rule out testicular torsion – if in doubt, the patient should be referred for urgent surgical exploration. Treatment of epididymo-orchitis is with bed rest and a long course of antibiotics (e.g. 6 weeks of oral ciprofloxacin). If an abscess develops, it requires drainage.

4. H – Testicular torsion

The development of sudden-onset pain and swelling in the testicle strongly suggests torsion of the testicle, which is a surgical emergency. Torsion accounts for 30% of cases of a painful scrotum. Patients may also suffer referred pain in the lower abdomen and groin (due to the T10 nerve, which supplies the lower abdomen as well as the testes) along with nausea and vomiting. The torsion occurs around the spermatic cord when there is an anatomically abnormal testicle, often following a history of mild trauma. An example of an anatomical anomaly is the 'bell-clapper' testis, where the testicle is not anchored to the scrotum by the gubernaculum ligament (as it should be normally), leaving it to swing freely like the clapper of a bell.

In testicular torsion, the testis may be riding high within the scrotum, although a normal lie of the testicle does not exclude torsion. Prehn's sign is negative and the cremasteric reflex may be lost. Irreversible infarction of a twisted testicle occurs within 6–12 hours, so affected patients should be taken to theatre for surgical exploration without further investigation. (Generally, to preserve spermatogenesis, torsion should be relieved within 4 hours.) Surgical management includes untwisting of the testicle and bilateral fixation of the testes to the tunica vaginalis to prevent further torsion. Bilateral fixation is required because anatomical abnormalities of the testes that predispose to torsion usually occur on both sides.

The *hydatid of Morgagni* is an embryological remnant on the upper pole of the testis. Torsion of this structure may affect boys just prior to puberty. It usually presents with pain that increases in intensity over 1–2 days. Sometimes, it can be seen as a blue dot on the superior aspect of the scrotal skin (the blue-dot sign). Torsion of the hydatid requires surgical excision.

Giovanni Battista Morgagni, Italian anatomist (1682–1771).

5. E – Orchitis

This boy's febrile episode with 'the glands up' is the parotid swelling of mumps infection. Mumps is caused by a paramyxovirus infection that is spread by saliva droplets and affects pre-adolescents. As well as constitutional symptoms, patients develop inflammation of the parotid glands (parotitis). Recognized complications of mumps include meningitis, pancreatitis and orchitis. Around 20% of postpubertal males with mumps will develop orchitis. Treatment is with bed rest, scrotal support and analgesia. Testicular atrophy is common, occurring in 50% of cases. If bilateral, this can cause infertility. The incidence of mumps has been drastically reduced by routine administration of the MMR (measles, mumps, rubella) vaccine.

Theme 2: Acid–base disturbances

The body normally controls serum pH within a tight range. One must always remember that pH is a logarithmic scale and so a change from 8 to 7 is a tenfold increase in H^+ concentration. A normal intracellular pH is required for the functioning of many enzyme systems. When blood becomes profoundly acidotic (pH < 7), cellular function becomes impossible and death ensues.

Simple interpretation of arterial blood gases is usually all that is required in final EMQs. The pH value shows if the gas is acidotic (<7.35) or alkalotic (>7.45). Next, you need to find out if the alkalosis or acidosis is due to a metabolic or respiratory cause – this is done by looking at the Pco_2 and bicarbonate levels. There are two things that you need to bear in mind before continuing: (1) carbon dioxide is acidic and bicarbonate is alkaline; and (2) bicarbonate equates to 'metabolic' and Pco_2 means 'respiratory'. Alkalosis can be due to either high bicarbonate ('metabolic alkalosis') or low Pco_2 ('respiratory alkalosis'). Conversely, acidosis can be caused by either low bicarbonate ('metabolic acidosis') or high Pco_2 ('respiratory acidosis').

In some cases of blood gas disturbance, the body has time to compensate. In other words, whichever chemical is causing the imbalance is counteracted by the opposite one. For example, if there is high bicarbonate (metabolic alkalosis) then Pco_2 starts to increase to bring in some acidity and counteract the alkalosis. If compensation is successful, the pH will return to within the normal range (7.35–7.45), even if the bicarbonate and Pco_2 levels are abnormal. It is important to know that the body can never overcompensate, i.e. if there is an initial acidosis, the body can never make that into an alkalosis, and the pH will always remain on the acidic side of normal (<7.40). Similarly, a compensated alkalosis will always have a pH >7.40, on the alkalotic side of normal.

1. H – Pyloric stenosis

This is difficult. Without a blood gas analyser, it would be difficult to say if this was definitely metabolic alkalosis with respiratory compensation. However, the history and results are strongly suggestive of pyloric stenosis. Pyloric stenosis is hypertrophy of the circular muscle of the pylorus causing gastric outflow obstruction. It presents in the first few weeks of life and it most commonly affects firstborn males. The presentation of non-bile-stained projectile vomiting soon after feeds in a hungry baby is characteristic of pyloric stenosis. A characteristic hypochloraemic, hypokalaemic, metabolic alkalosis results from vomiting stomach acid. Pyloric stenosis is diagnosed by giving the baby a 'test feed': when the baby is given milk, visible gastric peristalsis may be seen over the epigastrium, and the pylorus is felt as an olive-shaped mass in the upper abdomen. If the diagnosis is in doubt, an ultrasound scan can be performed. After initial rehydration, management is by Ramstedt's pyloromyotomy (where the muscle of the pylorus is cut longitudinally down to the mucosa). The baby can tolerate milk feeds a few hours after the operation.

2. G – Normal blood gas

The only abnormal result here is the Po_2; however, this is a venous blood gas, so a low Po_2 is expected. This is therefore a normal blood gas. It is important to rule out diabetic ketoacidosis (DKA) in children with diabetes who are unwell with high blood sugars. The learning point here is that blood gas analysis does not just have to be performed on arterial blood. A lot can be established from venous or capillary samples.

3. C – Metabolic acidosis with respiratory compensation

This girl most likely has diabetic ketoacidosis (DKA) and has metabolic acidosis with respiratory compensation. However, you do not have a result for ketones, therefore you cannot technically diagnose DKA. She will need aggressive management, as DKA is a life-threatening complication of type 1 diabetes.

4. D – Metabolic acidosis without respiratory compensation

This boy has meningococcal sepsis causing metabolic acidosis. In this case, the acidosis is relatively mild and there is no respiratory compensation. He will need intravenous fluids to correct his poor perfusion, as well as intravenous antibiotics, such as penicillin or a cephalosporin. Note the high oxygen level. This is because the emergency department doctor correctly approached this case in an ABC manner and commenced oxygen therapy.

5. E – Metabolic alkalosis with respiratory compensation

This history and acid–base disturbance are suggestive of bulimia. The teeth are pitted due to chronic acid exposure. Chronic vomiting is associated with metabolic alkalosis. The CO_2 is mildly elevated, suggesting a degree of compensation.

Theme 3: Sore throat

Most sore throats are simply viral infections that are self-limiting. It is always important to consider group A streptococcal infections because of the complications associated with scarlet fever and rheumatic fever.

1. C – Diphtheria

Diphtheria is a rare cause of sore throat, especially now with the uptake of the DTaP vaccine. Characteristically, there is a grey slough covering the mucosa of the tonsils and pharynx. Culture of the organism *Corynebacterium diphtheriae* and demonstration of its toxin are required to confirm the diagnosis.

2. E – Infectious mononucleosis

Infectious mononucleosis (glandular fever) is caused by Epstein–Barr virus (EBV). Symptoms are varied and include fever, malaise, pharyngitis, tonsillitis and lympadenopathy. Other features are petechiae on the soft palate, jaundice, splenomegaly and hepatomegaly. Symptoms may persist for as long as 3 months. Infectious mononucleosis is diagnosed by finding atypical lymphocytes on the blood film or by demonstrating the presence of heterophile antibodies (i.e. antibodies that agglutinate sheep or horse erythrocytes, but that are not absorbed by guinea-pig kidney extracts!). This is known as the monospot test or the Paul Bunnell test. Treatment is symptomatic.

In this case, the GP incorrectly prescribed antibiotics. Administration of ampicillin or amoxicillin in infectious mononucleosis causes a widespread maculopapular rash. This makes treatment of any form of tonsillitis or pharyngitis with these antibiotics difficult, as EBV cannot be ruled out clinically. Penicillin is difficult to administer due to its bitter taste, although it is better to use this than potentially to cause a drug reaction with amoxicillin or ampicillin.

3. A – Acute epiglottitis

Acute epiglottitis is a life-threatening emergency caused by *Haemophilus influenzae* type b. A toxic-looking child with stridor, drooling and fever is strongly suggestive of acute epiglottitis. The child sits upright and immobile in order to optimize the airway. Do not be reassured by a quiet stridor or a quiet wheeze. This is often a sign that the airway is almost closed and very little air can be moved. Examination of the throat should be performed only by an ENT surgeon in an ICU with facilities to intubate and protect the airway. *Do not* attempt to examine the throat yourself or make the child lie down, as this may precipitate airway obstruction. Treatment is with intravenous antibiotics (e.g. a cephalosporin), with rifampicin prophylaxis given to all contacts.

A differential diagnosis in this case would be a retropharyngeal abscess. A retropharyngeal abscess is often preceded by an upper respiratory tract infection. The child with a retropharyngeal abscess presents with a fever, drooling, dysphagia and stridor. Occasionally, the head may be tilted to one side and the neck may be stiff.

4. F – Quinsy

Quinsy (peritonsillar abscess) is a collection of pus outside the tonsil usually seen in older children as a complication of tonsillitis. Affected patients are unwell and may develop severe dysphagia, earache and trismus (lockjaw). As you inspect the pharynx, there will be a unilateral bulge of the soft palate, with deviation of the uvula to the opposite side. The tonsils will be inflamed and there is associated halitosis. Rupture of the abscess can result in aspiration pneumonia.

Treatment is with penicillin. There may be as many as five organisms in the pus found in the abscess. Six weeks after quinsy, it is conventional to perform tonsillectomy.

5. B – Candidal infection

This boy with white oral lesions and a sore throat has probably developed oesophageal candidiasis. Infection of the oesophagus by *Candida albicans* occurs most often in patients who are immunosuppressed (e.g. with acquired immune deficiency syndrome (AIDS)) or who have recently used antibiotics). Inhaled steroids can cause a candidal infection at the back of the mouth due to local immunosuppression. Asthmatic patients on inhaled steroids should be advised to keep their inhaler by their toothbrush. This will remind them to take their steroids and to rinse their mouth out afterwards. Patients often complain of dysphagia, odynophagia and a hoarse voice. Oesophageal candidiasis can be treated with antifungals such as fluconazole, nystatin or amphotericin.

Theme 4: Illnesses protected against by immunization

The illnesses protected against by immunizations are now becoming rare. This has resulted in a significant reduction in morbidity and mortality. However, cases do still present, and so a knowledge of the clinical features is required. Also, to counsel a family effectively regarding the protection given by immunization, one needs to be aware of the effects that these infections cause.

1. A – Diphtheria

Diphtheria is caused by the Gram-positive anaerobe *Corynebacterium diphtheriae*. It is a highly contagious droplet-borne infection. Affected children present with a flu-like illness, pharyngitis and neck swelling. The diphtheria toxin released by the bacterium can also cause severe hypotension. On examination, a greyish membrane can be seen to cover the tonsils and pharynx.

Diphtheria, from Greek *diphtheria* = leather, alluding to the leathery membrane that covers the pharynx.

2. J – Tetanus

Tetanus is caused by wound contamination by the Gram-positive anaerobe *Clostridium tetani*. It is not the organism itself but its neurotoxic exotoxin, tetanospasmin, that acts on the motor cells in the central nervous system to cause muscle spasm. Signs of tetanus include:
- trismus: lock jaw
- risus sardonicus: grinning face due to facial muscle spasm
- opisthotonus: arched body, hyperextended neck
- autonomic dysfunction: tachycardia/arrhythmias, low blood pressure and sweating

Death is eventually caused by aspiration, respiratory failure, cardiac failure or exhaustion. Treatment is with anti-tetanospasmin immunoglobulins.

Risus sardonicus, from Latin *risus* = smile + *sardonicus* = sardonic (mocking, scornful).

Trismus, from Greek *trismos* = grinding of teeth.

3. K – Tuberculosis

Tuberculous meningitis is rare, but does occur. The onset of symptoms is gradual, with lethargy, irritability, a low-grade fever and a change in personality. Headache, confusion and neck stiffness may then follow. The priority is to rule out pyogenic meningitis caused by more common bacteria and treat with broad-spectrum antibiotics. However, if there is no growth and the child continues to deteriorate then one must consider tuberculosis as a possible organism.

4. G – Polio

Poliomyelitis is an acute disorder of the anterior horn cells caused by the highly contagious RNA poliovirus. It affects lower motor neurones. Features include a flu-like illness associated with muscle pain, flaccid paralysis and areflexia. The infection can also cause cranial nerve dysfunction, resulting in deafness, blindness, dysarthria and dysphagia. Paralysis of the respiratory muscles historically warranted management in a non-invasive negative-pressure ventilator (iron lung). Although polio is now rare in the UK and other developed countries, it should still be included in your differential diagnosis for any patient presenting with an acute onset of flaccid paralysis of a single limb.

Poliomyelitis, from Greek *polios* = grey + *myelos* = spinal cord.

5. F – Pertussis

Whooping cough is caused by the bacterium *Bordetella pertussis*. The illness usually begins with coryza, and a dry cough develops a few days later. This cough becomes more pronounced and occurs in paroxysms. Repeated episodes of coughing classically then end with an inspiratory 'whoop'. Another name for pertussis is the '100-day cough', as the symptoms often continue for that duration. There is no treatment that will change the course of the illness, although erythromycin is said to reduce the period of infectivity. Complications are uncommon, but include pneumonia and bronchiectasis. Immunization does not give total protection, and protection is not necessarily lifelong.

Pertussis, from Latin *per* = throughout + *tussus* = cough ('intensive coughing').

Theme 5: The febrile child

1. K – Tuberculosis

Tuberculosis (TB) is the most common infection worldwide, occurring most often in poorer areas, in people with poor nutrition and in those infected with human immunodeficiency virus (HIV). It is caused by *Mycobacterium tuberculosis*. Primary infection is often asymptomatic and occurs through droplet inhalation. Re-infection or re-activation of TB causes post-primary disease, which presents with cough, haemoptysis, dyspnoea, fever, night sweats and anorexia. Skin lesions of TB are erythema nodosum (see below) and lupus vulgaris (nodular, painful, disfiguring lesions, predominantly on the face). Chest X-ray may show lesions in the upper lobes. Infection may be confirmed by skin tuberculin testing: either the Heaf test (multipuncture method, read at 5–7 days) or the Mantoux test (intradermal tuberculin injection, read at 2–4 days). Drug management is with antituberculous therapy for 6 months (four drugs for 2 months, then two drugs for 4 months). Common drugs include rifampicin, isoniazid, pyrazinamide and ethambutol.

In this case, recurrent fever without a source of infection along with erythema nodosum (a painful, inflamed rash on the lower limbs) suggest TB. Other causes of erythema nodosum include streptococcal throat infection, drug reactions (sulphonamide antibiotics or the oral contraceptive pill), inflammatory bowel disease, sarcoidosis and idiopathic.

2. C – Kawasaki's disease

Kawasaki's disease is an acute febrile systemic vasculitis affecting children. It is most common in Japanese boys. The diagnosis is made clinically as follows: patients must have a fever for 5 or more days *plus* four of the following:
- cervical lymphadenopathy
- oral mucosal erythema (red lips, strawberry tongue)
- conjunctivitis without exudates
- rash
- extremity changes such as oedema and desquamation (peeling)

There may also be thrombocytosis. Treatment is with anti-inflammatories and intravenous immunoglobulins. The main complication of Kawasaki's disease is the development of coronary aneurysms (which can result in heart attack and sudden death), and patients conventionally undergo coronary angiography after recovery to rule this out.

Tomisaku Kawasaki, Japanese paediatrician (described the condition in 1967).

3. D – Malaria

Malaria remains endemic in many parts of the world where the *Anopheles* mosquito that transmits the disease is present. Four species of the parasite *Plasmodium* are responsible: *P. falciparum*, *P. vivax*, *P. malariae* and *P. ovale*. *P. falciparum* and *P. vivax* cause the most severe illness. *P. vivax* and *P. ovale* can also remain dormant in the liver, with recurrence later in life (remember 'v & o do not go').

4. B – Cat-scratch fever

The wound on the back of this girl's hand is an infected cat scratch. Cat-scratch fever is caused by infection with the Gram-negative bacterium *Bartonella henselae*, which lives in cats' blood. The original scratch is followed 7–14 days later by painful, hot, regional lymphadenitis and flu-like symptoms. Some patients may suffer altered mental state and convulsions. Treatment is with antibiotics.

5. E – Malignancy

This child presents with widespread painless lymphadenopathy that is typical of lymphoma. Many children (30%) will also have systemic symptoms such as fatigue, weight loss, itching, fevers and night sweats. These are known as 'B' symptoms and indicate a worse prognosis.

Causes of generalized lymphadenopathy include:
- viral infection: EBV, cytomegalovirus (CMV), HIV
- bacterial infection: brucellosis, syphilis
- protozoal infection: toxoplasmosis
- malignancy: lymphoma, leukaemia
- inflammatory conditions: rheumatoid arthritis, systemic lupus erythematosus, sarcoidosis

Theme 6: Modes of inheritance

The inheritance of various conditions, diseases and syndromes comes up in exams time and time again. These have to be learnt. The mode of inheritance can be the key exam clue in determining which of two possible answers is correct, and so marks are there to be had or lost.

1. C – Autosomal recessive

Sickle cell disease is an autosomal recessive condition. These patients have defective globin genes. When exposed to hypoxia or acidaemia, the abnormal globin causes sickling of the red blood cells, resulting in a painful crisis. Other autosomal recessive conditions include cystic fibrosis, congenital adrenal hyperplasia, oculocutaneous albinism, thalassaemia, Tay–Sachs disease and galactosaemia.

2. E – Uniparental disomy (deletion mutation)

Children with Prader–Willi syndrome are hypotonic as infants and go on to develop learning difficulties and obesity (due to hyperphagia) in childhood. Angelman's syndrome (happy disposition, little speech, severe learning disabilities, poor attention span and epilepsy) is also inherited by uniparental disomy. Both these conditions are caused by 'imprinting', whereby the gene required for normal function comes from only one parent. If this gene is deleted (de novo deletion) or both genes come from the other parent (uniparental disomy) then the syndrome will ensue. In Prader–Willi syndrome, only the paternal copy of the Prader–Willi gene is active (chromosome 15q11–13).

Therefore either the paternal copy is deleted or both copies come from the mother.

Harry Angelman, British paediatrician (described the condition in 1965).

Andrea Prader and Heinrich Willi, Swiss paediatricians (described the condition in 1956).

3. B – Autosomal dominant

Marfan's syndrome is characterised by tall stature, high arched palate, mitral valve disease, lens dislocation, joint laxity and arachnodactyly. Other autosomal disorders include achondroplasia, Huntington's disease, neurofibromatosis, Noonan's syndrome and tuberous sclerosis.

Antoine Marfan, French paediatrician (1858–1942).

4. G – X-linked recessive

Duchenne muscular dystrophy is an X-linked recessive condition, though approximately 30% of cases are due to a new mutation. Children present in the first 5 years of life with delayed walking, frequent falling, difficulty climbing stairs, Gower's sign and pseudohypertrophy of the calves. Gower's sign describes a patient who uses their hands to 'walk up' their own body when standing from a sitting position. Other X-linked recessive conditions include colour blindness, fragile X syndrome, haemophilia A and B, and glucose-6-phosphate dehydrogenase deficiency.

Guillaume Benjamin Amand Duchenne, French neurologist (1806–75).

5. B – Autosomal dominant (deletion mutation)

Williams' syndrome is a form of microdeletion syndrome. It is caused by a loss of chromosomal material at 7q11 that can be inherited in an autosomal dominant fashion. Affected children characteristically have a short stature, elf-like faces, transient hypercalcaemia as infants, supravalvular aortic stenosis and mild-to-moderate learning difficulties. Other conditions arising from microdeletions include cri-du-chat and DiGeorge's syndromes.

J C P Williams, New Zealand cardiologist (described the condition in 1961).

Other forms of inheritance include X-linked dominant (vitamin D-resistant rickets), and mitochondrial disorders, which are inherited from the mother (Leber hereditary optic neuropathy).

Theme 7: Headaches

1. A – Acute sinusitis

Acute sinusitis is inflammation of the paranasal sinuses, which usually occurs following a bacterial or viral upper respiratory tract infection. Common bacterial causes are streptococci, staphylococci, and *Haemophilus* spp. The main features are pain and headache. The pain of acute sinusitis is worse on bending and coughing, and percussion or palpation over the affected area will elicit tenderness. The site of the pain depends on which sinus is affected. Acute maxillary sinusitis causes pain over the cheek, which may be referred to the teeth. Acute frontal sinusitis causes pain above the eyes. Acute ethmoid and sphenoid sinusitis can result in pain between or behind the eyes. In reality, however, the site of sinusitis may be very difficult to distinguish. In maxillary sinusitis, a skull X-ray may show a fluid level on the affected side. Treatment is with antibiotics (if bacterial infection is suspected, as this case where the child is systemically unwell) and analgesia. Vasoconstricting nose drops (1% ephedrine) aid drainage of the sinus.

2. F – Intracranial mass

This girl has an intracranial mass until proven otherwise (which requires neuroimaging by CT or MRI). The warning signs here are the focal neurological signs (tremor) and the behavioural changes. The right-sided tremor indicates a left-sided tumour. Headaches associated with intracranial masses tend to be worse in the morning, and are worse with coughing, bending and straining (these actions cause raised intracranial pressure). Examination may reveal papilloedema.

3. H – Meningitis and septicaemia

This is a case of meningitis with meningococcal septicaemia. The likely causative organism is *Neisseria meningitidis*. Rapid treatment of shock with intravenous fluids and the administration of intravenous antibiotics are required. Always administer oxygen (ABC) in cases such as this, as much of the damage caused is due to hypoxia.

4. B – Alcohol intoxication

This girl has a hangover, although encephalitis, meningitis and subarachnoid haemorrhage would certainly be differential diagnoses. A good history would prevent expensive and invasive investigations.

5. I – Migraine

This girl has a hemiplegic migraine associated with dysphasia. The headache associated with migraines is profound and disabling. Migraines are frequently associated with ataxia, nausea, vomiting and visual aura. Migraine, however, is a diagnosis of exclusion, and other causes of hemiplegia should be ruled out before making a formal diagnosis.

Features of concern when assessing headaches include an acute onset, exacerbation on lying supine, associated vomiting, changes in personality, unilateral pain, developmental regression, hypertension, papilloedema, increasing head circumference and focal neurological signs.

Idiopathic intracranial hypertension (previously known as benign intracranial hypertension) usually occurs in young women and is associated with obesity. There is raised intracranial pressure in the absence of a mass lesion. This can be idiopathic or precipitated by drugs (tetracyclines, oral contraceptive pills and steroid withdrawal). Features include headache, transient diplopia and bilateral papilloedema. A CT scan is normal and a lumbar puncture will confirm a raised cerebrospinal fluid pressure. Management options include weight loss, avoidance of precipitating drugs and repeated lumbar puncture. The aim of treatment is to prevent permanent visual loss.

Theme 8: Dysuria

1. E – Oral cephalosporin

This girl has an upper urinary tract infection (UTI) – pyelonephritis – involving the right kidney. Some patients can have pyelonephritis with a negative urine dipstick, but in this case the blood, nitrites and leucocytes confirm a UTI. This question is testing your knowledge of management, i.e. should the antibiotics be intravenous or oral, and which antibiotic should be used? NICE guidelines (August 2007) now suggest that a 7- to 10-day course of oral antibiotics should be used in patients with pyelonephritis once a culture has been sent. If the patient is septic or cannot tolerate oral antibiotics (due to vomiting) then intravenous antibiotics are given instead. In pyelonephritis, antibiotics that have a low resistance pattern should be used such as a cephalosporin or co-amoxiclav. The antibiotic of choice may depend on local guidelines/resistance patterns.

2. N – Topical oestrogen

Labial adhesions are relatively common in prepubertal girls. They are caused by recurrent irritation, trauma or infection. The prepubescent labia are prone to adhesions due to the lack of oestrogenized epithelium. Bleeding and dysuria are common with these adhesions. This condition has a high enough incidence to require all physicians in paediatrics and general practice to be familiar with and comfortable in diagnosing and managing it in their patients. Most cases will require no treatment. Treatment is required only if the patient is symptomatic with dysuria or frequent vulval or vaginal infections. Most cases respond with topical oestrogen therapy. If unsuccessful, symptomatic cases need surgical intervention.

3. E – Oral cephalosporin

This patient has a lower UTI – cystitis. A midstream urine (MSU) should be sent to obtain microscopy, culture and sensitivity to ensure that any organism found is sensitive to the empirical antibiotic that you have started. A dipstick positive for nitrites and leucocytes confirms the diagnosis of UTI. A 3-day course of relevant antibiotics (a cephalosporin, trimethoprim or co-amoxiclav) should be completed. Ciprofloxacin offers good antibiotic cover in community-acquired UTIs, but should be avoided in children and growing adolescents due to the risk of arthropathy (unless the benefit of using this drug outweighs the risk).

4. G – Oral erythromycin

This girl is pregnant and is therefore having unprotected sex. As a result, she is at risk of sexually transmitted infections (STIs). UTIs are also more common in pregnancy. In this case, she is systemically well and has grown an intracellular organism. *Chlamydia trachomatis* is an obligate intracellular organism that is sexually transmitted. (*Neisseria gonorrhoeae*, another common STI, is a Gram-negative diplococcus.) Oral ciprofloxacin or cephalosporins are used to treat gonorrhoea. Oral tetracyclines (e.g. doxycyline) can be used to treat chlamydial infection, but is contraindicated in this scenario as it is teratogenic in the first trimester and causes dental discoloration in the second and third trimesters. Erythromycin is therefore the drug of choice here. STIs should be treated in specialist GUM clinics to enable screening for further STIs and contact tracing.

5. D – No treatment required

Phimosis is the inability to retract the prepuce. Ninety per cent of boys will have a retractile prepuce by the age of 3 years. Phimosis should be diagnosed only at an age when one would expect the foreskin to be retractable. In this case, the non-retractile foreskin is causing a degree of pain on micturition. As it is infrequent, no management should be performed in this case. Only if the prepuce remains non-retractile, or if he has a UTI/balanitis secondary to the phimosis, should surgical correction be performed.

Paraphimosis is caused by retraction of a tight foreskin over the glans. The foreskin then acts as a tight band, impeding venous outflow from the glans and resulting in oedema, making it more difficult to reduce the skin. The management of paraphimosis is by administering a local anaesthetic ring block to the glans followed by simultaneous squeezing of the glans and reduction of the foreskin. After paraphimosis, formal circumcision should be performed to prevent recurrence.

Theme 9: Short stature

1. D – Cushing's syndrome

This boy has a chronic illness that in itself is a cause of short stature. However, he is obese, suggesting that his chronic illness is not causing a hypercatabolic state. Rather, he is having repeated exacerbations of asthma that require treatment with oral steroids, resulting in iatrogenic Cushing's syndrome.

2. C – Constitutional delay

Constitutional delay is a normal variant, which is seen more frequently in boys. Puberty is delayed, as is the growth spurt associated with it. Bone age would also be delayed, and mid-parental height will be achieved later than in peers. Laboratory tests will be normal. There is often a family history of delayed puberty.

3. J – Turner's syndrome

This girl is likely to have Turner's syndrome (45XO), as she is short, is in pubertal failure and has a murmur suggestive of coarctation of the aorta. Turner's syndrome needs to be excluded in all girls whose height is below that expected of their mid-parental height, as not all affected girls will show the classic phenotype of webbed neck, widely spaced nipples, wide carrying-angle, etc.

4. F – Growth hormone deficiency

Growth hormone deficiency can be either congenital or acquired. Acquired causes include head injury, irradiation and tumours. Congenital deficiencies can be inherited, idiopathic or associated with midline defects such as cleft palate. Babies with congenital growth hormone deficiency tend to have hypoglycaemias and prolonged jaundice in the neonatal period. Treatment is with growth hormone supplementation.

5. B – Congenital hypothyroidism

Most cases of congenital hypothyroidism are picked up on screening with the Guthrie card, which looks for an elevated thyroid-stimulating hormone (TSH) level (found in 90% of cases). Early treatment is required to prevent learning difficulties. Treatment is with lifelong oral thyroxine (T_4), titrating the dose to maintain normal hormone levels (TSH and T_4) and normal growth.

Theme 10: Petechiae and purpura

Petechiae are pinpoint, flat, red lesions that do not blanch on pressure. They are caused by capillary bleeding into the skin. Purpura comprises larger lesions that are red, brown or purple. They do not blanch with pressure, are raised and may be palpable.

1. B – Disseminated intravascular coagulation

This child is septic and the culture has grown Gram-positive cocci, which could be either staphylococci or streptococci. Meningococcal sepsis can present in a very similar manner, but this would have grown the Gram-negative coccus *Neisseria meningitidis* on culture. Disseminated intravascular coagulation (DIC) is a generalized consumption of clotting factors, platelets and anticoagulant proteins. This process can be triggered by severe illness, hypoxia, acidosis, tissue necrosis or endothelial damage. Clinical findings may include generalized bleeding, purpura and thromboembolism. Investigations may reveal fever, hypotension, proteinuria and hypoxia, with low platelets, increased prothrombin time (PT) and activated partial thromboplastin (APTT) and reduced fibrinogen. Fibrinogen correlates most closely with the severity of the event. DIC is often accompanied by shock.

2. G – Malignancy

The emergency department doctor is right to be concerned about physical abuse. Petechiae forming a ring around a limb can be a sign of a twisting injury. To make a diagnosis of non-accidental injury, one has to rule out pathological causes. In this case the key symptoms are lethargy, bruising, frequent infections and petechiae. The blood tests confirming a thrombocytopenia with a very high white cell count are indicative of underlying haematological malignancy.

3. F – Increased superior vena cava pressure

This boy has pertussis, which can often produce violent coughing and vomiting. Both coughing and vomiting can cause increased pressure in the superior vena caval region, resulting in bleeding from the superficial capillaries into the skin. The petechiae will be restricted to the drainage distribution of the superior vena cava (upper limbs, face and trunk above the nipple line).

4. E – Idiopathic thrombocytopenic purpura

Causes of thrombocytopenia in a well child are idiopathic thrombocytopenic purpura (ITP), systemic lupus erythematosus, HIV, drugs and congenital disorders (TAR syndrome, Wiskott–Aldrich syndrome and Fanconi's anaemia). ITP is the most common of these. It is characterized by autoantibody formation to platelets (specifically to the IIb/IIIa glycoprotein). Children present 2–3 weeks after a viral infection with sudden-onset purpura and epistaxis. The platelet count is low, but bleeding is only usually a problem if it is $<20 \times 10^9$/L. Management is symptomatic. The most severe complication of ITP is intracranial bleeding, which occurs in less than 1% of cases. Half the cases of ITP will re-establish a normal platelet count within 2 months.

Wiskott–Aldrich syndrome is an X-linked recessive disorder characterized by thrombocytopenia, immunodeficiency, eczema and a predisposition to haematological malignancies. Fanconi's anaemia is an autosomal recessive condition characterized by short stature, aplastic anaemia, skeletal anomalies and a predisposition to haematological malignancies.

5. D – Henoch–Schönlein purpura

Henoch–Schönlein purpura is an immunologically mediated diffuse vasculitis, often preceded by an upper respiratory tract infection (especially β-haemolytic streptococci). It usually occurs between 3 and 10 years of age, and is twice as common in boys. The child characteristically presents with a non-thrombocytopenic palpable purpura (usually on the buttocks and extensor surfaces of the lower limbs), arthralgia, periarticular oedema, colicky abdominal pain and glomerulonephritis. The rash is initially urticarial, rapidly becoming purpuric. Treatment is symptomatic.

Eduard Heinrich Henoch, German paediatrician (1820–1910).

Johann Lukas Schönlein, German paediatrician (1793–1864).

Practice Paper 9: Questions

Theme 1: Dementia

Options

A. Alzheimer's disease
B. Creutzfeldt–Jakob disease
C. Depression
D. HIV dementia
E. Huntington's disease
F. Lewy body dementia
G. Normal-pressure hydrocephalus
H. Parkinson's disease
I. Pick's disease
J. Vascular dementia
K. Wernicke–Korsakoff syndrome

For each of the following scenarios, select the most appropriate cause of dementia. Each option may be used once, more than once or not at all.

1. A 73-year-old man presents with a 6-month history of worsening forgetfulness and intellectual decline. He has, however, had frequent episodes of relative lucidity during this period. He tries to chase soldiers that he thinks he sees in the garden, but his gait has markedly slowed down. His sleeping pattern is now irregular.

2. A 58-year-old woman presents to the emergency department following her first-ever seizure. Her husband said that she had to leave her job because, over a period of 2 months, she has rapidly lost the ability to cope with its intellectual demands. A previous cryptic crossword fanatic, she cannot even fill out the simplest tabloid grid. On further questioning, she admits to muscle weakness and difficulty walking.

3. A 75-year-old man who is a lifelong smoker presents with a mild but sudden-onset loss of concentration and problem-solving ability. This has become progressively more severe on three separate occasions without recovery in between.

4. A 45-year-old man has been arrested by the police for stealing furniture and verbally abusing his neighbours. They took him to the hospital because he appeared confused. His family are concerned that he is behaving strangely and is unable to cope with his work and finances. His general demeanour is apathetic.

5. A 66-year-old woman presents with a fall, having been unsteady on her feet for some time. She has severe memory loss, but is relatively well orientated. She has recently developed urinary incontinence. On examination, she has a wide-based gait.

Theme 2: First-rank symptoms

Options

- A. Delusional perception
- B. Made actions
- C. Made feelings
- D. Made impulses
- E. No first-rank symptoms
- F. Running commentary
- G. Somatic passivity
- H. Third-person auditory hallucinations
- I. Thought broadcast
- J. Thought insertion
- K. Thought withdrawal
- L. Voices repeating the patient's thought

For each of the following scenarios, select the most appropriate first-rank symptom. Each option may be used once, more than once or not at all.

1. An 18-year-old man sees someone being given a parking ticket and, as a result, at that moment he realizes that it is the right time to begin his mission of revolutionizing the world of fashion.

2. A 27-year-old woman complains to her university lecturer that a fellow art student was deleting the ideas from her head before she had time to say them or write them down.

3. A 45-year-old man experiencing hallucinations quotes the voice as saying 'and he's calling a cab while he's having a smoke, and he's taking a drag, and he's going to bed, and his stomach is sick and it's all in his head, and he's touching his chest now ...'.

4. A 21-year-old woman has been acting out of character for several days. She is spending all the money available to her because she feels invincible and capable of anything.

5. A 38-year-old man has not slept for 3 days. He says that he is being kept awake by aliens incessantly poking and pinching him.

Theme 3: Causes of weight loss

Options

A. Anorexia nervosa
B. Bulimia nervosa
C. Depression
D. Hyperthyroidism
E. Hypothyroidism
F. Malignancy
G. Mania
H. Obsessive–compulsive disorder
I. Patient does not meet criteria for any of the above conditions

For each of the following scenarios, select the most likely cause of weight loss. Each option may be used once, more than once or not at all.

1. A 21-year-old woman presents to the GP complaining that her periods have stopped. She has lost 14 kg from her normal healthy weight over the past few months and is now 42 kg. She admits to dieting and running for 2 hours a day in an attempt to reduce her weight. Her motivation is to change the way that she looks; she says that she is embarrassed by her obesity.

2. A 28-year-old man reluctantly visits his dentist with dental caries. He admits to stealing his grandmother's senna tablets, and feels that his eating is out of control. Sometimes, he will not eat all day in order to lose weight and at other times, when he is alone, he eats two or three large pizzas in one go, followed by a family-size tub of ice-cream.

3. A 55-year-old woman presents to her GP with weight loss and tiredness. She has lost 10 kg in the last month, although she denies any desire to lose weight. She has not used any laxatives, but has noticed an increase in frequency of bowel movements over the last 6 months, with occasional blood.

4. An 18-year-old woman presents to her GP complaining of weight loss, and admits to not eating proper meals. She also complains of insomnia, but denies any worry about her weight. She does mention that she no longer takes pleasure dining out and visiting her friends, activities that she previously enjoyed, as she does not see the point.

5. A 19-year-old woman presents to her GP with her mother, complaining of gradual weight loss over 1 year. Her weight is now 69 kg, around what is expected of someone her size. She admits to thinking that she still needs to lose some more weight and is disgusted by her body shape. She eats very little, and occasionally makes herself vomit. She has not noticed any other symptoms and has no medical history. Her only medication is the oral contraceptive pill.

Theme 4: Mood disorders

Options

A. Atypical depression
B. Bipolar affective disorder
C. Cyclothymia
D. Depression – mild
E. Depression – moderate
F. Depression – severe
G. Dysthymia
H. Hypomania
I. Mania
J. Masked depression
K. Schizophrenia
L. Seasonal affective disorder
M. Somatic syndrome
N. This does not meet the criteria for any of the above

For each of the following scenarios, select the most appropriate diagnosis. Each option may be used once, more than once or not at all.

1. A 24-year-old man asks his GP for a sick note from work. He says that he feels down, is lethargic and has stopped enjoying playing the piccolo (his main hobby). He was admitted to a psychiatric hospital last year following an episode of mania.

2. A 19-year-old man has been happier and more positive than usual, with more energy than he has ever felt before for no particular reason. He has been getting more work done at the office today and has been socializing with his friends as usual.

3. A 60-year-old woman is admitted to hospital after a fall. She is noted to have poor eye contact. When asked how she is feeling, she admits to feeling low in mood, having very little energy and losing enjoyment in all her usual hobbies. She has also found it difficult to concentrate, feels that she is no good at anything, feels guilty over minor issues and feels very negative about the future.

4. A 55-year-old woman who attends the clinic has recently been diagnosed with a depressive episode. She complains of unintentionally waking early in the morning, a recent disinterest in sex and a loss of appetite, losing 5 kg in weight in the last month. She feels that her mood improves as the day wears on.

5. A 40-year-old woman presents to the GP with low mood. Of note, she has an increased appetite and has gone up two dress sizes. She also complains that she cannot get out of bed until the afternoon as she is so tired.

Theme 5: Descriptive psychopathology 1

A. Circumstantiality
B. Coprolalia
C. Delusion
D. Egomania
E. Eidetic image
F. Flight of ideas
G. Hypnagogic hallucination
H. Hypnopompic hallucination
I. Knight's move thinking
J. Neologism
K. Obsession
L. Overvalued idea
M. Pareidolia
N. Perseveration
O. Word salad

For each of the following scenarios, select the most appropriate description. Each option may be used once, more than once or not at all.

1. A 20-year-old man with mania is difficult to understand. He is declaring, 'I want to become a shawalawam maker. Shawalawams can help you all!'

2. A 69-year-old man being investigated for confusion asks, 'when can I go for a cigarette ... ette ... ette ... ette ... ette ... ette ... ette?'

3. A 25-year-old woman says that her mind is racing and that no one is intelligent enough to keep up with the speed of her thoughts. She speaks rapidly, frequently changing the subject without explaining her meaning.

4. A 45-year-old man with severe depression feels that he is a despicable human being because he ran over a cat in his car in the dark by mistake. Worry and guilt surround this incident and are dominating his thoughts and conversation. He occasionally reluctantly accepts that it could have happened to anyone, but he still continues to think that what happened is unforgiveable.

5. A 31-year-old woman who has no previous psychiatric history fell asleep on a train. She said that as she woke up she saw a scuba diver momentarily swimming through the carriage.

Theme 6: Sleep disorders

Options

A. Hypersomnia
B. Insomnia
C. Narcolepsy
D. Night terrors
E. Nightmares
F. Non-organic disorder of the sleep–wake cycle
G. Physical problem causing sleep disturbance
H. Psychiatric/psychological problem causing sleep disturbance
I. Psychoactive substance causing sleep disturbance
J. Sleep apnoea
K. Somnambulism

For each of the following scenarios, select the most likely sleep disturbance. Each option may be used once, more than once or not at all.

1. A 3-year-old girl wakes suddenly during the night screaming and seems very distressed. She is unable to explain why she is upset, and returns to sleep after 10 minutes. The next morning, she cannot remember any of it.

2. A 5-year-old boy wakes from his sleep after a terrifying dream, and he explains to his parents that he was being chased by a monster. He had a similar dream once before.

3. A 36-year-old woman presents with daytime tiredness and difficulty getting to sleep at night. Her mood is not affected, and she is usually fit and well.

4. A 55-year-old woman presents with difficulty sleeping, particularly waking up around 5am and being unable to get back to sleep. She also has a decreased appetite and, on examination, she is less well groomed than usual and difficult to engage with.

5. A 12-year-old girl on a residential school trip is found wandering the corridors during the night. She appears disorientated when questioned, but goes back to bed. In the morning, she cannot remember the events.

Theme 7: Suicide

Options

A. 1 in 1000000
B. 1 in 10000
C. 3 in 1000
D. 1%
E. 10%
F. 66.6%
G. 90%
H. 100%

For each of the following description, select the most appropriate proportion. Each option may be used once, more than once or not at all.

1. The likelihood that any member of the population will die as a result of suicide in the next year (taking no other factors into consideration).

2. The likelihood that a person who presents with deliberate self-harm will go on to complete suicide during the next year.

3. The proportion of people with completed suicide who have seen a GP in the last month.

4. The proportion of people with completed suicide who have a psychiatric illness.

5. The likelihood that any member of the population will present with an episode of self-harm in the next year (taking no other factors into consideration).

Theme 8: Psychiatric disorders relating to women's health

Options

A. Couvade syndrome
B. Cyclic psychosis
C. Dysmenorrhoea
D. Maternity blues
E. Not a psychiatric condition
F. Postnatal depression
G. Perimenstrual syndrome
H. Premenstrual syndrome
I. Postmenstrual syndrome
J. Pseudocyesis
K. Puerperal psychosis

For each of the following scenarios, select the most likely diagnosis. Each option may be used once, more than once or not at all.

1. A 30-year-old woman gave birth to her first child 3 days ago. It was a planned pregnancy and there were no physical problems with the delivery or baby. She has no past psychiatric history, but has become inconsolably tearful, anxious and low in mood today.

2. A 32-year-old man presents to his GP with abdominal distension, insomnia, urinary frequency, constipation and cravings for beetroot with ice-cream. His wife is pregnant at 39 weeks' gestation.

3. A 22-year-old woman complains of abdominal bloating, headache and breast tenderness accompanied by irritability and low mood for at least 1 week every month.

4. A 28-year-old woman who is 2 weeks post-partum was brought to the emergency department by her partner and parents. She is confused and upset, and is complaining of hearing voices telling her to kill her baby. Over the last few days, she has been having difficulty sleeping, despite the baby sleeping well.

5. A 25-year-old woman is pregnant for the first time. Her husband has noticed her walking around the house talking to her unborn baby. This began 3 days ago. She has no previous psychiatric history.

Theme 9: Substance use

A. Alcohol use
B. Alcohol withdrawal
C. Amphetamine use
D. Amphetamine withdrawal
E. Cannabis use
F. Cannabis withdrawal
G. Cocaine use
H. Cocaine withdrawal
I. Opiate use
J. Opiate withdrawal
K. Sedative use
L. Sedative withdrawal

For each of the following scenarios, select the most likely cause. Each option may be used once, more than once or not at all.

1. A 76-year-old woman is an inpatient on a surgical ward following a hip replacement. The nursing staff said that she vomited earlier and she has been unresponsive since her operation 12 hours ago. On examination, you notice that her pupils are small and she has a respiratory rate of 7 breaths/min.

2. An 18-year-old man presents to his GP complaining of a dry cough and tiredness. His mother said that he has become very suspicious of those around him. She adds that he has withdrawn himself socially and has not been the same since he met a new group of friends at university.

3. A 34-year-old man presents to the emergency department complaining of the sensation of insects crawling over his skin. He is tachycardic and hypertensive, and his pupils are noted to be large.

4. A 74-year-old woman has recently changed GPs and has moved into a nursing home. The doctor is called because she became unwell; she was sleeping poorly, complaining of nausea and sweating, and went on to have a seizure.

5. A 63-year-old man was admitted for an elective cholecystectomy. On the second postoperative day, he complains of sweating and tremor. On examination, he is confused, anxious and tachycardic, and appears to be responding to visual hallucinations. He says that he can see thousands of miniature country dancers running around the floor.

Theme 10: Syndromes in psychiatry

A. Capgras' syndrome
B. Cotard's syndrome
C. Couvade syndrome
D. de Clerambault's syndrome
E. Ekbom's syndrome
F. Folie à deux
G. Fregoli's syndrome
H. Ganser's syndrome
I. Munchausen's syndrome
J. Othello syndrome
K. Rett's syndrome
L. Pickwickian syndrome
M. Tourette's syndrome

For each of the following descriptions, select the most appropriate syndrome. Each option may be used once, more than once or not at all.

1. A 19-year-old man presents to the emergency department having been at a cocaine party. He complains that he has 'little parasites, like ants' running around inside his body.

2. A 2-year-old girl is brought to the GP by her parents. They say that her behaviour has changed drastically over the last 3 months; she is screaming and has stopped interacting with those around her. She is also finding it increasingly difficult to walk and feed herself. Previously, her developmental milestones were all normal.

3. A 34-year-old woman works in a sandwich bar near Downing Street. She is convinced that the Prime Minister is in love with her, which is why he lives so close to her place of work. (It is well known that the current Prime Minister does not eat sandwiches.)

4. A 28-year-old woman is in court charged with benefit fraud. When asked how many children she has, she replies 'seventy-three'. When asked to confirm her name, she says 'Mary Queen of Scots'. (This is not her real name!)

5. A 42-year-old woman who is estranged from her physically abusive former husband attends the GP in tears. She is upset because she thinks that her former husband is following her, in disguise as her sister.

Theme 1: Dementia

Dementia is defined as a progressive, irreversible decline in cognitive function *without* impaired consciousness. It can affect all aspects of higher brain function: concentration, memory, language, personality and emotional control.

Dementia, from Latin *de* = away + *mens* = mind.

1. F – Lewy body dementia

Lewy body dementia is the second most common dementia after Alzheimer's disease. Characteristic features of Lewy body dementia include day-to-day fluctuating levels of cognitive functioning, visual hallucinations, sleep disturbance, transient loss of consciousness, recurrent falls and parkinsonian features (tremor, hypokinesia, rigidity and postural instability). Although people with Lewy body dementia are prone to hallucination, antipsychotics should be avoided, as they precipitate severe parkinsonism in 60%. Lewy bodies are abnormalities of the cytoplasm found within a neurone, containing various proteins and granular material. They are found in the cerebral cortex in patients with Lewy body dementia, and are also found in patients with Parkinson's disease.

Frederick Lewy, German neurologist (1885–1950).

2. B – Creutzfeldt–Jakob disease

Creutzfeldt–Jakob disease (CJD) is a rapidly progressive dementia caused by prions (infectious agents composed only of protein). The prion proteins can be transmitted by neurosurgical instruments and human-derived pituitary hormones. Features of CJD include rapid cognitive impairment, which may be preceded by anxiety and depression. Eventually, physical features become prominent, including muscle disturbance (rigidity, tremor, wasting, spasticity, fasciculations, cyclonic jerks and choreoathetoid movements). Convulsions may also occur. The EEG is characteristic (showing stereotypical sharp wave complexes). Death occurs within 6–8 months.

New variant CJD (nvCJD) occurs secondary to ingestion of bovine spongiform encephalopathy (BSE)-infected beef. It is more common in younger adults. The features are as for CJD, but decline is slower, with mortality occurring within 18 months. There are no typical EEG changes in nvCJD, although there is a characteristic feature on MRI (symmetrical hyperintensity in the posterior nucleus of the thalamus – the pulvinar sign).

Other prion diseases include kuru (in Papa New Guinea, transmitted by cannibalistic consumption of human neural tissue) and Gerstmann–Straussler syndrome (an autosomal dominant mutation of the prion protein gene on chromosome 20).

Hans Gerhard Creutzfeldt, German neuropathologist (1885–1964).

Alfons Maria Jakob, German neurologist (1884–1931).

3. J – Vascular dementia

Vascular dementia is an ischaemic disorder characterized by multiple small cerebral infarcts in the cortex and white matter. When >100 mL of infarcts have occurred, dementia becomes clinically apparent. Vascular dementia begins in the 60s with a stepwise deterioration of cognitive function. Other features include focal neurology, fits and nocturnal confusion. Risk factors for vascular dementia are as for any atherosclerotic disease (male sex, smoking, hypertension, diabetes and hypercholesterolaemia). Death in vascular dementia often occurs within 5 years, due to ischaemic heart disease or stroke.

4. I – Pick's disease

Pick's disease is a form of frontotemporal dementia (it can only be differentiated from other forms at post mortem, so 'frontotemporal dementia' is the preferred term). Clinical features include disinhibition, inattention, antisocial behaviour and personality changes. Later on, apathy, akinesia and withdrawal may predominate. Memory loss and disorientation only occur late. Post mortem examination shows atrophy of the frontal and temporal lobes (knife-blade atrophy) and Pick's bodies (cytoplasmic inclusion bodies of tau protein) in the substantia nigra. In advanced cases, the atrophy may be seen on MRI.

Arnold Pick, Czechoslovakian neurologist and psychiatrist (1852–1924).

5. G – Normal-pressure hydrocephalus

Normal-pressure hydrocephalus is characterized by the triad of dementia (mainly memory problems), gait disturbance and urinary incontinence. It is caused by an increased volume of cerebrospinal fluid (CSF), but with only a slightly raised pressure (as the ventricles dilate to compensate). There is an underlying obstruction in the subarachnoid space that prevents CSF from being reabsorbed but allows it to flow from the ventricular system into the subarachnoid space. Diagnosis is by lumbar puncture (to demonstrate a normal CSF opening pressure) followed by head CT/MRI (showing enlarged ventricles). Treatment is with ventriculoperitoneal shunting.

HIV-related dementia (also known as AIDS dementia complex) occurs years after initial infection. It presents with reduced cognitive function, low energy and libido, general apathy, and eventually muscle spasticity with hyperreflexia, incontinence and ataxia. It is caused by the virus itself rather than an opportunistic infection. Diagnosis is based on clinical probability.

Pseudodementia is recognized in people with severe depression. Their apparent cognitive dysfunction is heavily affected by their lack of motivation. The mood disturbance precedes the cognitive impairment, and patients may not try during formal assessments, often providing 'don't know' responses to questions asked. They are more likely to complain of memory loss, whereas someone with true dementia is more likely to confabulate and try to hide it. Depressive pseudodementia is a diagnosis of exclusion in someone with depression, and management aims to treat the underlying mood disorder.

Huntington's disease is an autosomal dominant disorder with excess CAG trinucleotide repeats on chromosome 4. Onset is usually in mid-adulthood. Features include choreiform movements, with an increased rate of depression, schizophrenia and suicide. Seizures may be a late feature. Insight tends to be maintained for much of the early course. Diagnosis is clinical, but can be confirmed by DNA analysis. Treatment is symptomatic.

George Huntington, American physician (1850–1916).

Choreiform, from Greek *chorea* = dance.

Alzheimer's disease is the most common type of dementia. There is global brain atrophy, with deposition of β-amyloid protein in the brain. Features include gradual progressive cognitive decline, apathy/lability of mood, personality deterioration, paranoia and parkinsonian features. The diagnosis is made by excluding other causes of dementia. The mainstay of treatment is acetylcholinesterase inhibitors (donepezil, galantamine and rivastigmine), which increase concentrations of the neurotransmitter acetylcholine, although these may only be effective in a select proportion of cases. Early-onset Alzheimer's disease (<65 years) can occur in people with Down's syndrome and in those who inherit the amyloid precursor or presenilin proteins.

Wernicke's encephalopathy is a reversible condition caused by a severe deficiency of thiamine (vitamin B$_1$). It is often associated with alcohol abuse, the processes being the lack of adequate oral intake, hyperemesis and malabsorption caused by gastrointestinal lesions. The triad of features in Wernicke's syndrome is confusion, ataxia and nystagmus. Ophthalmoplegia is also an important feature. If untreated, Wernicke's encephalopathy can lead to the irreversible *Korsakoff's syndrome*, characterized by confusion, anterograde and retrograde amnesia, and confabulation.

Alois Alzheimer, German psychiatrist (1864–1915).

Sergei Korsakoff, Russian neuropsychiatrist (1854–1900).

Karl Wernicke, German psychiatrist (1848–1905).

Theme 2: First-rank symptoms

Kurt Schneider described the 'first-rank symptoms' as being highly suggestive of schizophrenia in the absence of organic brain disease. However, they are absent in 20% of people with schizophrenia and can be present in other psychiatric disorders, such as depression and mania. The presence of first-rank symptoms in schizophrenia is not an indicator of prognosis.

Kurt Schneider, German psychiatrist (1887–1967).

1. A – Delusional perception

2. K – Thought withdrawal

3. F – Running commentary

4. E – No first-rank symptoms (more indicative of mania)

5. G – Somatic passivity

The first-rank symptoms can be categorized as follows:
- auditory hallucinations: third-person, running commentary, repeating thought
- thought alienation: thought insertion/withdrawal/broadcast
- influences on the body: made feelings/actions/impulses
- other: somatic passivity and delusional perception

In *third-person auditory hallucinations*, the patient hears the voices of more than one person discussing matters between themselves. A *running commentary* is one voice describing the patient's every action. Finally, the patient can experience *thought sonorization* (hearing their thoughts out aloud). These 'audible thoughts' can occur either at the same time as the real thoughts (*gedankenlautwerden*) or just afterwards (*écho de la pensée*).

In *thought insertion*, the patient believes that thoughts are being put into the mind by an outside agency. In *thought withdrawal*, they feel as if their thoughts are being removed. *Thought broadcasting* is where the patient feels that their thoughts are being made accessible to others (i.e. others can hear them).

Made feelings, *actions* or *impulses* describe when the patient feels that their feelings/actions/impulses are under the control of a third party and that their free will is being taken away. In *delusional perception*, a real perceived event leads to a different idea or incorrect conclusion without logical reasoning. *Somatic passivity* is where the patient feels that they are receiving bodily sensations from an outside agency (e.g. an alien is twisting their intestines).

Theme 3: Causes of weight loss

1. A – Anorexia nervosa

A diagnosis of anorexia nervosa requires all four of the following:
- body weight 15% below expected, or body mass index < 17.5 kg/m^2
- self-induced weight loss (by dieting, exercising, vomiting, etc.)
- morbid fear of being fat (an overvalued idea rather than a delusion)
- endocrine disturbance (e.g. amenorrhoea, pubertal delay or lanugo hair)

The incidence of anorexia is 4 per 100 000, with a peak at age 18 years. Around 10% of cases of anorexia occur in males. Risk factors include being Caucasian, high social class, academic prowess, and interests such as ballet or modelling. Other common features are anaemia, expressing a high interest in preparing or buying food, feeling tired and cold, bradycardia, and hypotension. Treatment options include cognitive–behavioural therapy/supportive therapy and raising caloric intake. Hospitalization is indicated if there is a weight loss of over 35%. Around 50% of people with anorexia nervosa eventually recover completely. The mortality rate is 5%, usually from starvation or suicide.

Anorexia, from Greek *an* = without + *orexe* = appetite.

2. B – Bulimia nervosa

A diagnosis of bulimia nervosa requires all three of the following:
- binge eating
- methods to prevent gaining weight (e.g. vomiting, purging, laxatives, etc.)
- morbid dread of fatness (overvalued idea, not a delusion)

The incidence of bulimia is 12 per 100 000, with females being affected 10 times more commonly than males. Individuals tend to be of a normal or above-normal weight. Complications are caused by starvation and vomiting, and include hypokalaemia, dehydration, enlargement of the parotid glands, dental caries, Mallory–Weiss tear, osteoporosis and Russell's sign (thick skin on the dorsum of the hands due to repeated induced vomiting by stimulating the gag reflex with the fingers). Treatment is similar to that of anorexia, but selective serotonin reuptake inhibitors may improve bingeing behaviour. Seventy per cent of cases recover within 5 years and there is no increase in mortality.

Bulimia, from Greek *bous* = ox + *limos* = hunger.

3. M – Malignancy

Malignancy is a common cause of weight loss and should always be considered, particularly in older people who complain of tiredness and a reduced appetite. A full examination and systems review should be carried out to determine a possible site of malignancy.

Thyroid dysfunction is associated with weight change. *Hyperthyroidism* can lead to weight loss despite a good appetite, and *hypothyroidism* can cause weight gain without increased intake.

4. C – Depression

Many psychiatric conditions may indirectly result in weight loss. The woman in this scenario complains of weight loss, insomnia and anhedonia, features suggestive of biological depression. Other features of biological depression are early morning wakening, decreased libido and psychomotor retardation/agitation. It should be noted that atypical depression is associated with reverse neurovegetative symptoms, namely hypersomnia, hyperphagia and weight gain.

Patients with *obsessive–compulsive disorder* may present with weight loss. This may be influenced by large periods of time taken up by the repetitive rituals. Additionally, if there is a preoccupation with cleanliness and a fear of contamination, this may affect eating habits. People with *mania* can lose weight with overactivity. They may also neglect eating for fear of wasting time.

5. I – Patient does not meet criteria for any of the above conditions

This girl presents with weight loss, induced vomiting and a poor body image. Although she may be on the slippery slope to an eating disorder, she does not quite meet the criteria for anorexia or bulimia.

Theme 4: Mood disorders

1. B – Bipolar affective disorder

Bipolar affective disorder is characterized by two or more episodes in which mood and activity levels are significantly disturbed. This should include at least one episode of elevation of mood and increased energy and activity (hypomania or mania), although on other occasions there may be a lowering of mood and decreased energy and activity (depression). There is a 1% lifetime risk, with the average age of onset being in the mid-20s. Males and females have equal risk of developing bipolar disorder, and higher social classes have a greater risk.

Manic episodes present with elevated mood in 70% of cases and an irritable mood in 80%. Biological symptoms of mania are decreased sleep, increased energy and psychomotor agitation. Cognitive symptoms are decreased concentration, flight of ideas and lack of insight. Manic patients often display thought disorders, such as circumstantiality (where the speaker eventually gets to the point in a very roundabout manner) and tangential speech (where the speaker digresses further and further away from the initial topic via a series of loose associations). Psychotic features include grandiose or persecutory delusions, hyperacusis and hyperaesthesia. First-rank symptoms occur in 20% of cases. In extreme cases, there is manic stupor, in which the patient is unresponsive, akinetic, mute and fully conscious, with elated facies.

Acute episodes of mania are managed with neuroleptics drugs (e.g. olanzaipine or haloperidol), with benzodiazepines for agitation. Long-term prophylaxis (mood stabilization) is most often given in the form of lithium. (Carbamazepine and sodium valproate may also be effective.) Mood stabilizers are prescribed only if there has been more than one episode of mania. Lithium causes sustained remission in 80% of cases. Psychotherapies have a supportive role and can improve concordance with therapy. Electroconvulsive therapy (ECT) is used for manic stupor and resistant mania, but, if used during a depressive episode in a patient with bipolar disorder, it can precipitate mania.

2. H – Hypomania

Hypomania is distinguished from mania in that the mood elevation is mild and does not disrupt social activity, nor is there psychosis. In *rapid cycling* bipolar disorder, there are at least four affective episodes in a 12-month period. This is more common in women and is associated with a poor prognosis.

3. F – Depression – severe

The three core symptoms of depression are low mood, anhedonia (loss of pleasure) and anergia (low energy). The diagnostic criteria require there to be a history of two out of three core symptoms for at least 2 weeks. In addition, there should be at least two of the following seven symptoms:
- decreased concentration
- reduced self-esteem
- guilt
- pessimism about the future
- self-harm ideation
- disturbed sleep
- reduced appetite

The severity of depression is classified as mild (four symptoms in total), moderate (five or six symptoms in total) and severe (seven symptoms in total, including all three core symptoms).

Beck's cognitive triad describes types of negative thought that occur in depression. These are a negative view of oneself, a negative view of the world and a negative view of the future.

The lifetime risk of depression is 10–25% in females and 5–12% in males. Marital status affects the risk of depression: the highest-risk group are those who are divorced, followed by people who are separated, then single, then married. Other risk factors are having three or more children below the age of 14, unemployment, maternal death below the age of 11 and a lack of confiding relationships. An adverse life event in the previous 6 months, personality disorders and a family history of bipolar disorder predispose to depression. Coexisting medical conditions are a risk factor – some specific examples are discussed in 'Psychiatric signs of physical illness' (Paper 10 Answers, Theme 8, page 275). Examples of medications that increase the risk of depression include β-blockers, steroids, anticonvulsants, benzodiazepines, antipsychotics, opiates and non-steroidal anti-inflammatory drugs.

Aaron Beck, American psychiatrist (b1921).

4. M – Somatic syndrome

Biological features of depression include:
- anhedonia
- decreased emotional reactivity
- early morning wakening
- diurnal variation
- psychomotor retardation/agitation
- decreased appetite
- weight loss (>5% in 1 month)
- reduced libido

If a patient displays at least four of these eight biological symptoms, this constitutes the somatic syndrome.

5. A – Atypical depression

Atypical depression is characterized by reverse neurovegetative biological symptoms, i.e. hyperphagia, weight gain and hypersomnia. *Seasonal affective disorder* presents with depressive episodes in the autumn and winter months, with an improvement in spring. It tends to be associated with symptoms of atypical depression. In *masked depression*, the patient does not present with low mood. Some patients present with somatization of symptoms; others do not complain of any symptoms, and maintain a cheerful exterior despite having significant symptoms affecting their life.

Persistent mood disorders (*dysthymia* and *cyclothymia*) last longer than 2 years and usually start in early adulthood. Dysthymia is a mild reduction in mood, and cyclothymia is mild reduction in mood alternating with mild elevations of mood. 'Double depression' is when a depressive episode occurs in an individual with dysthymia.

Theme 5: Descriptive psychopathology 1

1. J – Neologism

2. N – Perseveration

Speech disorders

A *neologism* is a new word, or an old word used in a new way. In *perseveration*, mental operations are continued beyond when they are relevant. It is highly suggestive of organic brain disease. Examples are *palilalia*, which is repeating a whole word (e.g. 'knife ... knife ... knife ...') and *logoclonia*, which is repeating the last syllable of a word (e.g. 'pass the Yorkshire pudding ... ding ... ding ... ding'). *Word salad*, or *schizophasia*, is an incomprehensible mish-mash of words and phrases. *Dysprosody* is loss of the normal melody of speech. *Logorrhoea* describes fluent, rambling speech – an extreme version of verbal diarrhoea!

Expressive aphasia is a difficulty verbalizing thoughts, although comprehension is intact. It is seen in patients after a stroke. In *receptive aphasia*, there is difficulty understanding and, although the patient feels that they are speaking fluently, it is not usually possible to make out any words in their voice. In *global aphasia*, both expressive and receptive aphasias are present. *Dysarthria* is physical difficulty in controlling movements of the mouth in order to articulate words.

Mutism is complete loss of speech. *Poverty of speech* is reduced/restricted speech (e.g. monosyllabic answers). *Pressure of speech* is increased quantity and rate of speech. *Stammering* is when the flow of speech is broken by pauses and repetition. *Echolalia* is the imitation of another person (even if it is in a foreign language). *Coprolalia* is the explosive exclamation of obscenities, seen in Tourette's syndrome.

Coprolalia, from Greek *kopros* = dung + *lalein* = talk.

The following forms of speech give the examiner insight into the form of the patient's thoughts. *Knight's move thinking* is demonstrated when speech jumps from one subject to another with no link. *Flight of ideas* is accelerated thoughts with abrupt incidental changes of subject and no central direction. The connections between topics are based on chance relationships, such as rhyming words or alliteration. *Circumstantiality* is the incorporation of unnecessary trivial details into speech, but the eventual goal is reached.

3. F – Flight of ideas

4. L – Overvalued idea
Thought disorders

Schneider's three features of normal thought are constancy, organization and consistency. There are five features of Schneider's formal thought disorder:
- derailment: a thought derails on to a subsidiary thought
- drivelling: a disordered intermixture of constituent parts of a thought
- fusion: heterogeneous thoughts are interwoven
- omission: part of a thought is omitted
- substitution: a major thought is substituted with a subsidiary thought

A *delusion* is a belief held with absolute conviction, such that it is not changeable, even by compelling counterargument or proof to the contrary. A *primary delusion* has no obvious cause considering the patient's circumstances. *Secondary delusions* are more closely linked with the rest of the clinical picture; for example, grandiose delusions (the belief of inflated self-worth) are common in mania, and a persecutory delusion may be seen in paranoid schizophrenia. A *bizarre delusion* is one that would be seen as totally implausible within the patient's culture.

An *overvalued idea* is an unreasonable, sustained, intense preoccupation that is maintained with less than delusional intensity, i.e. the patient may accept that it might not be true. An *obsession* is a repetitive senseless thought that is recognized as irrational but is unsuccessfully resisted by the person. The motor equivalent of an obsessional thought is a *compulsion* – a repetitive, stereotyped, seemingly purposeful behaviour that is not actually useful and is recognized as such by the patient. *Ideas of reference* are thoughts that the events or objects in one's immediate environment have a particular or unusual significance. *Monomania* is a pathological preoccupation with a single subject, and *egomania* is a pathological preoccupation with oneself.

5. H – Hypnopompic hallucination
Sensory disorders

A *hallucination* is a false perception in the absence of a real external stimulus. It can be visual, auditory or tactile. Examples of hallucinations include *autoscopy* (the person sees their own image in front of them as if looking in a mirror), *extracampine hallucinations* (something may be seen out of the corner of one's eye, but on turning to look at it the object disappears), *functional hallucinations* (precipitated by another stimulus, e.g. a voice speaks to you every time you hear a toilet flushing), *reflex hallucinations* (a stimulus causes a hallucination in a different sensory field, e.g. a green monster is seen at the sound of a flushing toilet), *formication* (the sensation of insects crawling over or under the skin) and the *trailing phenomenon* (when moving objects appear as a series of pictures). *Hypnagogic* and *hypnopompic* hallucinations are visual images seen when falling into and waking up from sleep, respectively. They can be normal phenomena.

A *pseudohallucination* is an image seen in subjective space, as if within the person's mind. One form is an *eidetic image*, which is the vivid reproduction of a previous memory (much like a photographic memory). Another form is *pareidolia*, which describes the phenomenon when one can make out images while looking at a poorly structured background, e.g. seeing someone's face in a camp fire. An *illusion* is a false perception of a real external stimulus, e.g. thinking that a shadow of a post box is a person in the distance.

Sensory distortions are abnormal sensory experiences that are altered experiences of a real stimulus. Examples include hyper-/hypo-aesthesia (a non-organic increase or decrease in sensation), dysmegalopsia (the inability to judge the size of objects), chloropsia/erythropsia/xanthopsia (where all objects appear green, red or yellow, respectively), and macropsia and micropsia (objects seem much larger or smaller than normal).

Theme 6: Sleep disorders

Sleep disorders can be divided into primary and secondary. Secondary problems are further subdivided depending on whether they are caused by a physical or psychiatric illness, or whether they are caused by psychoactive substances.

1. D – Night terror

Night terrors are seen in children, affecting 6% of 4–12 year olds, and resolve by adolescence. The child usually awakes suddenly during the first third of the night in a state of panic and fearfulness. There are associated autonomic responses, e.g. tachycardia and dilated pupils. Affected children are not easily comforted, but, when they fully awake (usually the next morning), they have no recollection of the event.

2. E – Nightmare

Nightmares are frightening dreams in which the individual awakes suddenly and is then fully alert and can remember the dream very well. They usually occur during the second half of the night. Nightmares affect up to 50% of adults occasionally, while 3–5 year olds are more likely to experience repeated nightmares.

3. B – Insomnia

Insomnia is a condition describing a reduced quantity or quality of sleep for a prolonged period. This may involve difficulty getting to sleep/staying asleep and early morning wakening. It is a common symptom of other conditions, but, if it dominates the clinical picture, it can be considered a condition in its own right. Assessment involves careful history-taking for causes, including other illnesses and substances (including caffeine). Factors in the daily routine that may be unhelpful should be identified and advice given about sleep hygiene. This involves going to bed and getting up at the same time each day, doing relaxing tasks such as bathing, reading, drinking hot milk before bed, using the bed for sleep only (except for sex) and not watching television. If there is an underlying cause, this should be treated. Drug treatments are limited and include short-acting benzodiazepines such as temazepam (which have less of a hangover effect than longer-acting ones such as diazepam) or zopiclone (which is similar). However, these drugs should have a limited duration, and their use for longer than 2 weeks increases the risk of addiction. Ideally, they should not be taken every day. The diagnosis of insomnia can be made at any age, but it is more common in the elderly.

Hypersomnia is a condition defined as either excessive daytime sleepiness with sleep attacks or an abnormal length of time taken to reach full arousal after sleeping (in the absence of an organic disorder). It affects 0.3–4% of the population. The management includes looking for a physical cause, improving sleep hygiene, and occasionally stimulants such as dexamphetamine and methylphenidate.

4. H – Psychiatric/psychological problem causing sleep disturbance

This woman presents with insomnia, early morning wakening and a blunted affect. This could be indicative of underlying depression

5. K – Somnambulism

Somnambulism (sleepwalking) is a state of altered consciousness in which there are some features of wakefulness and some of sleep. The individual usually arises from bed (during the first third of nocturnal sleep) and begins walking, but with reduced awareness, reactivity and motor skill. Upon awakening, there is usually no recollection of the event. It is more common in children. Management is by reassurance, simple safety measures and gentle encouragement to return to bed by the family.

Narcolepsy forms a part of the differential diagnosis. It is less common, affecting <0.1% of the population. It is a neurological condition caused by a loss of inhibition of rapid eye movement (REM) sleep. It has four main features: irresistible attacks of sleep at inappropriate times, cataplexy (sudden loss of muscle tone when intense emotion occurs, leading to collapse), hypnogogic/hypnopompic hallucinations (hallucinations that occur on falling asleep and waking, respectively) and sleep paralysis. Not all cases of narcolepsy have all four features. When forming the diagnosis, factors that point to hypersomnia are sleeps that have a gradual onset, are worse in the mornings and rarely occur in unusual places. Factors that suggest narcolepsy are a short duration of sleep (10–20 minutes,) the inability to control sleep attacks and interrupted night-time sleep, as well as the four main features. Management falls under the remit of neurologists.

Sleep apnoea is a physical condition in which the upper respiratory tract becomes partially occluded during sleep. This can cause transient cessation in breathing, which causes the patient to wake repeatedly during the night, reducing the quality of sleep. Sleep apnoea results in daytime tiredness. It is more common in overweight males who snore. Treatment is by continuous positive airway pressure (CPAP) via facemask during sleep.

Non-organic disorder of the sleep–wake cycle is caused by a lack of synchrony with the desired sleep–wake pattern. The problem is often perceived as either insomnia or hypersomnia. Management is by attention to sleep hygiene.

Theme 7: Suicide

Suicide is important to consider because it is one of the most extreme negative outcomes in psychiatry. It is important to know the risk factors in order to identify and manage those at risk. A thorough assessment of an individual's risk should be made in the psychiatric history; this involves frank questioning about suicidal ideation, particularly after an act of self-harm. Discussing suicidal ideation with a patient does not increase their risk of suicide (as is sometimes feared). However, it is not always possible to accurately identify those most at risk.

Risk factors for suicide include:
- male sex
- age >45 years
- being divorced, single or widowed
- unemployed
- social classes I and V
- psychiatric illness
- previous episodes of self-harm
- chronic physical illness
- recent adverse life events

Protective factors include having children and being religious. In populations, the rate of suicide increases in summer months and decreases during times of war.

1. B – 1 in 10 000

The annual incidence of suicide is 1 in 10 000.

2. D – 1%

After an act of self-harm the risk of completed suicide within the next year is 1%, i.e. 100 times more than the risk in the general population. The following features of self-harm are indicators of strong suicidal intent: a more violent/ dangerous action, careful planning and preparation, making precautions to avoid being discovered, failing to seek help afterwards and final acts (e.g. making a suicide note or a will). It should be ascertained whether or not they intended to die at the time and, if so, what their reaction is to still being alive (do they regret being alive and still wish to die?). There is a high rate of recurrence in people who self-harm.

3. F – 66.6%

Two thirds of people who have completed suicide have seen a GP within the last month. Around 25% are psychiatric outpatients, and half of those will have seen their psychiatrist during the previous week.

4. G – 90%

Ninety percent of those who self-harm have a psychiatric illness; the most common of these are depressive episodes, alcohol dependence, other substance use, personality disorders, chronic neuroses and schizophrenia.

5. C – 3 per 1000

The annual incidence of self-harm is 3 per 1000. The nomenclature and definitions of self-harm are contentious. The term 'parasuicide' is now outdated, and use of the word 'deliberate' before self-harm is out of favour, because it implies blame or judgement (as does using the term to 'commit' suicide). Self-harm describes either self-injury (10%) or self-poisoning (90%) that is non-fatal. If a drug or poison is ingested that is not actually harmful, or at a dose that is not harmful, the term self-harm is still used if the patient *believed* it to be harmful. Risk factors for self-harm include female sex, age 15–25, lower social class, unemployment and living in an urban area. Individual risk factors are psychiatric illness, learning disability, death of a parent at a young age and childhood neglect/abuse. Predisposing factors at a particular time include physical illness (in the patient or a family member), relationship loss/difficulties and criminal proceedings. Additionally, in severe depression with psychomotor retardation, a recent improvement in symptoms is a risk factor for suicide, because patients gain enough motivation and energy to do it.

Theme 8: Psychiatric disorders relating to women's health

1. D – Maternity blues

Maternity blues affects two-thirds of women post-partum. It begins 3–5 days after birth, and lasts no longer than 10 days. It is characterized by low mood and tearfulness, and usually recovers spontaneously. Management is by reassurance. *Postnatal depression* starts within 3 months of giving birth, and usually lasts less than 6 months. It affects 10% of women. Features are similar to those of depressive episodes, but some symptoms of depression (insomnia, tiredness and low libido) are normal post-partum. There may be obsessional thoughts, particularly intrusive thoughts about harming the baby. There may be an excessive concern about the baby's health and the mother's own adequacy as a parent. Treatment may be solely supportive or include antidepressants.

2. A – Couvade syndrome

Couvade syndrome occurs in males around the time of the birth of their child. They experience symptoms similar to those of pregnancy, such as nausea and dyspepsia. They may even suffer abdominal distension and labour-like contraction pains. The cause is not well understood, but symptoms usually resolve soon after birth. *Pseudocyesis* is the presence of the signs and symptoms of pregnancy (e.g. amenorrhoea, breast enlargement and significant abdominal distension) in a non-pregnant woman.

Couvade, from Old French *couver* = to hatch.

Pseudocyesis, from Greek *pseudes* = false + *kyesis* = pregnancy.

3. H – Premenstrual syndrome

Premenstrual syndrome (PMS) describes the emotional and physical symptoms during the second half of the menstrual cycle, which increase in intensity until menstruation. Around 40% of women report symptoms at some time. Symptoms affecting mood include irritability, low mood, tiredness, tension and emotional lability. Management is supportive, and aims to identify and avoid psychological stressors. Antidepressants can be effective in reducing the psychological symptoms, and the oral contraceptive pill is effective at alleviating the physical symptoms. *Cyclic psychosis* can be seen as a rare complication of extreme PMS, with psychotic symptoms that are absent for most of the cycle. *Dysmenorrhoea* relates to pain during menstruation itself (or very slightly before).

Neither 'perimenstrual syndrome' nor 'postmenstrual syndrome' is a recognized medical condition, although there are outrageous allegations that these concepts exist.

4. K – Puerperal psychosis

The puerperium is defined as the first 6 weeks after childbirth. This is a high-risk period for developing psychiatric illness. Puerperal psychosis affects one pregnancy in 500 and has a rapid onset during the first 3 weeks after birth. There may be a prodrome of insomnia and irritability, followed by acute confusion and psychosis. It should be treated as a medical emergency in a specialist centre, because there is a suicide risk of 5% and an infanticide risk of 4%. Seventy per cent of cases recover fully. The aims of treatment are to keep the mother and child together in a safe environment, and ECT is sometimes required.

Puerperium, from Latin *puer* = child + *parere* = to give birth.

5. E – Not a psychiatric condition

Although this behaviour may be seen as eccentric, there is nothing in the history that suggests an underlying psychiatric disorder.

Theme 9: Substance use

1. I – Opiate use

This woman is likely to be suffering the effects of opiate use. Examples of opiates include morphine, heroin, methadone and codeine. Effects of opiates (in addition to analgesia) include euphoria, nausea and vomiting, constipation, anorexia, hypotension, respiratory depression, tremor, pinpoint pupils and erectile dysfunction. The treatment of overdose (after ABC) is with the antidote naloxone. This is ideally given intravenously (but can be given intramuscularly or by inhalation). An infusion of naloxone may be necessary, as the half-life is short. The effects of opiate withdrawal can be very extreme. They include dilated pupils, lacrimation, sweating, diarrhoea, insomnia, tachycardia, abdominal cramp-like pains, nausea and vomiting. Opiate dependence can be managed (once drug use has stopped) by methadone and buprenorphine (a partial agonist).

2. E – Cannabis use

Cannabis (Δ^9-tetrahydrocannabinol) has the following effects: dry cough, increased appetite, conjunctival injection and fatigue. Psychological effects include euphoria, relaxation, an altered perception of time, social withdrawal and paranoia.

3. G – Cocaine use

Cocaine intoxication may present with tachycardia, mydriasis, hypertension, nausea and vomiting, euphoria, increased interest in sex and formication (a tactile hallucination described as insects crawling over the skin). Cocaine withdrawal results in a dysphoric mood, cravings, irritability and paranoia. Cocaine use is a risk factor for cardiovascular disease.

4. L – Sedative withdrawal

This woman may be on long-term sedatives (benzodiazepines or barbiturates) that stopped being prescribed when she moved location. Symptoms of sedative withdrawal include nausea and vomiting, autonomic hyperactivity, insomnia, delirium and seizures. Features of sedative use include loss of coordination, slurred speech, decreased attention and memory, disinhibition, aggression, meiosis, hypotension and respiratory depression.

Amphetamines are available illegally, but are also prescribed in narcolepsy, hyperkinetic syndromes (e.g. attention-deficit hyperactivity disorder) and as appetite suppressants. Features of intoxication include euphoria, insomnia, agitation, hallucinations, hypertension and tachycardia. Symptoms of the withdrawal state include dysphoric mood, fatigue and agitation.

5. B – Alcohol withdrawal

Alcohol withdrawal usually occurs if blood alcohol concentration falls in someone with alcohol dependence. Symptoms usually start approximately 12 hours after the last intake and include anxiety, insomnia, sweating, tachycardia and tremor. Seizures may occur after 48 hours. Treatment is supportive with a reducing dose of regular benzodiazepines (e.g. chlordiazepoxide) and vitamin B supplements (intravenous or oral). The mortality rate is approximately 5%.

Delirium tremens may also be a feature of alcohol withdrawal, and occurs after 48 hours, lasting for 5 days. There is tremor, restlessness and increased autonomic activity, fluctuating consciousness with disorientation, a fearful affect and hallucinations. Hallucinations may be auditory, tactile or visual, and delusions may also be present. *Lilliputian hallucinations* (seeing little people) are characteristic.

Lilliputian, named after the island of Lilliput in Jonathan Swift's novel *Gulliver's Travels*, where the inhabitants were 'not six inches high'.

Alcohol intoxication presents with mood changes, loss of inhibition, cerebellar signs (dysdiadochokinesis, ataxia, nystagmus, intention tremor, slurred speech, hypotonicity and hyporeflexia) and decreased conscious level.

Alcohol consumption is measured in units: 1 unit is equal to 10 g alcohol. Safe levels are 28 units/week for men and 21 units/week for women, with not more than 4 and 3 units per day, respectively. Alcohol-free days are recommended.

Excessive drinking can lead to *alcohol-dependence syndrome*, which is characterized by the following seven features:
- increased tolerance (the drug produces less effect per gram ingested)
- repeated withdrawal symptoms
- subjective awareness of compulsion to drink, and cravings if resistance is attempted
- prioritization of alcohol over other aspects of life (e.g. career and family)
- avoidance of withdrawal by continued drinking
- narrowing of the drinking repertoire (habits develop, including the preference of one particular drink, often as part of a daily routine)
- rapid reinstatement of alcohol if a period of abstinence is successfully achieved

The *CAGE questionnaire* is a sensitive screening tool for alcohol dependence. There are four questions:
- Have you ever felt that you should **C**ut down?
- Have you ever been **A**nnoyed by criticism of your drinking?
- Have you ever felt **G**uilty about your drinking?
- Have you ever had an **E**ye-opener (morning drink)?

Examples of physical morbidity from alcohol use are vomiting, peptic ulcer disease, Mallory–Weiss tears, oesophageal varices, hepatic cirrhosis and liver failure, pancreatitis, repeated trauma, endocrine disturbances and aspiration pneumonia. Fetal alcohol syndrome is seen in children whose mothers had drunk excessive amounts of alcohol during pregnancy. Features include microcephaly, small nose, low IQ (mean 70), strabismus and long philtrum.

Theme 10: Syndromes in psychiatry

I. E – Ekbom's syndrome

Ekbom's syndrome is a delusional psychosis that one is infected with parasites. It may be accompanied by a physical sensation of parasites crawling around or burrowing into the skin (formication). *Cotard syndrome* is a nihilistic delusion that one is dead, has lost all one's possessions, does not exist or is decaying, etc. It can be a feature of severe depression.

Formication, from Latin *formica* = ant.

Jules Cotard, French neurologist (1840–89).

2. K – Rett's syndrome

Rett's syndrome is a neurodevelopmental disorder, similar to autism, where developmental decline occurs after 1 to 2 years of age following a normal initial development. Typical behaviours include screaming attacks, avoidance of eye contact, poor social interactions, loss of fine motor skills, development of stereotyped hand movements (especially hand-wringing) and ataxia. It is more common in females.

The *pickwickian syndrome* is the association of obesity with sleep apnoea and hypersomnia. It is named after a character in Dickens' novel *The Pickwick Papers* who was extremely obese and often fell asleep during the day. *Tourette's syndrome* is characterized by multiple vocal and motor tics.

Georges Gilles de la Tourette (1859–1904).

3. D – de Clerambault's syndrome

de Clerambault's syndrome (erotomania) is a delusional belief that someone of higher social status is in love with them. It is commoner in women.

Gaetan Gatian de Clerambault, French psychiatrist (1872–1934).

4. H – Ganser's syndrome

Ganser's syndrome is a factitious disorder in which people give approximate answers to simple questions that show that they understand the underlying theme of the questions asked. Individuals mimic what they believe to be psychotic behaviours e.g. when asked how many legs a donkey has, they will answer 'twelve' as opposed to 'chicken wing'. Ganser's syndrome was first described in prison inmates awaiting trial.

Munchausen's syndrome is a factitious disorder where people repeatedly feign illness or self-inflict pathology for the sole purpose of seeking medical attention (e.g. injecting faecal matter into the skin). In *Munchausen by proxy*, a different person is used for the same purpose (e.g. saying that a child has been repeatedly fitting).

Sigbert Ganser, German psychiatrist (1853–1931).

Karl Munchausen, German baron (1720–97). He acquired a reputation for telling exaggerated tales about his adventures in other countries, including travelling to the moon.

5. G – Fregoli's syndrome

Fregoli's syndrome is a delusion that a persecutor is able to change into many forms and disguise themselves to look like different people, much like an actor. It is named after Leopold Fregoli, an Italian actor (1867–1936) who was famous for being able to make quick changes of appearance during stage acts.

Othello syndrome (*delusional jealousy*) is a feeling of delusional intensity that one's partner is being unfaithful. It is named after Shakespeare's character Othello, who murdered his wife based on false beliefs of her disloyalty. *Capgras' syndrome* is a delusional belief that a close acquaintance has been replaced by an identical double. It is most commonly seen in schizophrenia. *Folie à deux* is when a delusion in one person becomes shared by someone close to them. A similar effect can occur in three or more people (*folie à trois, folie à plusieurs*).

Folie à deux, from French *folie* = madness.

Joseph Capgras, French psychiatrist (1873–1950).

Theme 1: Neurotic disorders

Options

A. Acute stress reaction
B. Agoraphobia
C. Dissociative (conversion) disorder
D. Generalized anxiety disorder
E. Grief reaction
F. Obsessive–compulsive disorder
G. Panic disorder
H. Post-traumatic stress disorder
I. Social phobia
J. Somatization disorder
K. Specific phobia
L. Undifferentiated somatoform disorder.

For each of the following scenarios, select the most likely diagnosis. Each option may be used once, more than once or not at all.

1. An 18-year-old woman prefers to spend time at home. She has started doing all her shopping online, and insists that her friends visit her at her own house, where she is quite happy. When she absolutely must go out anywhere, she dreads it for days, occasionally gets palpitations and finds the whole situation unbearable. The most frightening place is her busy college common room.

2. A 45-year-old man attends the GP with his wife because he is never able to relax. He worries excessively over trivial daily issues, with no obvious pattern, and his muscles always feel tense.

3. A 61-year-old woman presents to her GP, and appears very concerned about the cause of her abdominal pains. They have been present for 3 years, and fluctuate in intensity and exact position. She has had a gastroscopy, colonoscopy, ultrasound and CT scans and has also seen consultants privately.

4. A 21-year-old man presents to the emergency department with shortness of breath and chest pain. His symptoms started very suddenly while at a bus station, and were associated with light-headedness, dizziness and a fear that he was going to die. His symptoms resolved after 10 minutes. He has had four previous similar episodes.

5. A 22-year-old woman who describes herself as having always been generally anxious admits to having unpleasant thoughts over the past 6 months. She cannot control them, but recognizes that they are her own. She also admits to spending 3 hours a day packing and repacking her bag before leaving the house to avoid forgetting anything.

Theme 2: Side-effects of psychiatric medication

Options

   A. Acute dystonia
   B. Agranulocytosis
   C. Akathisia
   D. Cheese reaction
   E. Hyperprolactinaemia
   F. Lithium toxicity
   G. Neuroleptic malignant syndrome
   H. Parkinsonism
   I. Serotonin syndrome
   J. Tardive dyskinesia
   K. Weight gain
   L. Weight loss

For each of the following descriptions, select the most appropriate side-effect. Each option may be used once, more than once or not at all.

1. A 42-year-old man with paranoid schizophrenia has been taking chlorpromazine. He has developed symptoms of restless legs and is requesting treatment for this.

2. A 65-year-old man has been taking haloperidol for many years. On examination, he had unusual facial movements that look as though he is chewing or sucking his tongue.

3. A 40-year-old woman with schizophrenia has recently had an increase in her dose of clozapine. She presented to the emergency department unconscious with a temperature of 39.8°C and muscle rigidity. Initial blood tests revealed a raised white cell count and a creatine kinase of 5000 IU/L.

4. A 23-year-old woman presents to her GP because she and her partner are concerned about a noticeable change in her body habitus. She has been taking olanzapine for 6 months.

5. A 30-year-old woman was seen by her GP with symptoms of sweating and fever, which was thought to be caused by a viral infection. She later presents to the emergency department with agitation and confusion. On examination, she is shocked and has overactive reflexes. Routine observations reveal a heart rate of 130 beats/min and a blood pressure of 210/110 mmHg. She denies illicit drug use, but has recently started taking an over-the-counter preparation for depression. Her repeat prescription includes lansoprazole, salbutamol inhaler and fluoxetine.

Theme 3: Descriptive psychopathology 2

Options

- A. Agitation
- B. Amnesia
- C. Depression
- D. Dysphoria
- E. Echopraxia
- F. Echolalia
- G. Euphoria
- H. Fugue state
- I. Hyperamnesia
- J. Hyperkinesia
- K. Stupor
- L. Paramnesia

For each of the following scenarios, select the most appropriate descriptive term. Each option may be used once, more than once or not at all.

1. A 36-year-old woman has had a difficult day at work. She is now in an unpleasant mood.

2. An 80-year-old woman is asked about the events leading up to a fall she had earlier in the day. She explains exactly what she can remember, but the description that she gives is significantly different from the account of her carers who were present at the time.

3. A 60-year-old man with schizophrenia is copying the exact movements of his social worker during a multidisciplinary team meeting.

4. A 26-year-old woman is very unhappy that she has just been sectioned. She appears restless and is not keeping her hands still. She is also intermittently striding around the room.

5. A 55-year-old man with severe depression was found in his flat by police. He was sitting on the floor, absolutely still, not speaking at all.

Theme 4: Psychotic disorders

Options

A. Antisocial personality disorder
B. Catatonic schizophrenia
C. Delusional disorder
D. Hebephrenic schizophrenia
E. Organic psychotic disorder
F. Psychotic depression
G. Schizoaffective disorder
H. Schizoid-type personality disorder
I. Simple schizophrenia
J. Substance-induced psychotic disorder
K. Transient psychosis

For each of the following scenarios, select the most appropriate diagnosis. Each option may be used once, more than once or not at all.

1. A 45-year-old man presents with a 4-week history of low mood, lack of enjoyment in his usual activities and reduced energy. He feels unhappy with his own abilities and appearance. He says that he is also worried about how to keep his thoughts clean, 'especially as they have been all over the BBC website for the past six weeks.'

2. A 60-year-old woman with a long history of recurrent depression is complaining that she can smell rotting flesh and that it is coming from her legs. Peripheral vascular examination is normal.

3. A 54-year-old man with a 30-year history of mental health problems is found to be standing on one leg with his arm in the air. He did not move for 30 minutes until a nurse pulled his arm down. It then stayed in the new position. He has not said anything for an hour, but yesterday was noted to be repeating the same word incessantly.

4. A 19-year-old male student is admitted to a psychiatric ward after hearing voices and behaving strangely. He admits to spending half of his weekly food budget on 'skunk'.

5. A 21-year-old woman has always preferred to be by herself. She has no hobbies and finds it difficult to share her feelings with others. She was referred to a psychiatrist, and a thorough mental state examination revealed a blunted affect. There were no specific abnormalities of thinking.

Theme 5: Psychiatry of sexuality

Options

A. Exhibitionism
B. Fetishism
C. Loss of sexual desire
D. Male erectile disorder
E. Masochism
F. Non-organic dyspareunia
G. Premature ejaculation
H. Sadism
I. Sexual aversion
J. Transsexualism
K. Transvestic fetishism
L. Vaginismus
M. Voyeurism

For each of the following scenarios, select the most appropriate diagnosis. Each option may be used once, more than once or not at all.

1. A 45-year-old man has begun to gain sexual excitement from shiny materials such as PVC. He is now relying on it in order to become aroused.

2. A 19-year-old man was arrested after flashing his genitals to a group of teenage girls at a fairground.

3. A 35-year-old man has felt for a long time that he is a woman trapped in a man's body. He has changed his name from Fred to Freda and is saving money for an operation to change his anatomy. He usually wears a pink pinafore dress and says that he feels 'much more comfortable dressed like this'.

4. A 45-year-old woman is married but says that she has never enjoyed sex. She has no specific physical problems with the process of it, but she dreads it and feels emotionally uncomfortable during intercourse itself, as well as while talking and thinking about it.

5. A 27-year-old man has a new sexual partner, but has been finding it increasingly difficult to achieve an erection. The more he worries about it, the less likely he is to be successful.

Theme 6: Management of depression

Options

    A. Amitriptyline
    B. Cognitive–behavioural therapy
    C. Diazepam
    D. Electroconvulsive therapy
    E. Fluoxetine
    F. Imipramine
    G. Lithium
    H. Moclobemide
    I. Phenelzine
    J. Psychodynamic psychotherapy

For each of the following scenarios, select the most appropriate step in the management. Each option may be used once, more than once or not at all.

1. A 25-year-old woman presents to her GP with a 3-month history of low mood. She feels that her self-esteem has suffered since stopping her usual hobbies and social activities after the breakdown of a relationship.

2. A 64-year-old man had been an inpatient for 3 months with severe depression. His symptoms have been resistant to selective serotonin reuptake inhibitors, lithium and the supportive environment of the hospital itself. He has deteriorated further to the point that he is not communicating and not adequately feeding himself.

3. A 36-year-old woman presents to her GP with a 4-month history of low mood, poor appetite and tearfulness. She has had a previous episode of depression, which responded to a 6-month course of first-line drug treatment.

4. A 45-year-old man with severe depression is managed by a community psychiatry team. His depression has not responded to three different antidepressants and, although he and his wife are fairly reliable and are coping at the moment, they are very keen to see some improvement. The only food that he likes to eat is pizza.

5. A 59-year-old woman with depression had started a course of fluoxetine, but was forced to discontinue it due to side-effects. Poor sleep is a prominent feature of her illness.

Theme 7: Transcultural psychiatric disorders

Options

A. Amok
B. Depressive episode
C. Dhat
D. Generalized anxiety disorder
E. Koro
F. Latah
G. Piblokto
H. Susto
I. Windigo

For each of the following scenarios, select the most appropriate diagnosis. Each option may be used once, more than once or not at all.

1. A 28-year-old man living in Malaysia took a knife and ruthlessly murdered nine of his family members and neighbours in a 30-minute rampage before finally killing himself. He had no previous psychiatric history and there was no obvious motive.

2. A 19-year-old man of Chinese origin has developed symptoms of severe anxiety and has become preoccupied with the fear that his penis is going to disappear inside him. He has tried to clamp it to prevent this happening.

3. A 38-year-old woman living in the Arctic Circle had a sudden-onset episode of bizarre behaviour. She cannot remember it, but her family say that she began screaming and crying hysterically and started throwing furniture and eating the broken splinters. She had to be physically restrained when she became violent.

4. A 22-year-old Indian man presented to his doctor complaining of extreme fatigue and anxiety. On questioning about his ideas regarding the cause, he admitted to excessive guilt about masturbation, and felt that he was losing semen in his urine.

5. A 26-year-old woman living in Tunisia is involved in a road traffic collision. Soon after the accident, she appears very on-edge, with a markedly exaggerated startle response. She has started repeating the words of everyone around her.

Theme 8: Psychiatric signs of physical illness

Options

A. Cushing's syndrome
B. Delirium
C. Hyperthyroidism
D. Hypothyroidism
E. Multiple sclerosis
F. Neurosyphilis
G. Pellagra
H. Punch-drunk syndrome
I. Space-occupying lesion
J. Systemic lupus erythematosus

For each of the following scenarios, select the most likely underlying physical cause. Each option may be used once, more than once or not at all.

1. A 58-year-old woman presents to the emergency department hearing voices. Her partner had noticed increased irritability, restlessness, change in behaviour and loss of libido over the past 2 months. On examination, she has a fine tremor, is underweight and has an irregular pulse.

2. A 45-year-old woman presents with low mood and tearfulness. She is upset about severe pains in her knees and hands and an embarrassing red rash over her face. She also complains of worsening shortness of breath.

3. A 42-year-old man presents with memory loss, and his wife says that he has been pointing at things in the room that are not there. He has also had a headache for over a month, which is worse in the mornings.

4. A 77-year-old woman was found by her carers confused and disorientated. She is usually lucid. The carers notice that she has been incontinent of urine.

5. A 34-year-old woman presents to her GP complaining of feeling sad all the time, difficulty sleeping and weight gain. She has a history of Crohn's disease and is taking medication regularly for frequent exacerbations.

Theme 9: The Mental Health Act

Options

- A. Section 2
- B. Section 3
- C. Section 4
- D. Section 5(2)
- E. Section 5(4)
- F. Section 12
- G. Section 17
- H. Section 35
- I. Section 36
- J. Section 37
- K. Section 135
- L. Section 136

For each of the following scenarios, choose which section of the Mental Health Act is most likely to be used. Each option may be used once, more than once or not at all.

1. A 46-year-old woman is accosted by the police after a member of the public alerted them to her strange behaviour. She has been playing on the swings all day and singing to the birds in her pyjamas, despite it being December. The police decide that it is best to take her to hospital.

2. A 19-year-old man presents with his first episode of psychosis and is seen by a consultant psychiatrist. He needs to be admitted for formal assessment, but the man is adamant that he wants to go straight home.

3. A 36-year-old woman, who is an inpatient on a psychiatry ward with depression, had agreed to her admission 1 week ago. She is now trying to leave. She has told a care assistant that she is following the devil's instructions to her, and will jump off a bridge once she has left. The psychiatry medical team are all away on a conference.

4. A 55-year-old man with known chronic severe depression is being managed in the community. He has recently deteriorated and is not currently safe at home. The community psychiatrist decides that he needs admission for treatment, although it is against the patient's wishes.

5. A 25-year-old man presents to the emergency department on a Saturday night, behaving strangely. His only speech is an impersonation of a rap artist, which he does while breakdancing. He has a history of bipolar affective disorder. His mother is concerned that he has stopped sleeping, and thinks that this is a manic episode. His usual consultant will be available on Monday morning, but the attending doctor decides that he needs to be admitted until then.

Theme 10: Personality disorders

Options

A. Anankastic
B. Antisocial
C. Anxious (avoidant)
D. Dependent
E. Emotionally unstable (borderline type)
F. Emotionally unstable (impulsive type)
G. Histrionic
H. Paranoid
I. Schizoid

For each of the following scenarios, select the most appropriate personality disorder. Each option may be used once, more than once or not at all.

1. A 19-year-old factory worker has no friends and has been experiencing difficulty with relationships at work. People have complained that he has aggressive outbursts and has no regard for anyone else's feelings. He himself does not feel guilty, but blames those around him who have made him feel frustrated. At school, he was diagnosed with conduct disorder.

2. An 18-year-old woman agrees to have a baby with her boyfriend, because he is extremely keen to do so and she wants to make him happy. She fears that he will leave her if she does not. She hates spending time alone and has difficulty making her own decisions.

3. A 35-year-old woman presents to the emergency department following an overdose. She has had 17 similar presentations this year, usually after an argument, and this time it was an attempt to stop her boyfriend from leaving her. They have an intense relationship, but her attitude towards it is variable, and sometimes she does not want to be a part of it.

4. A 50-year-old man is known as the local 'loner'. He has no interest in other people, nor does he enjoy any activities. If directly addressed, he appears detached and shows little emotion.

5. A 45-year-old woman has racked up enormous debt buying clothes and make-up. Her teenage children cringe at how she wears excessively revealing clothes and makes uninhibited advances towards male strangers. She behaves dramatically and can become very upset if she is not the centre of attention.

Practice Paper 10 Answers

Theme 1: Neurotic disorders

Generally, neurotic disorders in childhood do not lead to neurosis in later life. Neuroses in children are more common in males, but are dominant in females after adolescence.

1. B – Agoraphobia

Agoraphobia is an example of a phobic anxiety disorder. The other two types are social phobias and specific phobias. Phobias usually relate to specific situations or triggers. There is anxiety even in anticipation of the trigger, and avoidance behaviour ensues. The fear in a phobia is out of proportion to the actual risk, but is not relieved by reasoning and is beyond voluntary control. Avoidance behaviour is reinforced because it temporarily relieves the anxiety.

Agoraphobia is the general term for fear of situations such as public places, open spaces, crowds, shops and public transport. It is often seen as a fear of the inability to escape. The fear is usually worse when the person is alone. The condition can be disabling, because severe avoidance can lead to the patient being housebound, and there is a predisposition to developing panic attacks.

Social phobia is the fear of scrutiny and criticism from others. It usually co-exists with low self-esteem and may cause problems especially with speaking to strangers, answering the phone and public speaking. There may be problems with tremor, blushing and urinary urgency.

Specific phobias relate to one specific trigger. Examples include animals (zoophobia), small spaces (claustrophobia), heights (acrophobia), strangers (xenophobia) and inanimate objects such as buttons (koumpounophobia).

Management of phobic anxiety disorders is by graded exposure therapy, which involves gradually increasing the intensity and proximity of the source of phobia. Antidepressants also have a role.

Phobia, from Greek *phobos* = fear.

Agoraphobia, from Greek *agora* = a place of gathering, marketplace.

2. D – Generalized anxiety disorder

Generalized anxiety disorder is defined as generalized, excessive worry for more than 6 months. It is twice as common in females and occurs frequently in early adulthood. Sufferers of generalized anxiety disorder feel anxious or nervous most of the time. There is no single particular trigger, and it can be described as 'free-floating'. There is an underlying worry that 'something bad may happen'. Physical symptoms include trembling, sweating, light-headedness, palpitations, dizziness, abdominal discomfort and muscle tension. Genetic predisposition overlaps with the predisposition to depression. Management options include psychological therapies, selective serotonin reuptake inhibitors (SSRIs), benzodiazepines for rapid anxiolysis and β-blockers for autonomic symptoms. The disease course is usually chronic and fluctuating.

3. J – Somatization disorder

The patient has somatization disorder. This is characterized by the following:
- over 2 years of multiple, variable physical symptoms of no underlying cause
- refusal to accept doctors' reassurance
- impairment of social function
- symptoms not intentionally produced

Patients often see doctors of several different specialties and undergo investigations with negative outcomes. There is often social/family disruption. There is some evidence that somatization disorder is more common in people who experienced parental physical illness as children. Management is difficult, and the development of a physical illness needs to be excluded. In *undifferentiated somatoform disorder*, the diagnostic criteria for somatization disorder are not met. Symptoms may last less than 2 years and they are likely to be even more generalized and varied. Somatization disorders are much commoner in females.

4. G – Panic disorder

Panic disorder is characterized by sudden-onset, severe panic attacks that are not limited to one particular situation. Panic attacks last a few minutes and are often accompanied by a fear of going mad or dying. Physical symptoms include nausea, hyperventilation, palpitations, chest pain, sweating and light-headedness. Affected people are symptom free between attacks. Panic disorder is diagnosed only if there is no underlying disorder such as depression. First-line management is with cognitive–behavioural therapy. Panic disorder is most common in young female adults.

5. F – Obsessive–compulsive disorder

Obsessive–compulsive disorder (OCD) is characterized by persistent obsessional thoughts and compulsive acts despite conscious resistance. Obsessions are images or ideas that are recognized as the patient's own thoughts, but are unwanted. Attempts to resist them are usually unsuccessful. Compulsions are the irresistible urge to perform tasks or rituals that are stereotyped behaviours from which the patient derives no pleasure. They may appear to have the purpose of preventing harm, but are objectively useless (and recognized as such by the patient). OCD is associated with simultaneous anxiety. OCD is equally common in males and females. Psychological therapies include response prevention (learning how to cope with tension), mass practice (where the patient is forced to repeat their rituals) and thought-stopping (blocking the undesired thoughts). OCD may respond to antidepressants, although severe, intractable cases with major life disruption may respond to psychosurgery (cingulotomy).

Acute stress reaction is a transient phenomenon that occurs secondary to exceptional physical or mental stress in people without a pre-existing psychiatric disorder. It can start a few minutes after the trigger and may last for a few days. The typical features are an initial 'daze' followed by disorientation and the inability to process external stimuli. There may later be amnesia of the event. If the duration exceeds 3 days, an alternative diagnosis should be considered.

Post-traumatic stress disorder ('shell shock') occurs secondary to a traumatic stressor (i.e. one that any 'normal' person would find stressful). Diagnostic features include:
- experience of a major traumatic event
- re-experiencing the trauma (nightmares or flashbacks)
- avoidance behaviour
- increased arousal (hypervigilance, insomnia or enhanced startle reaction)
- onset is delayed (but within 6 months) and the features should last ≥1 month

The usual course is recovery, but occasionally symptoms become chronic. An *adjustment disorder* is defined as a state of emotional distress that interferes with social functioning occurring within 1 month of a significant life event.

The stages of *normal grief* (described by the Swiss-born psychiatrist Elisabeth Kubler-Ross in 1969) are denial, anger, bargaining, depression and acceptance. This process usually lasts less than 6 months. Complicated grief is suggested by duration above 6 months, suicidal ideation, hallucinations and functional impairment.

Dissociative disorders are characterized by a loss of normally integrated concepts such as self-identify, memories of the past, awareness of the present and even control of bodily movements. There must be some form of traumatic or interpersonal stress and the absence of a pre-existing physical or psychiatric disorder in order to make the diagnosis. The term *conversion* describes the unconscious change of intrapsychic anxiety into physical symptoms of symbolic significance.

Theme 2: Side-effects of psychiatric medication

1. C – Akathisia

2. J – Tardive dyskinesia
Typical antipsychotics block dopamine D_2 receptors in the central nervous system in various pathways. This accounts for both their therapeutic activity and their side-effects. The effect on the mesolimbic pathway improves psychotic symptoms, but action on the mesocortical pathway worsens negative symptoms. The effect on the tuberoinfundibular pathway causes the side-effect of hyperprolactinaemia (leading to gynaecomastia, galactorrhoea, reduced sperm count, amenorrhoea and reduced libido). Action on the chemoreceptor trigger zone has an antiemetic property.

Extrapyramidal side-effects are a consequence of nigrostriatal pathway blockade. These include parkinsonism (rigidity, bradykinesia and tremor, which can begin within 1 month and are treated with anticholinergics, e.g. procyclidine), acute dystonias (which occur within 72 hours of treatment and include trismus, tongue protrusion, spasmodic torticollis, opisthotonus, oculogyric crisis and grimacing), akathisia (which occurs within 60 days and features a subjective feeling of inner tension and restless leg syndrome, but can be treated with β-blockers and benzodiazepines) and tardive dyskinesia (which affects 20% in the long term and presents with chewing, grimacing, sucking and a darting tongue).

Other side-effects of typical antipsychotics are anticholinergic effects, which cause an increased QT interval, arrhythmias and cardiac arrest. Alpha-adrenoreceptor blocking action causes postural hypotension, and antihistamine activity causes sedation and weight gain. Chlorpromazine specifically causes greying of the skin in response to sunlight, and a reduced seizure threshold.

3. G – Neuroleptic malignant syndrome

Neuroleptic malignant syndrome is a life-threatening neurological condition that can occur with the use of typical and atypical antipsychotics, particularly after an increase in dose. Symptoms include pyrexia, fluctuating consciousness, muscle rigidity and autonomic dysfunction. Investigations may reveal a raised creatine kinase, raised white cell count and abnormal liver function tests. Treatment is with dantrolene to stop muscle spasm and bromocriptine to reverse dopamine blockade.

4. K – Weight gain

Two examples of atypical antipsychotics are clozapine and olanzapine. These act on dopamine D_1 and D_4 receptors. They generally have fewer extrapyramidal side-effects and cause less worsening of negative symptoms. Olanzapine does cause weight gain, diabetes and sedation. Clozapine causes agranulocytosis in 1% of cases, and must be withdrawn if the leucocyte or neutrophil count falls significantly. Risperidone and amisulpride are other examples of atypical antipsychotics.

5. I – Serotonin syndrome

This woman has taken an over-the-counter preparation for depression, which is likely to be St John's wort. The combination of this herb with SSRIs (fluoxetine in this case) is associated with the development of serotonin syndrome. Signs include severe hypertension, tachycardia, high pyrexia, myoclonus, sweating and hyperreflexia. Management is initially symptomatic, followed by removal of the offending drugs.

Theme 3: Descriptive psychopathology 2

1. D – Dysphoria
Description of mood and feeling

The *affect* refers to a snapshot of a patient's emotional state. It tends to be used to describe the observer's impression of a patient's mood at one particular time. A *blunted/flattened affect* describes reduced emotional reactivity. *Inappropriate affect* is emotion that is inappropriate to the associated speech or thought, e.g. laughing when talking about death.

Mood refers to a patient's sustained emotional state. *Dysphoria* is an unpleasant mood and *elation* is an abnormal exaggeration of the feeling of well-being. *Euphoria* is the feeling of contentment and lack of concern. It can be caused by opiates and is a late complication of head injury. *Apathy* is the loss of emotional tone (detachment or indifference) and *alexithymia* is difficulty in understanding and describing one's emotions.

Anxiety is apprehension and tension due to anticipation of an internal or external danger. In *phobic anxiety*, there is a clear focus on the danger and it is avoided. In *free-floating anxiety*, the anxiety is pervasive and unfocused. *Fear* is anxiety due to a realistic danger at a conscious level. *Tension* is an unpleasant increase in psychological stress. *Agitation* describes the excess motor activity associated with feelings of inner tension. *Depressive retardation* is psychomotor retardation in depression. *Hyperchondriasis* is the fear of a serious illness that is not based on any real organic pathology, but on unrealistic interpretations of physical signs. *Depersonalization* is the feeling that you are not real, or are altered in some way. *Derealization* is the feeling that the surroundings do not seem real.

2. L – Paramnesia
Description of memory, intellect and attention

Amnesia is an inability to recall past experiences. *Hypermnesia* is exaggerated retention of detail about past experiences. *Paramnesia* is a distorted recall of events, such that falsification of memory occurs. *Confabulation* is verbal evidence of unconscious filling of gaps in memory with false memories. A *fugue state* is an abandonment of personal identity and a loss of memory, often associated with travel/wandering to unexpected locations. It is important to determine a patient's *insight* into their psychiatric condition, because it has a high impact on their concordance with treatment. This can be done by asking: 'Are you ill? Is it psychiatric? Do you need treatment?'

Learning difficulty is categorized according to IQ. Mild retardation is defined as an IQ between 50 and 70, moderate retardation is defined as an IQ between 35 and 49, severe retardation is defined as an IQ between 20 and 34, and profound retardation is defined as an IQ less than 20. *Distractibility* is a state when the patient's attention is drawn to unimportant stimuli. In *selective inattention*, anxiety-provoking stimulants are ignored.

3. E – Echopraxia

4. A – Agitation

5. K – Stupor

Description of movement

Stupor describes the state of being unresponsive, akinetic and mute, but fully conscious. Stupor can occur in depression, mania, catatonia, epilepsy and hysteria. *Obsessional slowness* is a reduced rate of activity due to repeated doubts and compulsive rituals in OCD. *Hyperkinesis* is often seen in children and teenagers. It comprises overactivity, distractibility, impulsivity and excitability. *Motor tics* are repeated involuntary movements involving a group of muscles. *Parkinsonism* describes a group of characteristic movements that occur in Parkinson's disease and other conditions. These include resting tremor, cogwheel rigidity, festinant gait (an involuntary tendency to making short, accelerated steps when walking) and posture abnormalities.

Movements seen in schizophrenia

Ambitendency involves making tentative incomplete movements, apparent when shaking hands. *Echopraxia* is copying of another person's movements, even when asked to stop. *Mannerisms* are repeated involuntary movements that appear goal-directed (e.g. flicking hair). *Stereotypies* are repeated patterns of movement that are not goal directed (e.g. moving the head from side to side). *Negativism* is a motiveless resistance to commands and attempts to be moved. *Posturing* is where a bizarre body position is adopted for an inappropriately long time. *Waxy flexibility* is when the patient remains motionless, but allows their limbs to be moved by someone else. The limbs will remain in the new posture.

Theme 4: Psychotic disorders

Schizophrenia is characterized by distortions in thought and perception, with a blunted, inappropriate affect. Intellect and clear consciousness are usually maintained. The most important features are first-rank symptoms, thought disorder and negative symptoms. Example of negative symptoms include apathy, poverty of thought, reduced speech, blunted affect, psychomotor retardation, social isolation, poor self-care and cognitive deficit.

There is a lifetime risk of 1%, with a peak age of onset of 25–30 years in females and 18–25 years in males. There is a slightly higher incidence in males. Risk factors include low socioeconomic status and exposure to a high level of expressed emotion (over 35 hours/week). There is also a higher incidence in those with a family history, winter/spring birthdays, maternal influenza infection during the second trimester of pregnancy, decreased brain volume and increased ventricle size, adverse life events and lack of social interactions. The dopamine hypothesis is a theory regarding the mechanism of schizophrenia. Briefly, it says that the symptoms are caused in part by central dopaminergic hyperactivity in the mesolimbic–mesocortical system.

Psychosis should lead to the diagnosis of schizophrenia only if symptoms have been present for 1 month, and there is an absence of significant mood disorder, overt brain disease and drug intoxication/withdrawal. Important differential diagnoses are organic psychotic disorder, substance-induced psychotic disorder, delusional disorder, schizoaffective disorder, transient psychosis and schizotypal disorder.

First-line management of schizophrenia is with an atypical neuroleptic (e.g. olanzapine). Response takes 3–4 weeks. Monthly depot injections can improve compliance. All antipsychotics are similar in efficacy, except for clozapine. Benzodiazepines are given for aggression. In treatment-resistant cases (i.e. where two different antipsychotics have been tried for 6–8 weeks), antidepressants and lithium are used for augmentation. Electroconvulsive therapy (ECT) is used for catatonic schizophrenia only.

Schizophrenia, from Greek *schitz* = split/shattered + *phrenes* = mind/heart.

1. G – Schizoaffective disorder

Schizoaffective disorder is diagnosed when the patient meets the full criteria for both a mood disorder and schizophrenia. It can be divided into manic-type and depressed-type.

2. F – Psychotic depression

This woman is having a nihilistic delusion – the delusion that parts of her body are rotting away. This is a recognized psychotic symptom associated with severe depression.

3. B – Catatonic schizophrenia

Catatonic schizophrenia has a prominence of catatonic symptoms. These are stupor, excitement, posturing, negativism, rigidity, waxy flexibility, perseveration of words and mutism.

The most common subtype of schizophrenia is the *paranoid subtype*, in which there are predominantly positive symptoms (delusions and hallucinations) with an increased suicide risk. Paranoid schizophrenia has the best prognosis. *Hebephrenic schizophrenia* has an earlier age of onset and a worse prognosis, and the main features are negative symptoms, thought disorders and an incongruent affect. *Simple schizophrenia* is a gradual decline in functioning. There are negative symptoms without positive symptoms. Chronic schizophrenia can be diagnosed if negative symptoms persist 1 year after positive symptoms. In *delusional disorder*, it is delusions alone that make up the clinical picture, although very occasional and transient hallucinations do not exclude the diagnosis. It usually starts in middle age. *Transient psychotic disorder* usually reaches a crescendo of symptoms within 2 weeks, with complete resolution within 3 months. It may be precipitated by a stressful life event.

4. J – Substance-induced psychotic disorder

If there is a potential organic or drug-related cause for someone's psychotic symptoms, this should be suspected above a true psychiatric condition. In this case, it is likely that excessive cannabis consumption has resulted in psychotic symptoms.

5. H – Schizoid-type personality disorder

Schizoid personalities have a preference for their own company over that of others. They lack emotional expression and may consequently be perceived by others as cold and disinterested. They may not gain pleasure from many activities, and have little interest in forming sexual or confiding relationships. Thought disorders and psychoses, which are features of schizophrenia, are not present in schizoid personalities. However, people with schizoid personalities are not exempt from developing schizophrenia.

Theme 5: Psychiatry of sexuality

Psychosexual disorders are non-organic problems preventing an individual from participating in a satisfactory sexual relationship. However, there is frequently a combination of physical and psychological factors contributing to an impairment of function.

1. B – Fetishism

2. A – Exhibitionism

Paraphilias are defined as disorders of sexual preference. Fetishism focuses on inanimate objects as a source of sexual stimulation, e.g. shoes or leather. Transvestic fetishism is the use of cross-dressing in order to gain sexual excitement. Exhibitionism is the tendency to expose genitalia to strangers in public places with subsequent gratification, particularly if there are reactions of shock or horror. Type 1 exhibitionism (80% cases) occurs often in young men, showing a flaccid penis. There is often remorse afterwards. Type 2 exhibitionism is the exposure of an erect penis. This is more common in those with dissocial personality types and there is often a lack of remorse. Voyeurism is the tendency to watch other people engaging in sexual activity. Sadism involves gaining pleasure from inflicting pain or humiliating someone else. Masochism involves gaining sexual excitement from having pain or humiliation inflicted on oneself by another. Sadomasochism is a term comprising both sadism and masochism.

Sadism, from the French novelist Marquis de Sade, whose writings describe it.

Masochism, from the Austrian writer Leopold von Sacher-Masoch, whose stories describe it.

3. J – Transsexualism

Transsexualism, a gender identity disorder, is the persistent desire to live and be accepted as a member of the opposite sex. There is a feeling that the physical body is inconsistent with the sense of self. There may be a desire to have surgery or hormonal treatment in order to change it. Dual-role transvestism is the intermittent desire to dress as the opposite sex that is not for the purpose of arousal or for any permanent change. The male-to-female ratio is approximately 3:1. Management is usually by specialists, and surgery/hormone treatments can be given, although the long-term outcome is uncertain. There is usually a requirement to live as the opposite sex for a year before starting treatment.

4. I – Sexual aversion

5. D – Male erectile disorder

Sexual aversion is an example of sexual dysfunction. There are four stages of sexual arousal – desire, excitement, orgasm and resolution – and problems with each will be dealt with in order. *Loss or lack of sexual desire* can be diagnosed when it is the principal problem, not caused by another factor (e.g. pain). *Sexual aversion* is the tendency to avoid sex due to negative feelings or associations. There may not be a specific problem with one of the four stages of the cycle, but there is an overall lack of enjoyment. *Dyspareunia* is pain during intercourse. It can occur at any stage, in either party. It may be caused by organic pathology, or may be psychogenic in origin. *Vaginismus* describes spasm of muscles in the outer third of the vagina making intercourse painful or impossible. Failure of the genital response interferes with the excitement stage. This includes *male erectile disorder* – a difficulty in achieving or maintaining an erection – or a lack of lubrication in women. Problems at the stage of orgasm can be *premature ejaculation* in men, and *anorgasmia*, which is more common in women.

Theme 6: Management of depression

In recent-onset mild depression, an acceptable first step is 'watchful waiting' with review in approximately 2 weeks. This is particularly appropriate if the patient is reluctant to have any intervention and if it appears likely that it might resolve spontaneously.

1. B – Cognitive–behavioural therapy

In mild depression, antidepressants are not the first-line intervention, because the risk–benefit ratio is poor. The first-line approach is cognitive–behavioural therapy (CBT). There is some evidence for internet-based self-help CBT programmes, which may become more readily available. CBT has been shown to be as effective as drug treatments in mild-to-moderate depression.

Talking therapies are broadly split into two groups: variations on psychodynamic psychotherapy, and CBT. *Psychodynamic psychotherapy* is based on the theory that subconscious ideas/conflicts can lead to emotional and interpersonal difficulties. During therapy, if these ideas can be identified and insight gained then they can be addressed and interpretations made. Important concepts include *transference*, which is the feelings and attitude of the patient towards the therapist, and *countertransference*, which is the feelings and attitudes of the therapist towards the patient. Traditionally, a great deal of time is needed (up to five 50-minute sessions per week, continuing for 2–5 years). Psychodynamic psychotherapy is mainly used for personality and long-standing relationship difficulties. The NICE guidelines for depression do not currently include psychodynamic psychotherapy.

CBT employs a more structured approach, with a limited course of sessions. It is based on the theory that thoughts, beliefs, behaviours and emotions are linked. In the context of depression, negative thoughts (frequently relating to low self-esteem) are exacerbated by unhelpful behaviours, which compound the thoughts and lead to unpleasant emotions. Clear goals are set to challenge specific beliefs and modify behaviour in order to break the cycle and improve mood.

2. D – Electroconvulsive therapy

ECT is the administration of an electric shock to the head (under general anaesthesia) in order to induce a seizure. The indications are severe depressive illness, especially if there is life-threatening behaviour, puerperal depressive illness, mania and catatonic schizophrenia. The absolute contraindication is raised intracranial pressure. Relative contraindications include high anaesthetic risk and known cerebral aneurysm. Long-term side-effects of ECT are unknown, but some patients have complained of long-term memory loss. Short-term side-effects are headache, temporary confusion and some short-term memory loss.

3. E – Fluoxetine

The first drug treatment of depression should be a selective serotonin reuptake inhibitor (SSRI), typically fluoxetine, paroxetine or citalopram. These drugs enhance the effect of the neurotransmitter serotonin (5-hydroxytryptamine, 5-HT) by inhibiting the 5-HT transporter on the presynaptic membrane. There is typically a 2-week delay before an improvement is noted, and it is usually recommended to continue treatment for 6 months after remission. The most common side-effects are hyponatraemia, gastrointestinal disturbance (nausea, vomiting, diarrhoea or pain), insomnia, sexual dysfunction and agitation. Patients should be told that, although the drug does not lead to tolerance or craving, stopping abruptly can lead to withdrawal effects. This is the *SSRI withdrawal syndrome* (characterized by transient dizziness, lethargy, nausea and headache).

4. G – Lithium

The mechanism of action of lithium is unknown, but it possibly acts on neuronal second-messenger systems. Indications for lithium therapy are augmentation of antidepressants in resistant depression and treatment/prophylaxis of mania. Side-effects at therapeutic levels include fine tremor, dry mouth, a metallic taste, mild polyuria, nausea and weight gain. Fetal abnormalities can occur if lithium is given during pregnancy. It can also cause hypothyroidism and renal impairment. At toxic levels (which can occur in mild dehydration), there can be twitching, polyuric renal failure, seizures, coma and death. Patients must have a physical examination before treatment is initiated, along with blood tests for thyroid and renal function, and a baseline ECG. Lithium levels should be measured every week until stable and every 3 months thereafter. Tests for renal function and thyroid function and a full blood count should be repeated after 6 months.

5. A – Amitriptyline

Amitriptyline was the drug of choice in this case because it has more sedating effects than imipramine. Taken at night, it can help people with initial insomnia. Amitriptyline is an example of a tricyclic antidepressant (TCA). The mechanism of action of TCAs is similar to that of SSRIs – inhibition of serotonin reuptake at the presynaptic membrane – but there is also inhibition of the reuptake of noradrenaline, histamine and acetylcholine, and stabilization of the membrane. The extent of the effect on each receptor depends on the individual drug, which is why the side-effects vary among them. TCAs are no longer first-line antidepressants, due to their side-effect profile, particularly in overdose. Their side-effects can be categorized according to which receptor is inhibited:

- anticholinergic: dry mouth, constipation, blurred vision, urinary retention
- antihistamine: weight gain, drowsiness
- membrane stabilization: reduced seizure threshold, cardiotoxicity

Other side-effects include sexual dysfunction, postural hypotension and haematological dysfunction (agranulocytosis, leucopenia, eosinophilia and thrombocytopenia). Routine checks such as blood pressure and ECG should be done before initiating treatment. In overdose, the patient may present with decreased conscious levels, tachycardia, dry skin and dilated pupils (there may also be a divergent squint). ECG changes include sinus tachycardia, but there may be a prolonged QRS interval with a risk of ventricular tachycardia.

TCAs can be used in low doses for neuropathic pain. The anticholinergic effects can be made use of in the treatment of children with nocturnal enuresis.

Monoamine oxidase inhibitors (MAOIs) are occasionally used for depression. They prevent breakdown of the neurotransmitters serotonin, dopamine and acetylcholine. Indications include treatment-resistant depression in secondary care, particularly in women with features of atypical depression. Phenelzine is the most commonly prescribed MAOI. The enzyme MAO metabolizes tyramine, a substance found in many foods (cheese, Marmite, red wine, game, pickled herrings and broad beans). If a patient on an MAOI eats tyramine, this can cause a hypertensive crisis (the 'cheese reaction'). The features are headache, palpitations, fever, convulsions and coma. Moclobemide is a *reversible inhibitor of MAO* and is less strongly associated with the cheese reaction. Before starting MAOIs, it is important to 'wash out' any previously used antidepressants from the body (i.e. have an antidepressant-free period: 5 weeks for SSRIs and 2 weeks for TCAs). This is to avoid the risk of serotonin syndrome, which most commonly occurs when MAOIs are used in combination with other antidepressants. Signs include severe hypertension, tachycardia and high pyrexia. There may be shock and agitated delirium. Earlier signs are myoclonus, overactive reflexes and sweating.

Other antidepressant agents include *tetracyclics* (e.g. mianserin). These are less cardiotoxic than TCAs, but can cause more severe haematological and hepatic reactions. *Serotonin–noradrenaline reuptake inhibitors* (SNRIs, e.g. venlafaxine) are more effective than other antidepressants when given in high doses. The side-effect profile is similar to that of the SSRIs, but adverse effects occur less frequently. Other agents are *selective noradrenaline reuptake inhibitors* (NARIs, e.g. reboxetine) and *noradrenergic and specific serotoninergic antidepressants* (NaSSAs, e.g. the tetracyclic mirtazapine). Benzodiazepines are not recommended for the treatment of depression.

Theme 7: Transcultural psychiatric disorders

There are some conditions that are described only within certain cultures. There are other conditions that have a higher incidence in certain cultures, e.g. there is a ninefold increase in schizophrenia in second-generation African–Caribbean immigrants in Britain. Dissociative disorders are more common in developing countries. Depressive disorders associated with guilt are higher in Christian cultures. Presentations of similar underlying pathology may also differ between cultures. For example, non-western immigrants in Britain are more likely to complain of abdominal pain or erectile dysfunction instead of low mood when the underlying diagnosis is depression.

1. A – Amok

Amok is seen in south-east Asia, usually in Malaysian men. The features are acquisition of a weapon followed by a series of frenzied attacks, killing or seriously injuring anyone within reach. The attacks can last several hours and are frequently terminated only by the attacker being killed by someone else or himself. If he is not killed, amok is followed by a stupor/sleep lasting 1 day, followed by amnesia of the event. It is thought to be a form of dissociative disorder.

Amok, from Malay *amuk* = mad with rage. It is the origin of the phrase 'to run amok'.

2. E – Koro

Koro is seen in Asian men, especially in Chinese cultures. It is the fear that the penis is retracting into the abdomen. Some have a secondary worry that full retraction will lead to death. Koro is more common in people who have limited access to education.

Koro, from Malay *koro* = turtle head – retraction of the turtle's head is seen as similar to koro.

3. G – Piblokto

Piblokto is described in Inuit women living within the Arctic Circle. There is sudden-onset hysteria (screaming, crying, etc.) and bizarre behaviour. This may include removal of clothes, coprophagia (ingestion of faeces) and violence. Attacks last a couple of hours and there is often amnesia after the event.

4. C – Dhat

Dhat occurs in young Indian males. It is associated with anxiety and a belief that semen is being lost in the urine. It often accompanies excessive guilt about masturbation. There may be a belief that semen is 'vital fluid', more so than blood, and that its loss leads to fatigue.

5. F – Latah

Latah is a culture-bound condition found in women in North Africa and the Far East. There is an exaggerated startle response, in which women sometimes start repeating the words of another person (echolalia) or obeying their commands. There is frequently amnesia after the event.

Susto usually occurs in people living in South America. It is a severe depressive episode usually occurring after a traumatic event. There are often physical symptoms such as diarrhoea and nervous tics. It is thought (within the culture in which it exists) to be caused by separation of the soul from the body. It has some features in common with acute stress reaction. *Windigo* is recognized in native North American tribes. Affected people believe that their body is possessed by a spirit that craves human flesh. This results in obsessive thoughts and compulsions regarding violence and cannibalism.

Theme 8: Psychiatric signs of physical illness

1. C – Hyperthyroidism

Thyroid disease is one of the most common endocrine disorders. Thyroid dysfunction results in systemic symptoms. Psychological symptoms of hyperthyroidism include irritability, behaviour changes, restlessness, loss of libido, weight loss despite an increased appetite and, in extreme cases, psychosis (mania). Psychological symptoms of hypothyroidism include depression, tiredness, reduced libido, cognitive impairment, and occasionally psychosis or coma. The accompanying physical symptoms of tremor, weight loss and atrial fibrillation in this case confirm hyperthyroidism. Investigations should proceed with measurement of thyroid hormones, expecting to find a raised thyroxine (T_4) with low levels of thyroid-stimulating hormone (TSH).

2. J – Systemic lupus erythematosus

Systemic lupus erythematosus is an autoimmune connective tissue disease. There is a very broad range of physical signs and symptoms. It can also cause depression, seizures and psychosis. A few of the possible physical manifestations mentioned in this case are malar (butterfly) rash, arthralgia and shortness of breath, which could be caused by lung fibrosis or several other pulmonary conditions.

3. I – Space-occupying lesion

Cerebral tumours should be considered as a differential diagnosis of psychiatric illness. Such space-occupying lesions present with headache that is worse in the morning and exacerbated by bending, straining and coughing. Possible psychological and psychiatric manifestations include impaired consciousness, irritability, apathy, hallucinations, seizures, neuroses and psychosis.

4. B – Delirium

This woman has a urinary tract infection causing delirium. Delirium is characterized by fluctuating impairment of consciousness, mood changes and abnormal perceptions. It affects 10–25% of people aged over 65 years on medical wards. The patient may be obviously confused, with disruptive behaviour and expressing bizarre ideas, but it is important to recognize that delirium can also cause a decreased level of activity and speech. It develops over a short period of time and is due to an underlying physical condition. Common causes are infection, hypoxia, electrolyte disturbances, constipation, drugs and central nervous system (CNS) disease. The main principle of management is to investigate and treat the cause, and to concurrently help relieve distress to the patient by optimizing their ability to orientate themselves. There should be a calm environment with adequate lighting, even at night. Patients should be wearing their glasses and hearing aids (if applicable), have continuity of staff contact where possible, and ideally have family members or familiar belongings around them. In some circumstances, oral or intramuscular haloperidol or benzodiazepines can be used to relieve severe agitation, but these should be avoided where possible. The average duration of delirium is 7 days. Around 40% of patients with delirium die of the underlying condition and 5% go on to develop dementia.

5. A – Cushing's syndrome

The features of Cushing's syndrome are caused by raised levels of glucocorticoids from any sources. Causes include steroid use, ectopic adrenocorticotropic hormone (ACTH) secretion and a pituitary tumour (Cushing's disease). In addition to the physical features (hirsutism, striae, acne, plethora, bruising, thin skin and cataracts), psychological features include depression, insomnia, reduced libido and occasionally psychosis.

Multiple sclerosis is a disorder of the myelin-producing oligodendrocytes in the CNS. Psychological disturbance can occur, including depression, abnormal affect, and occasionally disinhibition, aphasia and psychosis.

Neurosyphilis is infection of the CNS by the sexually transmitted parasite *Treponema pallidum*. Before the advent of antibiotics, it occurred in 25–30% of those infected. Features of neurosyphilis are cranial nerve palsies, meningitis and eventually tabes dorsalis. Another late manifestation is general paralysis of the insane, which causes chronic cognitive impairment and personality change, depression, psychosis and mania. Death usually occurs within 3 years.

Punch-drunk syndrome (also known as post-traumatic dementia or boxing encephalopathy) occurs after repeated blows to the head. Brain atrophy is a feature. Clinical features are cognitive impairment and personality deterioration, with cerebellar, extrapyramidal and pyramidal signs. Occasionally, pathological jealousy and rage reactions are associated.

Pellagra is a disorder caused by niacin (vitamin B$_3$) deficiency. It is most common in South America, where maize forms the staple diet. The main physical features are weakness, dermatitis and diarrhoea. There can also be personality change progressing to dementia. Treatment is with niacin. Death can occur within a few years if untreated.

Theme 9: The Mental Health Act

These are all sections from Part II of the Mental Health Act for England and Wales 1983. They relate to compulsory detention in hospital of patients with a psychiatric disorder that requires treatment. Around 90% of psychiatric admissions to hospital are on a voluntary (informal) basis. Patients and their nearest relatives have the right to appeal against their section. This may go to Mental Health Act managers or a mental health review tribunal, which has the authority to discharge patients.

The Mental Health Act was updated in 2007, specifying one small alteration to this section: '... it will not be possible for patients to be compulsorily detained or their detention continued unless medical treatment which is appropriate to the patient's mental disorder and all other circumstances of the case is available to that patient ...'.

1. L – Section 136

Sections 135 and 136 allow police to take someone from the community to a hospital or another safe place. The detention lasts 72 hours and is granted by a magistrate. Section 135 applies when a patient is in private property, and allows the police to break in. Section 136 applies if the patient is in a public place.

2. A – Section 2

Section 2 is compulsory detention for assessment, when the exact diagnosis and response to treatment are unknown. Its duration is 28 days. It must be agreed by two doctors (one of whom must be Section 12 approved). To become approved under *Section 12(2)*, one has to attend a specific Section 12 training course and be recommended to do so by two psychiatry consultants. Before attending training, doctors must usually hold membership of the Royal College of Psychiatrists or have at least 3 years' experience in psychiatry.

3. E – Section 5(4)

Section 5(4) is nurse's holding power. This allows detention of informal psychiatry inpatients by nurses if there is no doctor available. It lasts 6 hours, allowing time for a more permanent Section to be administered. *Section 5(2)* is doctors' holding power. It allows the detention of a hospital inpatient (under any speciality) by the doctor responsible for their care. It lasts 72 hours (long enough to arrange a Section 2). Note that, in even more acute situations, patients can be stopped under common law for a short time if there is an immediate threat to their health.

4. B – Section 3

Section 3 allows compulsory detention for treatment when the diagnosis is already known. It lasts for 6 months, but may be renewed if necessary. It must be agreed by two doctors (one of whom must be Section 12-approved).

5. C – Section 4

Section 4 allows an emergency admission to hospital when there is not enough time to organize a Section 2. Its duration is 72 hours and there is no right of appeal against it. It can be arranged by one doctor.

Sections 35–37 can be requested by a court on advice of a Section 12-approved doctor when a patient has been charged with an offence that may lead to imprisonment. *Section 35* is for the purpose of producing a medical report on the psychiatric illness of the offender. The duration is 28 days. *Section 36* allows treatment of the patient. It also lasts 28 days, but requires two doctors to agree on it. *Section 37* is for the detention and treatment of a patient already convicted of an imprisonable offence. This also requires two doctors' agreement and lasts 6 months.

Section 17 allows for set periods of leave (with a responsible adult) to be granted by the responsible medical officer.

Theme 10: Personality disorders

The International Classification of Diseases (ICD)-10 definition of a personality disorder is 'a severe disturbance in the characterological constitution and behavioural tendencies of the individual, usually involving several areas of the personality, and nearly always associated with considerable personal and social disruption'. These often become apparent during childhood or adolescence, and continue into adulthood. The prevalence of personality disorders is probably under-reported. They are likely to affect around 10% of the population, but the prevalence is higher in psychiatric settings. There are several theories regarding personality and personality disorders; the dimensional approach suggests that people with personality disorders exhibit traits that feature as a spectrum in the population, but to an exaggerated degree.

1. B – Antisocial

Antisocial personalities often display little feeling towards others. There is a tendency to be aggressive, commit crimes and lack remorse. Affected persons have difficulty in forming intimate relationships, and the diagnosis is supported by a previous childhood conduct disorder.

2. D – Dependent

Dependent personality types are often passive, relying on others to make decisions. They fear abandonment and find it difficult to cope with daily chores. Such personalities may excessively give priority to the needs and wishes of others, over their own, in an attempt to maintain their close relationships.

3. E – Emotionally unstable (borderline-type)

The emotionally unstable personality disorder (borderline-type) is characterized by emotional instability, disturbed views of self-image, feelings of emptiness and intense, but easily broken, relationships. Self-harm is a common feature, often in an attempt to avoid abandonment. The *emotionally unstable (impulsive-type)* personality disorder is similar, but a lack of self-control and violent outbursts are more prominent features.

4. I – Schizoid

Schizoid personalities have a preference for their own company over that of others. They lack emotional expression and may consequently be perceived by others as cold and disinterested. They may not gain pleasure from many activities and have little interest in forming sexual or confiding relationships. Thought disorders and psychoses, which are features of schizophrenia, are not present in schizoid personalities. However, schizoid personalities are not exempt from developing schizophrenia.

5. G – Histrionic

Histrionic individuals crave attention, are preoccupied with appearance and are inappropriately flirtaceous. They may display theatrical expressions of emotions, from excessive excitement to unexpected, manipulative tantrums.

Histrionic, from Latin *histrionicus* = pertaining to an actor

People with a *paranoid personality disorder* are often suspicious of others (including their own partners) and are very sensitive to rejection. They often bear grudges and misinterpret the actions of others as malicious. *Anxious (avoidant) personality disorder* is characterized by a tendency to worry, extreme anxiety, feelings of inferiority and a fear of criticism/disapproval to the point of avoiding people/situations where this might happen. People with *anankastic personality disorder* frequently display an inflexible preoccupation with rules, order and attention to detail. They may be very cautious and stubborn, and may try to enforce their ways with others.

In DSM-IV, two further personality disorders are categorized: the *narcissistic personality* (arrogant with a grandiose sense of self-importance, often lacking empathy for others) and the *schizotypal personality* (eccentric behaviours, thinking, speech and appearance, and lacking social confidence and close relationships.

Personality disorders may be categorized into clusters (according to the *Diagnostic and Statistical Manual of Mental Disorder (DSM-IV-TR)*, American Psychiatric Association):

- Cluster A (paranoid, schizoid, schizotypal): odd or eccentric
- Cluster B (antisocial, borderline, histrionic, narcissistic): emotional or dramatic
- Cluster C (avoidant, dependent, anankastic): anxious or fearful

Narcissism, from the Greek legend *Narcissus*, who was cursed into falling in love with his own reflection after breaking the heart of the shy nymph *Echo*. (Incidentally, *Echo* loved the sound of her voice so much, she was herself cursed into only being able to repeat what others said.)

Anankastic, from Greek *Ananke*, the goddess of necessity.